AF697397

Clinical Nurse Leader® Certification Review

Cynthia R. King, PhD, NP, MSN, RN, CNL, FAAN, is an owner and consultant of Special Care Consultants. She specializes in consulting in healthcare and nursing as well as writing and editing. Previously, Dr. King was a full professor and developed a clinical nurse leader program while at Queens University of Charlotte, North Carolina. She has presented numerous times at the American Association of Colleges of Nursing Clinical Nurse Leader (AACN CNL) conference on the template she developed for a CNL review course on how to best study for the CNL® certification exam. Dr. King has worked as a clinician (staff nurse, clinical nurse specialist, nurse practitioner), educator, administrator, and researcher. She presents nationally and internationally and has been a keynote speaker at several major meetings. Dr. King has published extensively, including four books and numerous articles in peer-reviewed journals, and she has served as editor-in-chief of two nursing journals. She serves on numerous local, regional, and national committees and boards of nursing associations, nonprofits, and foundations.

Sally O'Toole Gerard, DNP, RN, CDE, CNL, is an associate professor and track coordinator of the nurse leadership graduate program at Fairfield University, Fairfield, Connecticut. Dr. Gerard has been in nursing for over 25 years and has a background in critical care and hospital education. She specializes in diabetes as a certified diabetes educator. Her publications and research focus on diabetes and improvement of patient-related outcomes, and include five articles published in peer-reviewed journals. Dr. Gerard has been involved in a number of academic collaborations with local hospitals to introduce evidence-based practice and improve quality care in the acute care setting. She has completed training in a national partnership for healthcare improvement practices with the Dartmouth Institute for Health Policy and the American Association of Colleges of Nursing. Dr. Gerard presents nationally and internationally on the subjects of nursing leadership and improvement science.

Clinical Nurse Leader® Certification Review

Second Edition

Cynthia R. King, PhD, NP, MSN, RN, CNL, FAAN
Sally O'Toole Gerard, DNP, RN, CDE, CNL

Editors

SPRINGER PUBLISHING COMPANY

Copyright © 2016 Springer Publishing Company, LLC

All rights reserved.

No part of this publication may be reproduced, stored in a retrieval system, or transmitted in any form or by any means, electronic, mechanical, photocopying, recording, or otherwise, without the prior permission of Springer Publishing Company, LLC, or authorization through payment of the appropriate fees to the Copyright Clearance Center, Inc., 222 Rosewood Drive, Danvers, MA 01923, 978-750-8400, fax 978-646-8600, info@copyright.com or on the Web at www.copyright.com.

Springer Publishing Company, LLC
11 West 42nd Street
New York, NY 10036
www.springerpub.com

Acquisitions Editor: Margaret Zuccarini
Senior Production Editor: Kris Parrish
Composition: diacriTech

ISBN: 978-0-8261-7219-8
ebook ISBN: 978-0-8261-7224-2

16 17 18 19 20 / 5 4 3 2 1

Publisher's Acknowledgment

Springer Publishing Company recognizes that the Clinical Nurse Leader® Certification Exam is a registered service mark of the American Association of Colleges of Nursing (AACN) and has applied this service mark to the first mention of the exam in each of the chapters in this book and on its cover.

The author and the publisher of this Work have made every effort to use sources believed to be reliable to provide information that is accurate and compatible with the standards generally accepted at the time of publication. The author and publisher shall not be liable for any special, consequential, or exemplary damages resulting, in whole or in part, from the readers' use of, or reliance on, the information contained in this book. The publisher has no responsibility for the persistence or accuracy of URLs for external or third-party Internet websites referred to in this publication and does not guarantee that any content on such websites is, or will remain, accurate or appropriate.

Library of Congress Cataloging-in-Publication Data
Names: King, Cynthia R., editor. | Gerard, Sally O'Toole, editor.
Title: Clinical nurse leader certification review / Cynthia R. King, Sally Gerard, editors.
Description: Second edition. | New York, NY : Springer Publishing Company, LLC, [2016] | Includes bibliographical references and index.
Identifiers: LCCN 2015051155 | ISBN 9780826172198 | ISBN 9780826172242 (ebook)
Subjects: | MESH: Nurse Clinicians | Leadership | Certification | Nurse's Role | Outlines
Classification: LCC RT55 | NLM WY 18.2 | DDC 610.73076--dc23 LC record available at http://lccn.loc.gov/2015051155

Special discounts on bulk quantities of our books are available to corporations, professional associations, pharmaceutical companies, healthcare organizations, and other qualifying groups. If you are interested in a custom book, including chapters from more than one of our titles, we can provide that service as well.

For details, please contact:
Special Sales Department, Springer Publishing Company, LLC
11 West 42nd Street, 15th Floor, New York, NY 10036-8002
Phone: 877-687-7476 or 212-431-4370; Fax: 212-941-7842
E-mail: sales@springerpub.com

Printed in the United States of America by Gasch Printing.

To all the clinical nurse leaders and clinical nurse leader students who are working hard to make all aspects of our healthcare system a model that will exceed expectations of quality and safety for all Americans. We gratefully recognize the dedication of faculty and healthcare organizations who are working collaboratively to support these master's-prepared nurses to lead change in this important era of healthcare.

Contents

Appendix A has been updated to reflect the spring 2017 changes made to the Clinical Nurse Leader® Certification Exam Blueprint.

Contributors

Katherine A'Hearn, MSN, RN-BC, CCRN
Clinical Instructor
Stamford Hospital
Stamford, Connecticut

Jonathan P. Auld, RN, CNL, MS, MAT
Nurse Educator
Oregon Health and Science University
Portland, Oregon

Audrey Marie Beauvais, DNP, MSN, MBA, RN, CNL
Associate Dean
Fairfield University School of Nursing
Fairfield, Connecticut

Denise M. Bourassa, MSN, RNC-OB, CNL
Assistant Clinical Professor
University of Connecticut
Storrs, Connecticut

Grace O. Buttriss, DNP, RN, FNP-BC, CNL
Assistant Professor
Presbyterian School of Nursing at Queens University of Charlotte
Charlotte, North Carolina

Stephanie Collins, MSN, RNC-MNN, CNL
Clinical Nurse Leader
Stamford Hospital
Stamford, Connecticut

Jodi A. Erickson, MSN, RN, CNL
Manager of Patient Care Services
MultiCare Good Samaritan Hospital
Puyallup, Washington;
Nursing Instructor
Pacific Lutheran University
Tacoma, Washington

Carol A. Fackler, DNSc, RN
Director of Nursing Programs
Maine College of Health Professions
Lewiston, Maine

Sally O'Toole Gerard, DNP, RN, CDE, CNL
Associate Professor
Fairfield University
Fairfield, Connecticut

Bonnie Haupt, DNP, RN, CNL, CHSE
Clinical Nurse Leader
South Texas VA Healthcare System
San Antonio, Texas

Deborah C. Jackson, MSN, RN, CCRN, CNL
Retired Adjunct Faculty
Sacred Heart University
Fairfield, Connecticut

Cynthia R. King, PhD, NP, MSN, RN, CNL, FAAN
Principal and Consultant
Special Care Consultants
New Hartford, New York

Dawn Marie Nair, DNP, RN
Assistant Professor
St. Vincent's College
Bridgeport, Connecticut

September T. Nelson, MS, RN, CNL
Director
Learning Resource Center
University of Portland School of Nursing
Portland, Oregon

E. Carol Polifroni, EdD, CNE, NEA-BC, ANEF
Professor
University of Connecticut School of Nursing
Storrs, Connecticut

Kathryn B. Reid, PhD, APRN, FNP-BC, CNL
Associate Professor
University of Virginia School of Nursing
Charlottesville, Virginia

Soraya Rosenfield, MSN, RN, CNL
Staff Nurse
Stamford Hospital
Stamford, Connecticut

Catherine Winkler, PhD, MPH, RN
Adjunct Faculty
Fairfield University
Fairfield, Connecticut

Teri Moser Woo, PhD, RN, CNL, CPNP-PC, FAANP
Associate Professor
Associate Dean for Graduate Nursing Programs
Pacific Lutheran University
Tacoma, Washington

Coordinator of Item Writers

Carla Gene Rapp, PhD, RN
Adult Gerontology Nurse Practitioner and Consultant
Durham, North Carolina

Item Writers

Chris Blackhurst, MS, RN, CNL
Adjunct Faculty
The University of Portland;
Pediatric Nurse
Providence Center for Medically Fragile Children
Portland, Oregon

Laura Carmichael Blackhurst, MS, RN, CNL
Adjunct Nursing Instructor
Clark College
Vancouver, Washington;
Inpatient RN
Peace Health
Longview, Washington

Stephanie Collins, MSN, RNC-MNN, CNL
Clinical Nurse Leader
Stamford Hospital
Stamford, Connecticut

Deborah Foll, MSN, RNC-MNN, CNL
Clinical Nurse Leader
Stamford Hospital
Stamford, Connecticut

Heather Helton, MSN, RN, CMSRN, CNL
Clinical Nurse Leader
Carolinas Medical Center
Charlotte, North Carolina

Valerie Short, MSN, RN, CMSRN, CNL
Clinical Nurse Leader
Carolinas Medical Center
Charlotte, North Carolina

Joselyn Wright, MSN, RN, CMSRN, CNL
Clinical Nurse Leader
Carolinas Medical Center
Charlotte, North Carolina

Foreword

I am pleased to provide a foreword for the second edition of the *Clinical Nurse Leader® Certification Review* by Cynthia R. King and Sally O'Toole Gerard. Drs. King and Gerard continue to provide an excellent review, reinforcing major skills and responsibilities of this advanced nursing practice role. This book will be most useful for students as they prepare for certification. The new revision provides an in-depth review, illustrated by examples on content that underpin the clinical nurse leader role. Competencies and curricular expectations for clinical nurse leader education and practice are integrated in the presentation of key areas of focus, including risk mitigation, lateral integration, interprofessional skills, care coordination, and evidence-based practice. I know that students and faculty will appreciate the authors' attention to detail as they continue to reach for this text as a resource for successful certification preparation.

Linda Roussel, PhD, RN, NEA-BC, CNL
Co-Author, Initiating and Sustaining the Clinical Nurse Leader Role: A Practical Guide

Preface

Clinical Nurse Leader® Certification Review is written by experts on the new clinical nurse leader (CNL) role. The book is written for nurses who have completed a qualified CNL program and are ready to take the certification exam, as a guide for faculty on how to design a review course, and as a resource for use during the CNL program. Because of the changes and additions to the "new" topics in the certification exam, this book may be especially helpful for faculty preparing the CNL curriculum and CNL review courses. This second edition has been enhanced to serve as a quality resource for all of these purposes, with new chapters, a glossary, and new multiple-choice questions and case studies. In spring 2017, after a thorough job analysis, the Commission on Nurse Certification (CNC), which oversees the CNL® certification exam, made minor changes to the exam content outline. The new exam content outline appears in Appendix A.

Chapter 1 describes the history and journey of developing the CNL role. Chapter 2 helps individuals and groups make the best use of this book, while Chapters 3 and 4 provide information on the actual certification exam and how to prepare for it. The remaining chapters cover the key topics outlined in the updated examination outline (Appendix A). Chapters 5 through 9 are grouped in the content outline under Nursing Leadership. Chapters 10 through 14 are grouped under Clinical Outcomes Management. The last chapters, 15 through 21, fall under Care Environment Management.

Of those chapters more specifically related to nursing leadership, Chapter 5 focuses on topics related to horizontal leadership, while Chapter 6 describes interdisciplinary collaboration and communication skills. Chapter 7 identifies key concepts related to healthcare advocacy and how CNLs serve as advocates. Chapter 8 outlines the specifics of how CNLs must integrate their new role into their healthcare setting. Chapter 9 is the last chapter related to nursing leadership in this section and describes the CNL's role in lateral integration of care services.

In the section devoted to clinical outcomes management, Chapter 10 discusses management of illnesses and diseases, while Chapter 11 focuses on knowledge management as a role for CNLs. Other areas of importance for CNLs are health promotion and disease prevention, which are outlined in Chapter 12. Chapter 13 describes the importance of using the latest evidence in practice by learning about and implementing evidence-based practice (EBP) in any of the key roles in which CNLs might be serving. The key components of advanced clinical assessment that CNLs need to be able to implement in practice are included in Chapter 14.

Care environment management is the last major section of the exam outline for CNLs. This section opens with Chapter 15, which focuses on team coordination. CNLs have a key role as members of a variety of interdisciplinary teams, influencing outcomes and managing costs. Chapter 16 describes health finance and economics, while Chapter 17 identifies health systems versus the specific microsystems in which CNLs work. In addition to being involved in outcomes, it is expected that CNLs be involved in healthcare policy (Chapter 18). The CNL role was developed specifically to help with quality and safety issues related to patient care. Chapter 19 focuses on quality management, which is equal in importance to healthcare informatics, the topic of Chapter 20. Finally, Chapter 21 discusses ethics and ethical principles.

Clinical Nurse Leader® Certification Review also includes four appendices. Appendix A contains the overall exam content. This new content outline *still validates* the need for all the chapters, questions, case studies, and glossary in this book. Currently, there is no need to revise the content of this book or the new CNL app. The changes in the exam content outline involved: (a) moving some content around under the three major headings, (b) making slight changes to chapter titles, and (c) minor changes in weighting of the three major headings. All of our faculty and student followers will still find the material in this book high quality, appropriate, and accurate.

Appendix B contains reflection questions to help nurses prepare for this exam. Appendix C includes multiple-choice questions and unfolding case studies, while Appendix D contains the correct answers for these questions and the rationale for the correct answers. In this new edition, a glossary of key terms has been added.

Cynthia R. King
Sally O'Toole Gerard

Acknowledgments

Cyndy King would like to thank her parents, Martha R. King and the late Dr. John A. King, for encouraging a career in nursing and for their love and support. She would also like to thank all her mentors, colleagues, students, and the patients and their families, who have added to her love of nursing and lifelong learning. Cyndy also thanks her late husband, Michael A. Knaus, who believed in this book and who always provided love and support. Lastly, special thanks to Dr. Carla Gene Rapp, who worked collaboratively with the editors to oversee the multiple-choice questions and case studies in this second edition.

Sally O'Toole Gerard would like to acknowledge the generosity of her colleagues who have mentored her in the wonderful journey of interprofessional improvement work. She would especially like to thank her CNL graduates, who are wonderful ambassadors of what this education was envisioned to create: creative, intelligent, collaborative leaders. In addition, she acknowledges that the support of her husband, Bill, and her children, Jack, Christian, and Holly, is the key to all good things.

Cynthia R. King
Sally O'Toole Gerard

I

Becoming Familiar With the CNL Role and Certification Exam

1

The Clinical Nurse Leader Journey for Clinicians and Academics

Teri Moser Woo

The clinical nurse leader (CNL) role evolved out of a partnership between nursing education and practice leaders to address the need for master's-educated nurses in a complex, changing healthcare delivery environment. This was developed in the early 2000s and was the first new nursing role in 35 years.

Background

In order to understand the need for a new nursing role, it is critical to understand the healthcare environment and where the profession of nursing was in the late 1990s and early 2000s. This section will describe the healthcare background and the need for the CNL role.

The Healthcare Environment

To Err Is Human, a landmark report published in 1999 by the Institute of Medicine (IOM) proposed that the healthcare system was not as safe as it should and could be (Table 1.1). The IOM report suggested that between 44,000 and 98,000 people died in hospitals annually due to medical errors (1999). Faulty systems, processes, and conditions that lead to errors were identified as the cause of most errors and the IOM called for a nationwide focus on leadership, research, tools, and protocols to improve patient safety.

In 2001, the IOM published a second report focusing on quality titled *Crossing the Quality Chasm: A New Health System for the 21st Century*, which proposed the U.S. healthcare system was too focused on acute and episodic care, when the aging population required care for complex chronic conditions. The 2001 IOM report noted the healthcare system

TABLE 1.1 Timeline of the Clinical Nurse Leader Role Development

1999	Institute of Medicine (IOM) *To Err Is Human: Building a Safer Health System* published.
	American Association of Colleges of Nursing (AACN) forms Task Force on Education and Regulation for Professional Nursing Practice #1 (TFER #1) committee in response to IOM report and the nursing shortage to explore new educational models and nursing roles.
2000	Buerhaus, Staiger, and Auerbach publish a RN workforce study projecting a 20% shortage of RNs by 2020.
2002	American Association of Colleges of Nursing (AACN) formed Task Force on Education and Regulation for Professional Nursing Practice #2 (TEFR #2) to continue the work of TEFR #1. TEFR #2 outlined the competencies of the "New Nurse" which led to the development of the draft white paper *The Role of the Clinical Nurse Leader* in May 2003.
2003	American Association of Colleges of Nursing (AACN) published a draft white paper *The Role of the Clinical Nurse Leader* based on the work of TEFR #2.
	American Association of Colleges of Nursing (AACN) hold a meeting of education and practice partners to further define and refine the role of the clinical nurse leader.
2004	AACN Clinical Nurse Leader Implementation Task Force formed to further define the skills and competencies of the CNL role.
	AACN sends a request for proposal (RFP) to all member schools, inviting them to submit a proposal to develop a CNL master's curriculum. Pilot programs were required to include a plan by their practice partner to implement the CNL role.
2005	First pilot CNL programs begin.
2006	Initial pilot programs grow to 70 in the 2006–2007 academic year, enrolling 1,270 students.
2007	AACN published *White Paper on the Education and Role of the Clinical Nurse Leader* which outlined CNL competencies and provided a curricular framework for schools to utilize when developing a program.
	First Clinical Nurse Leader® certification exam is offered.
2008	First meetings of Clinical Nurse Leader Association (CNLA).
	First national AACN-CNL Partnership Conference in Arizona, which evolved into an annual CNL Summit.
2013	AACN publishes *Competencies and Curricular Expectations for the Clinical Nurse Leader℠ Education and Practice* updating the CNL competencies based on the 2011 *Essentials of Master's Education in Nursing*.

was too complex and uncoordinated, leading to a waste of resources, poor quality, and safety issues (Table 1.1). The *Quality Chasm* report identified six aims to improve healthcare quality, stating that care should be: (a) safe, (b) effective, (c) patient-centered, (d) timely, (e) efficient, and (f) equitable. Ten rules or principles were proposed in the *Quality Chasm* report to guide healthcare redesign:

1. Care is based on continuous healing relationships.
2. Care is customized according to patient needs and values.

3. The patient is the course of control.
4. Knowledge is shared and information flows freely.
5. Decision making is evidence based.
6. Safety is a system property.
7. Transparency is necessary.
8. Needs are anticipated.
9. Waste is continuously decreased.
10. Cooperation among clinicians is a priority.

These new expectations for healthcare to improve patient safety, quality, and satisfaction provided the backdrop for the development of a new nursing role with the skills to meet the challenge of healthcare in the 21st century.

Nursing at the Turn of the 21st Century

The nursing profession was experiencing its own pressures at the turn of the century. Buerhaus, Staiger, and Auerbach (2000) published a report predicting another 20% decrease of RNs by 2020. The average age of RNs in 2000 was 44, and the number of students enrolled in baccalaureate programs was not enough to replace the aging RN workforce (American Association of Colleges of Nursing, 2007; U.S. Department of Health and Human Services, 2010). The Joint Commission weighed in on the looming nursing shortage, stating "the impending crisis in nurse staffing has the potential to impact the very health and security of our society" (p. 5). The Joint Commission recommended that the workplace be transformed, that nursing education and clinical experience align, and healthcare organizations invest in high-quality nursing care (2002).

Nursing Responds With a New Role

In a response to the IOM report and in recognition of declining enrollments in baccalaureate nursing programs, the leadership of the American Association of Colleges of Nursing (AACN) formed the Task Force on Education and Regulation for Professional Nursing Practice #1 (TFER #1) to explore new educational models and nursing roles (Long, 2003) (Table 1.1). The TEFR #1 committee recommended a new nursing role with a different scope of practice and license from the RN. The recommendations of TEFR #1, including creating a new license, were not accepted by the National Council of State Boards of Nursing (NCSBN), and the AACN convened the Task Force on Education and Regulation for Professional

Nursing Practice #2 (TEFR #2) in 2002 to continue the work of TEFR #1 (Long, 2003; Table 1.1). TEFR #2 outlined the competencies of the "New Nurse" which led to the development of the draft white paper *The Role of the Clinical Nurse Leader* in May 2003.

Practice/Education Partnership in Developing the CNL Role

From the beginning, the CNL role has evolved out of a strong partnership between nursing education and practice. In October 2003, the AACN convened a meeting of education and practice partners to further define and refine the role of the CNL (Table 1.1). The only requirement to attend the meeting was that each educational program was required to bring a practice partner to the meeting and over 100 potential education/practice partnerships attended (Stanley, 2014). The Clinical Nurse Leader Implementation Task Force formed in January 2004 was tasked with the development of the skills and competencies of the CNL role and comprised of members from both education and practice, including the American Organization of Nurse Executives and the Veterans Health Administration (Tornabeni & Miller, 2008). In 2004, the AACN sent a request for proposal (RFP) to all member schools, inviting them to submit a proposal to develop a CNL master's curriculum and were required to include a plan by their practice partner to implement the CNL role on at least one unit in the practice setting (Stanley, 2014). The requirement for every CNL program to have a committed practice partner continues into the present (AACN, n.d.).

The strong alliance between practice and education has been crucial to the success of implementing the CNL role. The academic partner solicits and incorporates input from the practice partner when developing the curriculum to educate CNL students. Likewise, the practice partner utilizes input from their academic partner to redesign care and implement the CNL role (Harris, Stanley, & Rosseter, 2011). Sherman (2008) interviewed chief nursing officers (CNOs) to identify the five factors that influence the CNO decision to involve their organization in the CNL project. The five factors are: (a) organizational needs, (b) desire to improve patient care, (c) opportunity to redesign care delivery, (d) promote professional development of RN staff, and (e) enhance physician–nurse relationships. One major nationwide practice partner has been the Veterans Health Administration (VHA), who was an early adopter of the CNL role with 50 Veterans Affairs Medical Centers (VAMC) sites participating in the initial pilot projects in 2004 (Ott et al., 2009). Based on the positive practice outcomes, the VHA developed a plan to implement the CNL role in all VAMCs by 2016 (Ott et al., 2009).

CNL Education

The first pilot CNL master's degree programs began in the 2005–2006 academic year, with rapid growth to 70 programs in the 2006–2007 academic year enrolling 1,270 students (Fang, Htut, & Bednash, 2008). The number of CNL degree programs has grown steadily from the first pilot programs to 130 programs and 190 practice settings in 2015 (Commission on Nurse Certification [CNC], 2015a). There are programs in all regions of the United States and online programs available for students who are place bound.

CNL Education Models

CNL education is at the graduate level in master's or post-master's programs. There are five curricular models for educating the CNL:

1. Model A for BSN graduates.
2. Model B for BSN graduates with a post-BSN residency that awards master's credit toward the CNL degree.
3. Model C for students with a degree in another discipline. These are also known as second-degree or entry-level programs.
4. Model D for ADN graduates. These are also known as RN to MSN (master of science in nursing) programs.
5. Model E are post-master's certificate programs.

As of 2015, approximately half (49%) of CNLs were educated in Model C programs, followed by Model B graduates, who represent 35% of CNLs (CNC, 2015b).

CNL Curriculum

The AACN (2007) outlined CNL competencies and provided a curricular framework for schools to utilize when developing a program. The CNL curriculum builds on a liberal education as the basis for developing clinical judgment and professional values as the foundation for practice. The values deemed essential for the CNL include altruism, accountability, human dignity, integrity, and social justice. The 2007 white paper outlined the competencies for the CNL to include (AACN, 2007):

- Critical thinking
- Communication
- Assessment
- Nursing technology and resource management
- Health promotion

- Risk reduction
- Disease prevention
- Illness and disease management
- Information and healthcare technologies
- Ethics
- Human diversity
- Global healthcare
- Healthcare systems and policy
- Provider and manager of care
- Designer/manager/coordinator of care
- Member of a profession

To assist with the design and implementation of CNL curriculum, AACN provided a "CNL Toolkit" with resources for schools and their practice partners.

In 2013, an update of the CNL competencies and curricular expectations was published based on the 2011 *Essentials of Master's Education in Nursing* and the changing healthcare environment, and replaced the original 2007 document (AACN, 2013). The competencies align with the *Master's Essentials* and guide curriculum development and revision.

CNL Certification

After completion of formal CNL education, which includes 400 hours of clinical practicum including a 300-hour immersion experience, graduates are qualified to take the CNL® Certification Exam. The exam is administered by the CNC, and the first exams were administered in 2007. In 2007, CNL became a registered trademark of the AACN to protect the title, with only those who pass the exam entitled to use the CNL title (CNC, 2014). The certification exam was updated in 2012 to reflect a job analysis study of the essential knowledge and skills required of the CNL. As of May 2015, there were 3,820 clinical nurse leaders reported by CNC (CNC, 2015b).

CNL Association

In 2008, a group of CNLs from Portland, Oregon, and Maine Medical Center joined forces to form the Clinical Nurse Leader Association (CNLA). Bylaws were written and approved, and the first board officers were elected from the original steering committee. According to its mission statement, "The mission of the Clinical Nurse Leader Association is to provide a forum for members in all practice settings to collaborate, collect data, publish results, network, promote high standards of practice, maintain a professional presence and stay abreast of issues affecting their practice." (CNLA, 2015). By 2011, CNLA had become a fully functioning association with 503(c)3 status, holding an annual conference and providing regional continuing education offerings. In 2015, there were 411 members of CNLA throughout the United States (B. R. Shirley, personal communication, July 15, 2015).

Growth of the CNL Role

The development and implementation of the CNL role involved a partnership between education and practice, providing a practice environment to operationalize the CNL role. The nation's largest employer of nurses has made a commitment to implement the CNL role in all of the VAMCs nationwide by 2016 (CNC, 2015a; Ott et al., 2009). The majority of CNLs are employed in acute care settings, working to decrease readmissions, improve patient outcomes, and smooth care transitions across the continuum of care (Harris et al., 2011). CNL also practice in specialty areas such as pediatrics (O'Grady & VanGraafeiland, 2012), oncology (Murphy, 2014), in community or public health, and in long-term care (Harris et al., 2011). The broad skill set of the CNL is particularly valuable in the rural, critical-access setting where underserved and poor patients can challenge the healthcare system (Jukkala, Greenwood, Ladner, & Hopkins, 2010). As more outcomes data have been published, it is clear the implementation of the CNL role leads to improved patient outcomes.

As the CNL role has matured, the AACN has provided support and structure to foster the role. The first national AACN–CNL Partnership Conference was in January 2008 in Tucson, Arizona, bringing education and practice partners together to share outcomes of the early pilot programs. This early meeting has evolved into an annual CNL Summit conference which provides a forum for individuals from academic and healthcare settings who are exploring or have fully implemented the CNL role. The CNL Summit provides a setting for healthcare partners to share CNL successes in quality and safety initiatives and for education to present innovations in CNL education. The CNL Summit is preceded by the CNL Research Symposium, a 1-day preconference workshop focused on the CNL's role in data collection that provides a venue for reporting clinical outcomes.

The CNL Role and Patient Care Outcomes

The CNL role evolved out of a growing concern for patient safety and the need to improve the quality of care delivered. From the beginning, the importance of measuring the impact of the CNL role on patient care outcomes was stressed. This measurement of the role was not only to document the improvement in care but also to demonstrate the cost effectiveness of adding a role devoted to improving quality and safety. Improved patient care outcomes have been disseminated at the CNL annual meetings (podium and poster presentations) and in publications. In a 5-year review of the impact of the CNL role in a tertiary care center in the Northeast, the CNL role demonstrated decreased: (a) readmission rates, (b) rapid response and code blue rates, (c) bloodstream infections, (d) length of stay, and (e) pressure ulcers (Wilson et al., 2013). The CNL role has also demonstrated improvement in fall rates, patient satisfaction, pain management, restraint use, and staff turnover (Bender, 2014). The Veterans Health Administration has tracked the impact of the CNL closely since its implementation and has reported improvement in pressure ulcer rates, ventilator-associated pneumonia, and the number of cancelled gastrointestinal procedures (Ott et al., 2009). Research is ongoing and there is an early body of evidence suggesting the CNL has met the goal of improving patient care quality, safety, and satisfaction.

Resistance to the CNL Role

Change as significant as introducing a new role into the healthcare team is bound to have some resistance. The clinical nurse specialist (CNS) role has some similarities with the CNL role and leaders in the CNS field have been vocal regarding the introduction of the CNL role (Goudreau, 2008). Goudreau proposes using educational resources to increase the number of CNSs rather than developing a new nursing role (2008).

Resistance to the CNL role may come at the administration or system level. In a qualitative analysis of 22 CNLs in practice, the CNO and/or middle nurse manager were identified as putting up roadblocks to the success of the CNL. Most frequently, they cited the cost of hiring CNLs rather than more bedside nurses as the reason for resistance (Moore & Leahy, 2012). Sherman (2008) identified resistance to the CNL role by unit managers was one barrier CNOs had to overcome to implement the initial CNL pilots. Organizations with less resistance to the CNL role are those with the following: (a) organizational needs, (b) desire to improve patient care, (c) opportunity to redesign care delivery, (d) desire to promote professional development of RN staff, and (e) methods to enhance physician–nurse relationships (Sherman, 2008).

The Future of the CNL

The CNL role is in its infancy, with the early programs less than 10 years old. The change the Affordable Care Act is demanding of the healthcare system calls for all healthcare team members to be focused on achieving maximum outcomes for patients and families. The CNL competencies are well matched with the need for high-quality, cost-effective care across the care continuum (Jeffers & Astroth, 2013). The CNL is educated to work in a team to provide high-quality integrated care in an accountable-care environment. The patient-centered medical home team can benefit from a CNL working with the patient and family to address health issues surrounding chronic illness. The nurse shortage is looming and the need for nurses educated to improve quality and safety will grow as the shortage deepens.

The CNL role will likely spread globally as the need to improve quality and decrease cost is universal. Coordinating, managing, and evaluating care across the care continuum are nursing competencies that are needed worldwide (Baernholdt & Cottingham, 2011). The AACN and CNC are working with a group of faculty from Japan to develop a CNL education program at Tsukaba University (AACN, 2015).

Conclusion

In a short 15 years, the CNL role evolved out of an identified crisis in healthcare to an active part of the healthcare team. Integrating CNLs into healthcare settings has demonstrated improved patient care outcomes across the care continuum. The clinical nurse leader role is fulfilling the vision of becoming the "new nurse" of the 21st century.

Resources

American Association of Colleges of Nursing. (n.d.). *Join the Clinical Nurse Leader (CNL) initiative*. Retrieved from http://www.aacn.nche.edu/leading-initiatives/cnl/cnl-certification/pdf/RFP.pdf

American Association of Colleges of Nursing. (2007). *White paper on the education and role of the clinical nurse leader*. Washington, DC: American Association of Colleges of Nursing.

American Association of Colleges of Nursing. (2013). *Competencies and curricular expectations for the clinical nurse leader*SM *education and practice*. Washington, DC: American Association of Colleges of Nursing.

American Association of Colleges of Nursing. (2015). *CNL & CNC news: CNL faculty preparing for CNL exam in Japan*. Retrieved from http://www.aacn.nche.edu/cnl

Baernholdt, M., & Cottingham, S. (2011). The clinical nurse leader—New nursing role with global implications. *International Nursing Review*, *58*, 74–78.

Bender, M. (2014). The current evidence base for the clinical nurse leader: A narrative review of the literature. *Journal of Professional Nursing*, *30*(2), 110–123.

Buerhaus, P., Staiger, D. O., & Auerbach, D. I. (2000). Implications of an aging registered nurse workforce. *Journal of the American Medical Association*, *283*, 22, 2948–2954.

Clinical Nurse Leader Association. (2015). *CNLA history*. Retrieved from http://www.cnlassociation.org/CNLA-history

Commission on Nurse Certification. (2014). *History of CNL certification*. Retrieved from http://www.aacn.nche.edu/leading-initiatives/cnl/cnl-certification/pdf/History.pdf

Commission on Nurse Certification. (2015a). *Certified Clinical Nurse Leader (CNL®) talking points*. Retrieved from http://www.aacn.nche.edu/cnl/pdf/CNL-Talking-Points.pdf

Commission on Nurse Certification. (2015b). *CNL certification exam data*. Retrieved from http://www.aacn.nche.edu/leading-initiatives/cnl/cnl-certification/pdf/CNLStats.pdf

Fang, D., Htut, A. M., & Bednash, G. D. (2008). *2007–2008 enrollment and graduations in baccalaureate and graduate programs in nursing*. Washington, DC: American Association of Colleges of Nursing.

Goudreau, K. A. (2008). Confusion, concern, or complimentary function: The overlapping roles of the clinical nurse specialist and the clinical nurse leader. *Nursing Administration Quarterly*, *32*(4), 301–307.

Harris, J. L., Stanley, J., & Rosseter, R. (2011). The clinical nurse leader: Addressing healthcare challenges through partnerships and innovation. *Journal of Nursing Regulation*, *2*(2), 40–46.

Institute of Medicine. (1999). *To err is human: Building a safer health system*. Washington, DC: National Academy Press. Retrieved from: http://iom.nationalacademies.org/Reports/1999/to-err-is-human-building-a-safer-health-system.aspx

Institute of Medicine. (2001). *Crossing the quality chasm: A new health system for the 21st century*. Washington, DC: National Academy Press. Retrieved from http://iom.nationalacademies.org/Reports/2001/Crossing-the-Quality-Chasm-A-New-Health-System-for-the-21st-Century.aspx

Jeffers, B. R., & Astroth, K. S. (2013). The clinical nurse leader: Prepared for an era of healthcare reform. *Nursing Forum*, *48*(3), 223–229.

Joint Commission on Accreditation of Healthcare Organizations. (2002). *Health care at the crossroads: Strategies for addressing the evolving nursing crisis*. Chicago: Author. Retrieved from http://www.jointcommission.org/assets/1/18/health_care_at_the_crossroads.pdf

Jukkala, A., Greenwood, R., Ladner, K., & Hopkins, L. (2010). The clinical nurse leader and rural hospital safety and quality. *Online Journal of Rural Nursing and Health care*, *10*(2). Retrieved from http://rnojournal.binghamton.edu/index.php/RNO/article/view/45

Long, K. A. (2003). *Brief history of the CNL*. American Association of Colleges of Nursing. Retrieved from http://www.aacn.nche.edu/cnl/about/history

Moore, L. W., & Leahy, C. (2012). Implementing the new clinical nurse leader role while gleaning insights from the past. *Journal of Professional Nursing*, *28*(3), 139–146.

Murphy, E. A. (2014). Healthcare reform—A new role for changing times: Embracing the clinical nurse leader role—A strategic partnership to drive outcomes. *Nurse Leader*, *12*(4), 53–57.

O'Grady, E. L., & VanGraafeiland, B. (2012). Bridging the gap in care for children through the clinical nurse leader. *Pediatric Nursing*, *38*(3), 155–167.

Ott, K. M., Haddock, K. S., Fox, S. E., Shinn, J. K., Walters, S. E., Hardin, J. W., ... Harris, J. L. (2009). The Clinical Nurse Leader℠: Impact on practice outcomes in the Veterans Health Administration. *Nursing Economics*, *27*(6), 363–383.

Sherman, R. O. (2008). Factors influencing organizational participation in the Clinical Nurse Leader℠ project. *Nursing Economics*, *26*(4), 236–249.

Stanley, J. M. (2014). Introducing the clinical nurse leader: Past, present, and future. In J. L. Harris, L. Roussel, & P. L. Thomas (Eds.), *Initiating and sustaining the clinical nurse leader role: A practical guide* (2nd ed.). Burlington, MA: Jones & Bartlett.

Tornabeni, J., & Miller, J. F. (2008). The power of partnership to shape the future of nursing: The evolution of the clinical nurse leader. *Journal of Nursing Management, 16*, 608–613.

U.S. Department of Health and Human Services. (2010). *The registered nurse population: Findings from the 2008 National Sample Survey of Registered Nurses*. Washington, DC: U.S. Department of Health and Human Services Health Resources and Services Administration. Retrieved from http://bhpr.hrsa.gov/healthworkforce/rnsurveys/rnsurveyfinal.pdf

Wilson, L., Orff, S., Gerry, T., Shirley, B. R., Tabor, D., Caiazzo, K., & Rouleau, D. (2013). Evolution of an innovative role: The clinical nurse leader. *Journal of Nursing Management, 21*, 175–181.

2

Making the Best Use of This Book

Cynthia R. King and Sally O'Toole Gerard

In the nursing profession, national certification is a distinction for those nurses who have reached beyond their required knowledge and competency to achieve more. Certifications in nursing are generally related to the specific practice specialty of the nurse and can range from somewhat general content such as medical surgical nursing to very specific subspecialties such as oncology, psychiatric-mental health, or home health nursing. National certification as a clinical nurse leader reflects a standard of knowledge and professional practice acquired in the academic setting and implemented in the practice setting. The range of content is immense.

Nurses, perhaps more so than other disciplines, are test phobic. They understand exactly why. The national licensure exam to enter the profession as a registered nurse sets nurses up for this fear very early on in their careers. Despite years of developing clinical expertise, many nurses revert to an overly developed fear of any form of exam. As the first new academic degree in nursing in more than 45 years, a national certification required to practice as a CNL proved very anxiety provoking for nurses. It was clear that a certification review book would be a welcome resource.

Original Purpose of This Book

Clinical Nurse Leader® Certification Review is a book that was originally proposed as the first review book for the clinical nurse leader (CNL) certification exam. The CNL role is a new role to nursing and, therefore, there were no books on the market for reviewing for this certification exam. The book was published in 2013 with chapters on test-taking strategies, reflection questions, content containing the specific topics covered in the exam, and 200 multiple-choice questions. Both the first and second editions of the book are strictly based on the test blueprint provided by the AACN on the website. The intent is to present a complete reference for the individual nurse (or group) studying for the certification exam. The layout of this new edition still contains the key essentials required to cover the content included in the exam. Each content item of the test blueprint has a book chapter dedicated to the topic, written by leading experts in the field. It is also composed of chapters featuring information for the exam, test-taking strategies, and reflection questions, as well as new material. The new information includes a glossary as well as a history (journey) of the CNL role and new multiple-choice questions and unfolding case studies.

Current Uses of This Book

Clinical Nurse Leader Certification Review is a book that has evolved over time. It still is widely used by individual students (or groups) to study for the certification exam; this remains the main purpose of the book. The editors are committed to this main purpose as there still remains no competitive comprehensive review book for the CNL® exam. However, several new uses for this book have evolved quickly, including its use by faculty to design and conduct review sessions for CNL students, as well as its use in CNL courses.

For some individuals, there is an advantage to attending a formal review session. This session can serve multiple purposes. A formal review may help a student with structured study time to review for the exam. It also may decrease test anxiety, especially if test-taking strategies are covered. One of the editors (CRK) actually had a unique review session that was designed to help students pass the exam; this book evolved from this editor's unique review session. Faculty from other institutions who have tried creating review courses have ended up relying on the *Clinical Nurse Leader Certification Review* because of the organization and thorough coverage of topics. For instance, the book provides detailed information on the specifics of the exam from the Commission on Nurse Certification (CNC) that is otherwise located in several different locations. Moreover, the multiple-choice questions and unfolding case studies have rationales for the correct answers. This, combined with the chapter on test-taking strategies, can help faculty to improve student scores on practice questions.

An unexpected result of developing the *Clinical Nurse Leader Certification Review* has been the decision of certain CNL programs to use this book throughout the core CNL courses that have clinical components (e.g., physical assessment and two to four key CNL core courses). Students read the appropriate chapter (e.g., Advanced Clinical Assessment for the physical assessment course). After reading the chapter and attending clinical time, the students frequently cite this book in the discussion forum. This new and unique way to use the *Clinical Nurse Leader Certification*

Review is a sensible way to use the book throughout the entire CNL program and also incorporate the multiple-choice questions and unfolding case studies as practice items throughout the program. Because the book follows the exact exam content outline for the certification exam, students have thoroughly reviewed each topic by the end of their courses. A designated review session may then still be added at the end of the courses. Students now have access to an online exam review course through AACN at http://www.aacn.nche.edu/cnc/exam-prep. This can provide extra review materials at the end of the courses if the CNL student desires additional review materials.

Keys to Success

This book has been designed to provide individuals and groups with a successful journey to help them pass the CNL® certification exam. In order to make the journey effective, individuals (or groups, classes) should continue with the following steps:

- Read each chapter carefully and several times for key content.
- Spend time on reviewing and learning the test-taking strategies.
- Take the practice tests at the back of the book.
- Understand the rationale for the correct answer for each practice question and case study.
- Identify your strengths and weaknesses as you go through the chapters, questions, and case studies.
- Spend more time on your weak areas.
- Do not rely solely on this book as your resource (review the AACN white paper and AACN website thoroughly as well as other resources).

Conclusion

Clinical Nurse Leader Certification Review was first developed out of necessity as support for those taking a challenging exam. As this new role in nursing has established itself, CNLs have become valuable in the rapidly changing outcome-focused healthcare environment. The CNL's role is associated with quality academic preparation, opportunities emerging in healthcare, and a successful national certification program. It is hoped that this text will continue to be a valuable resource and used in innovative ways as nurses, prepared at the master's level, achieve a prestigious professional achievement.

3

Information for Taking the Certification Exam

Cynthia R. King

Who Provides the Certification Exam?

The Clinical Nurse Leader (CNL^{SM}) certification program is managed by the Commission on Nurse Certification (CNC), an autonomous arm of the American Association of Colleges of Nursing (AACN). This exam is overseen by the CNC board of commissioners. CNC recognizes individuals who have demonstrated professional standards and knowledge through CNL certification. CNC promotes lifelong learning through CNL recertification requirements. The CNC board of commissioners and staff are the only ones who decide the policies and administration of the CNL certification program (http://www.aacn.nche.edu/cnl-certification).

Information for Taking the Certification Exam

The CNL certification review prepares master's-prepared nurses to take the national CNL® certification exam offered by the CNC, a division of the AACN. For some nurses completing a master's degree in a CNL program, it is required by their employer to complete and pass the CNL certification exam. However, by obtaining CNL certification, nurses gain power, credibility, and trust similar to other certified advanced practice nurses and board-certified physicians. It also demonstrates commitment and credibility. It acknowledges that a CNL has a certain amount of knowledge and skills.

In some organizations, there is an incentive, bonus, or differential pay raise given to those who become certified in a particular area of expertise. Many hospitals that have achieved and maintain Magnet® status further support and recognize certification as a part of professional development.

It is up to employers whether or not they will reimburse candidates for the fee required to take the CNL certification exam. It is important to inquire before taking the exam whether you will be compensated.

The purpose of this chapter is to explain:

- Who provides certification
- Information about taking the exam
- The new exam format
- The exam content outline
- Total time
- Exam results
- Who is eligible
- The application process
- What to bring to the exam
- Resources

Certification Exam Format

As of April 2012, the CNC exam is one inclusive exam, with multiple-choice questions and unfolding case studies. However, for each section of the unfolding case study, there is only one multiple-choice question with one correct answer. More information in this regard is located in the Certification Guide at http://www.aacn.nche.edu/cnc/exam-prep.

The multiple-choice format allows examinees to test in one sitting and to receive automatic score results immediately following completion of the exam. In addition, the exam reflects the CNL job analysis that has recently been conducted and will continue to be conducted periodically. The format and content of the exam are robust, along with the unfolding case study items. The content outline is now part of the Certification Guide and is also listed separately as an Exam Content Outline. Both of these are available at http://www.aacn.nche/edu/cnc/exam-prep and a part of this content outline appears at the back of this review book (Appendix A).

The exam is only offered as a computer-based exam. The multiple-choice questions have an option of choosing one of four possible answers. Only one of the four answers is correct (even under the unfolding case studies), so examinees do not have to worry about choosing multiple correct answers out of the four choices. The exam has approximately 140 questions (between regular multiple-choice questions and unfolding case studies).

Of the approximately 140 questions, 130 will count toward the examinee's score. The remaining 10 questions are "trial" or "pretest" questions that are interspersed throughout the exam. Pretesting questions allow the exam committee and CNC to collect meaningful statistics about new questions that may appear as scored questions on future exams.

The exam is based on three major content areas composed of 7 to 23 subcontent areas. These are listed in the Examination Content Outline in the Certification Guide. In addition, the percentage of exam questions devoted to each major content area is indicated. This can help the examinee decide what areas to emphasize when studying. Additionally, each question of the multiple-choice and unfolding case study sections is also categorized by a cognitive level that a candidate would likely use to respond. These categories are:

- Recall—the ability to recall or recognize specific information.
- Application—the ability to comprehend, relate, or apply knowledge to new or changing situations.
- Analysis—the ability to analyze and synthesize information, determine solutions, and/or evaluate the usefulness of a solution.

The questions are developed by item writers and based on the AACN white paper and a list of resources and bibliography. The purpose of the exam is to assess whether nurses are competent to work as CNLs in any healthcare setting. There is a CNL self-assessment exam and review course that may be purchased at http://www.aacn.nche.edu/cnc/exam-prep. There are also multiple-choice questions and unfolding case studies at the end of this review book that should be used to practice for the certification exam. Completing practice questions is strongly recommended. Additionally, it is helpful to review test-taking skills, as described in the next chapter.

Detailed Test-Content Outline

This book is organized chapter by chapter according to the AACN/CNC Exam Content Outline (http://www.aacn.nche.edu/cnc/exam-prep). The Certification Guide (used to be Exam Handbook) with content outline, along with many other resources, may be found at http://www.aacn.nche.edu/cnc/exam-prep. This is the main resource section for the certification exam.

Total Time for the Test

The format of the certification exam is now scheduled as a 3-hour exam without any breaks. It is anticipated that most individuals will not need a full 3 hours for the exam, but all individuals may take the full 3 hours. You may go back and change your answers at any time. It is recommended that you arrive 20 minutes before the test begins. Any individual who arrives 15 or more minutes late will not be allowed to take the exam.

Exam Results

Candidates who take the CNL certification exam will receive automatic information as to whether they have passed immediately after the exam. Currently, individuals who pass the exam will only receive an e-mail that they have passed. Individuals who were unsuccessful will receive their exam scores and a diagnostic report.

In order to see the results, the successful examinee must click on the link that reads "View Results." In addition, exam results will be sent to the examinee's e-mail address that was provided on the certification application. The results will include scores in different content areas of the exam (the content areas outlined in the Certification Guide, at http://www.aacn.nche.edu/cnc/exam-prep). The final report of results will also show the examinee's scores in comparison with the highest possible score in each content area. The faculty contact for the institution/school will receive aggregate pass/fail reports within approximately 2 weeks, following completion of the testing period (not the exam date).

Who Is Eligible to Take the Exam?

An individual who meets the CNL eligibility requirements and passes the CNL certification exam will be awarded the CNL designation. In order to register for the certification exam, each individual must meet the requirements that follow (http://www.aacn.nche.edu/cnc/apply-exam).

RN Licensure

The individual must hold a current and active RN license in the United States. Any individual will be ineligible if currently being disciplined by a state nursing board.

CNL Education

Graduation from a CNL master's or post-master's program, accredited by a nursing accrediting agency recognized by the U.S. Secretary of Education, which prepares individuals with the competencies delineated in the AACN (2013), is required. All individuals scheduled to graduate from a CNL education program are encouraged to sit for the CNL certification exam. Students may apply to take the certification exam, but they must be in their last academic term. Students enrolled in a Model C program may sit for the exam before earning RN licensure. Students must then submit documentation of RN licensure to the CNC after successful completion of the CNL certification exam and meet all requirements to be awarded CNL certification.

Process for Enrolling for the Exam

All CNL certification application materials and resources provided by the CNC are located at http://www.aacn.nche.edu/cnc/apply-exam. There are a number of steps that the student/candidate and faculty contact must take. The list of steps includes:

1. Candidates must meet eligibility requirements established by the CNC and that are previously listed in this chapter.
2. The institution or school is required to schedule the testing date(s) within the testing period offered by the CNC. Then the institution must notify the CNC of the scheduled testing date, time, and proctor and contact information. Additionally, the school or institution must submit (a) the Site Registration Form (http://www.aacn.nche.edu/cnl/exam-site-registration) and (b) School of Nursing CNL Education Program Verification Form (which needs to be signed by the dean/chief academic officer). This form is submitted only once for each school, but must be approved and on file in the CNC office for candidates to be eligible to sit for the exam. A list of schools with forms on file is posted on the website.
3. The CNC will confirm proctor via e-mail and send a proctor manual to the faculty serving as proctor. If an online student or graduate is not near a CNL education program, he or she may take the exam at a testing center affiliated with Schroeder Measurement Technologies, Inc. (SMT). In this case, the proctor will be provided.
4. Another alternative is to take the test at one of several testing centers provided by SMT. These are sites that are available for CNL graduates and online students.
5. The candidate must also submit documents and a fee to CNC to register for the exam, whether he or she will be taking the exam at a school of nursing or a site sponsored by SMT. Documents are located at http://www.aacn.nche.edu/cnc/exam-application and include:
   a. CNL Certification Examination application
   b. Application attestation
   c. CNL Education Documentation Form (signed by CNL program director)
   d. Request for special exam accommodations and documentation
   e. Disability-Related Needs forms (if applicable)

6. Once the application is received, CNC sends electronic notification confirming receipt to the applicant; CNC also notifies candidates of outstanding documents.
7. CNC reviews the application.
8. The candidate confirms testing date, time, and location with the faculty contact/proctor or testing site.
9. Once the candidates are confirmed, CNC sends a list of scheduled examinees to the faculty contact of the exam site or the site sponsored by SMT.
10. At least 2 days prior to the exam date, CNC sends an electronic notification to the faculty contact or testing site with names of eligible candidates and pass codes for each candidate to access the exam.
11. On the testing date, the exam is administered at the institution/school or testing site as scheduled.
12. Exam results and detailed scoring are electronically available to the candidate immediately after the exam.
13. Once the exam is over, the faculty contact may receive aggregate pass/fail results. This will occur approximately 2 weeks following completion of the testing period.
14. After the exam, CNC also mails official notification and a certificate to each successful candidate. It is important to know that an individual is not officially certified until he or she receives a formal letter and certificate. Certification will be withheld from candidates who have outstanding documentation or payment.
15. The current exam fees are listed in the Certification Guide.

The Day of the Exam: What to Bring and What Not to Bring

On the day of the certification exam, the candidate must bring ONLY a current government-issued photo ID to the test site. The candidate will be required to sign in for verification of identity. *Any candidate without proper identification is not permitted to take the certification exam. Proper identification may include a valid driver's license with a color photograph and signature or a valid passport or military-issued identification card with a color photograph and signature.*

It is recommended that all examinees report to the scheduled designated testing site no later than 20 minutes before the scheduled testing time. *You will not be allowed to take the exam if you arrive more than*

15 minutes after the scheduled testing time, and your exam fees will be forfeited.

- EXCEPT for your photo ID, no personal materials including purses, briefcases, hats, food/drink, paper, pen, books, or reference materials may be taken into the testing center. Car keys are permitted.
- No electronic devices are allowed in the testing room, including cameras, cell phones, pagers, tablets, iPads, Blackberrys, laptop computers, or calculators.

Conclusion

Taking the certification exam is an important step for graduates of CNL programs. Tests and exams always provide some anxiety and fear. However, when provided with concrete objective information about the exam and places to find resources, it can make taking the exam much easier and less anxiety provoking. It is hoped that this chapter and the entire review book will be helpful for CNL students now and in the future.

Resources

American Association of Colleges of Nursing. (2013). *Competencies and curricular expectations for Clinical Nurse Leader℠ education and practice.* Retrieved from http://www.aacn.nche.edu/publications/white-papers/cnl

American Association of Colleges of Nursing. (2016a). *Apply for the Exam.* Retrieved from http://www.aacn.nche.edu/cnc/apply-exam

American Association of Colleges of Nursing. (2016b). *CNL recommended reading.* Retrieved from http://www.aacn.nche.edu/cnc/exam-prep/recommended-reading

American Association of Colleges of Nursing. (2016c). *CNL certification guide.* Retrieved from http://www.aacn.nche.edu/cnc/exam-prep/CNL-Certification-Guide.pdf

American Association of Colleges of Nursing. (2016d). *CNL job analysis study.* Retrieved from http://www.aacn.nche.edu/cnl/publications-resources/job-analysis-study

American Association of Colleges of Nursing. (2016e). *Commission on nurse certification.* Retrieved from http://www.aacn.nche.edu/cnl/cnc

American Association of Colleges of Nursing. (2016f). *Self-assessment exam.* Retrieved from http://www.aacn.nche.edu/cnc/exam-prep/self-assessment

Commission on Nurse Certification. (2014). *Clinical Nurse Leader (CNL®) certification exam blueprint.* Retrieved from http://www.aacn.nche.edu/leading-initiatives/cnl/cnl-certification/pdf/ExamContentOutline11.pdf

Commission on Nurse Certification and Schroeder Measurement Technologies, Inc. (2014). *Exam content outline.* Washington, DC: Author.

4

Test-Taking Skills

Cynthia R. King

Taking any type of test or exam may provoke significant anxiety. This is also true for many individuals taking the clinical nurse leader (CNL®) certification exam. There are a number of strategies that can be used to help individuals prepare for a test or exam. These strategies may help an individual decrease his or her anxiety and ultimately increase his or her score. Unfortunately, test-taking strategies are not always taught in nursing school. Consequently, it is important for CNL students to learn these skills by reading or attending workshops.

Preparation Strategies for the CNL® Certification Exam

When preparing for the exam, it is important for CNL students to remember they are experienced nurses and have completed all of the required courses for the certification exam. Thus, you are already prepared for the exam in many ways. However, this may not be enough to decrease anxiety and fear about taking the certification exam. What is most important to learn before the exam is how to analyze and dissect the exam questions.

For Those With Test Anxiety

Test anxiety is considered a psychological condition that can cause stress related to preparing for an exam. Test anxiety is a type of performance anxiety, because the individual is under pressure to do well in order to pass. Different individuals may experience tension and stress before, during, and maybe even after a test. Symptoms may include butterflies in the stomach, stomachache, nausea, vomiting, diarrhea, headaches, excessive sweating, rapid heart rate, and rapid breathing. If you feel you have an overwhelming test anxiety, you should talk to a faculty member or health professional.

There are ways to prevent and alleviate test anxiety. These may include the following:

- Be prepared for the exam (with time management and study plan).
- Prior to the exam, ask family and friends for help so that you may manage your time, study plan, and anxiety.
- Use relaxation, meditation, and breathing.
- Engage in positive pampering—take care of yourself the day before with exercise, fun, relaxation, good nutrition, and massage.
- Do not cram the night before the exam—rest your body and mind.
- Get up 15 to 30 minutes early to be relaxed for the test.
- If anxious during the test, do deep breathing exercises.

Preparation Before the Exam

Before taking the CNL certification exam, there are specific resources to access and ways to prepare. Many of the resources are found in the Publications and Resources section of the American Association of Colleges of Nurses (AACN) website at http://www.aacn.nche.edu/cnl/publications-resources. Other ways to prepare include the following:

- Go to review sessions and pay attention to hints that the instructor may give about the test. Take notes and ask questions about items you may be confused about.
- Ask the instructor to specify the areas that will be emphasized on the test.
- Go over any material from practice tests, sample problems, and review materials.
- Set up a regular study schedule (daily schedule, weekly schedule).
- It is recommended that you not study for more than 1 to 2 hours without a break. The break should be about 10 minutes.
- Increase your self-confidence (use guided imagery/visualization to decrease anxiety). Worry about how much you know and not how much others know.
- Try studying in a group.
- Focus first on the subjects that you find most difficult as these will take the most time.
- Avoid distractions while studying. Turn off the television, telephone, and music.
- Manage your anxiety—different things work for different people—do *not* cram the day or night before, but do get enough rest and arrive early for the exam.

- Minimize discomfort—dress comfortably, take a sweater (in case the air conditioning is too cold), sit near the front or wherever there are fewer distractions, or sit away from windows if distracting.
- Get to the test site early to relax (do muscle relaxation or visualization); arrive at least 20 to 30 minutes before the test starts.
- Be careful about taking too much sleeping medication the night before or drinking too much coffee before the exam.
- If given a piece of paper, write down quick notes of things you are afraid you might forget.
- Eat before the test. Having food in your stomach will give you energy and help you focus; however, avoid heavy foods, which can make you groggy.
- Do not try to pull an "all-nighter." Get at least 6 to 8 hours of sleep before the test (normally 8 hours of sleep a night is recommended, but if you are short on time, get at least 6 hours, so that you will be well-rested enough to focus during the test).
- Put the main ideas/information/formulas onto a sheet that can be quickly reviewed many times; this makes it easier to retain the key concepts that will be on the test.
- Set your alarm and have a backup alarm set as well.
- Go to the bathroom before walking into the exam room. You do not want to waste any time worrying about your bodily needs during the test.

The Day of the Exam

There are also key ways to help decrease your anxiety and fear and be successful on the day of the certification test. Among these are the following:

- Bring a watch to the test, so that you can better pace yourself.
- Keep a positive attitude throughout the whole test and try to stay relaxed. If you start to feel nervous, take a few deep breaths to relax. Repeat these actions throughout the test. This process will help you to stay relaxed and to make more energy available for remembering, thinking, and writing.
- Read directions carefully—do not overanalyze questions or instructions.
- Do a quick "mind dump" of information you do not want to forget. Write it down on the paper or in the margin provided for the CNL® exam.
- Look for tricky or key words (e.g., the best answer, the first step).
- At the end, go over the question and answers to make sure you have read the question accurately.
- Do not change answers erratically.

- Look for clues in the question.
- Look for clues in the answer choices.
- If you have a tough question—answer it and keep it in the back of your mind; as you go along you may return to it, as something else may trigger a different response.
- If all else fails, eliminate as many choices as you can and then make an educated guess.
- Generally, questions proceed from easy to difficult, so if you think you have a difficult question at the beginning, you are probably reading too much into it.
- If two answers look correct, give the most obvious answer.
- If no answer seems correct, choose the one that is most nearly correct.
- Look for clues within the questions. For example, if the question is in the past tense, but three of four of the multiple-choice answers are in the present tense, the one answer in the past tense is likely to be the correct answer.
- Do not stay on a problem that you are stuck on, especially when time is a factor.
- Pace yourself, so you do not rush.
- Read the entire question and pay attention to the details.
- Always read the whole question carefully. Do not make assumptions about what the question might be.
- Use good strategies for answering objective questions versus essay questions.
    - Look for the central idea of each question. What is the main point?
    - Statements that begin with *always*, *never*, *none*, *except*, *most*, or *least* are probably NOT the correct answer.
    - Try to supply your own answer before choosing an alternative listed on the test.
    - Mark an answer for every question.
- When problem solving, ask yourself:
    - What am I being asked to find?
    - What do I need to know in order to find the answer?
    - What information has been provided that will help me to find the answer?
    - How can I break the problem down into parts? What steps should I follow to solve the problem?
    - Does the answer make sense? Does it cover the whole problem?

- Keep an eye on the clock.
- If you do not know an answer, skip it. Go on with the rest of the test and come back to it later. Other parts of the test may have some information that will help you out with that question.
- Do not worry if others finish before you. Focus on the test in front of you.
- If you have time left when you are finished, look over your test. Make sure that you have answered all the questions.
- Change an answer only if you misread or misinterpreted the question, because the first answer that you put is usually the correct one. Watch out for careless mistakes.

Strategies for Analyzing Multiple-Choice Questions

It is essential for all students or nurses taking tests to understand the different parts of a question. In the CNL certification exam, all of the questions are essentially multiple choice. There are multiple-choice questions with four possible answers, only one of which is the correct answer. The unfolding case studies provide information on a case study and then generally have five multiple-choice questions that occur after new information is added to the case study. Each of these questions also has only four possible answers, only one of which is the correct answer. Consequently, it is helpful to understand strategies for analyzing multiple-choice questions. These include the following:

1. There are different parts to the question and answers. Various terms are used for these in different textbooks. The *case event* or *background statement* is the "heart" of the question. This portion provides the information that you need to think about to answer the question. The *question query* or *stem* follows the case event and asks something specific about the background statement. This is the element that contains the specific problem or intent of the item. Lastly, the *options* are all the potential answers presented with the question. Among the options, the correct answer is called the *keyed response*, whereas the other options are called *distractors*.
2. If the question asks for the *most correct answer*, remember it is not what you believe is the most correct that counts, but what the CNC/test writers believe is the most correct.
3. Read every word that counts. If the entire question has several sections that include several complicated statements, isolate each of them. Then, when you have picked an answer, check it against each complicated segment. Your answer has to satisfy every part of the question.

4. When reading the question, carefully look for strategic words or phrases in the case event and query of the question. Strategic words or phrases should focus your attention on specific points that you should consider when answering the question.
5. Certain strategic words and phrases indicate there is *only one correct option*. Examples of these include: *early sign, late sign, understands goal has been achieved, goals have not yet been fully met, has not met the outcome criteria, adequately tolerating, inadequate, unable to tolerate, ineffective, avoid, needs additional instructions,* and *lack of understanding*.
6. Strategic words and phrases that may indicate the need to prioritize to select the correct option include the following examples: *best, first, initial, immediately, most likely* or *least likely, most appropriate* or *least appropriate, highest* or *lowest priority, order of priority, at highest risk, at lowest risk,* and *best understanding*.
7. Some strategic words and phrases indicate a positive or negative event question query that may indicate there is one correct option. Words or phrases that may indicate a positive event question/query include: *early sign, late sign, best, first, initial, immediately, most likely, most appropriate, highest priority, order of priority, all nursing interventions that apply, goal has been achieved,* and *adequately tolerating*. On the other hand, the words or phrases that indicate a negative event question/query include examples such as: *least likely, least appropriate, least priority, least helpful, at lowest risk, avoid, needs additional instructions, needs additional teaching, lack of understanding, goals have not yet been fully met, has not met the outcome criteria, ineffective, inadequate,* and *unable to tolerate*.
8. In a multiple-choice question, in addition to the case event there are *always* distractors (usually three or five) and a single correct answer. There may also be descriptive items, labels, an introductory sentence to be completed, or case studies.
9. Try reading the case event and question query with each response.
10. Be sure you understand what the question is asking.
11. Often all of the choices will seem somewhat plausible. In this case, there will probably be at least one clue or strategic word in the case event that makes one answer obviously better than the rest. Go back and read the case event looking for the strategic word.
12. Discard as many ridiculous choices for answers as you can. Some answers are obviously wrong, so move quickly on to the next choice. Many answers are partly wrong. If they are wrong in *any* way, then they are not the right choice.

13. Many answers are correct statements by themselves, but they have nothing to do with the case event part of the questions.
14. A positive choice is more likely to be true than with a negative one.
15. A correct answer is often (not always) the choice with the longest and most precise information.
16. Options or answers that are closed-ended are often incorrect. As you read the options available, eliminate any closed-ended words such as: *all, always, cannot, every, must, never, none, not, only,* and *will not*. On the other hand, if an option has an open-ended word, then that may be the correct option. Examples of open-ended words include: *generally, may, possibly,* and *usually*.
17. Choose answers that include qualifying terms such as *often* and *most*.
18. If you have time to go over the questions and answers, check the one you were concerned about first and then go over the rest of the answers if you have enough time.
19. If you have eliminated two of four of the options, then how do you select the correct answer? Follow these steps to try to make the correct choice: read the case event and question again, identify the case event from the query of the question, look for strategic words or phrases, identify the subject of the question, ask yourself, "What is the question asking me?," read all the options again, and make your final choice by focusing on what the question is asking.
20. There is no guessing penalty, so always take an educated guess.

Conclusion

For some individuals, test taking comes easily. Other individuals learn these skills early on. However, for the majority, proper coaching and practice can increase their test-taking abilities. This chapter provides tips to help all individuals taking the CNL certification exam so they can be successful. The tips for preparing for the exam, what to do the day of the exam, and tips for dissecting multiple-choice questions will hopefully decrease anxiety and fear for all CNL students.

Resources

Kesselman-Turkel, J., & Peterson, F. (2004). *Test-taking strategies*. Madison, WI: University of Wisconsin Press.

Macdonald, V. (2014). *Test taking strategies for everyone*. Retrieved from http://www.amazon.com/Vernon-Macdonald/e/B00HP4ESGG/ref=dp_byline_cont_pop_book_1

Nugent, P., & Vitale, B. (2008). *Test success: Test-taking techniques for beginners.* Philadelphia, PA: F. A. Davis Company.

Rozakis, L. (2003). *Test taking strategies & study skills for the utterly confused.* New York, NY: McGraw-Hill.

Sides, M. B., & Korchek, N. (1998). *Successful test-taking* (3rd ed.). Philadelphia, PA: Lippincott-Raven Publishers.

Silvestri, L. A., & Silvestri, A. (2014). *Strategies for test success.* St. Louis, MO: Elsevier Saunders.

II

Key Certification Topics: Nursing Leadership

5

Horizontal Leadership

Jodi A. Erickson and Teri Moser Woo

Clinical nurse leader (CNL) education provides the graduate with the ability to assume horizontal leadership within the healthcare team (American Association of Colleges of Nursing [AACN], 2007). A *horizontal organization* is one of decentralization of power and/or control, at least within specific departments. The emphasis is placed on horizontal collaboration. *Horizontal leadership* is where there may be multiple individuals who assume leadership of a team or teams in order to achieve a common goal. In contrast, vertical leadership is when there is always one team leader. Horizontal leadership is a philosophy of organizational leadership whereby the structure promotes equality and an open-door policy. This allows team members to voice their opinions and to provide feedback freely. This is different from vertical leadership, which is a top-down style of leadership whereby team members are not encouraged to question or provide feedback. In order to provide horizontal leadership, the CNL must understand and apply leadership theories, work within the patient care team to plan and guide care, and promote an environment where nurses feel supported and empowered.

Theories of Leadership and Change

To provide horizontal leadership, the CNL is required to understand and apply theories of nursing, leadership, and change to practice:

- Nursing theories such as Orem's self-care or Leininger's culture care diversity and universality enable the planning of nursing care to be systematic, predictable, and purposeful.
- Leadership theories assist the CNL to function within a microsystem by understanding leadership styles and grow as a leader.
- Complexity theory is used to understand a rapidly changing, unpredictable healthcare environment. It has its origins in the chaos model (e.g., changes are rapid, random, and frequent; Cannon & Boswell, 2010).

- Systems theory is used "in the design, delivery, and evaluation of effective health care" (AACN, 2007, p. 24).
- Change theory is critical to guiding clinical practice improvement. Using a theory such as Kotter's 8-Step Change Model provides and explains that there is a predictable process to practice improvement change. Another common change theory was developed by Kurt Lewin. Lewin's model described three stages of change: unfreezing, moving, and refreezing (Cannon & Boswell, 2010).

The Practice of Horizontal Leadership

In order to practice horizontal leadership, the CNL needs a "tool kit" of skills. These critical skills include guiding evidence-based practice, healthcare outcomes, lateral integration, use of feedback, coaching, and leading teams. The horizontal leadership may be formal or informal.

Evidence-Based Practice

The CNL uses evidence-based practice (EBP) to guide decisions regarding care and leadership decisions and to improve the quality of patient care in the microsystem. In order for EBP to be integrated into care, the CNL may need to educate the staff on the definition of EPB and how it can be applied to practice. The CNL may personally use or assist nursing staff in using EBP principles to design care for individuals or populations. Likewise, the steps of the EBP process can be used in making clinical decisions and assessing outcomes, such as preventing pressure ulcers or falls in the population (Thomas, 2014).

Healthcare Outcomes

As leaders in the healthcare system, CNLs have a vital role in healthcare outcomes. For example, the Veterans Administration (Ott et al., 2009) has discovered numerous outcomes where CNLs have a positive effect. The outcomes may be financial (nursing hours per patient day), quality processes (e.g., pressure ulcers, discharge teaching, ventilator-associated pneumonia), patient and staff satisfaction, or changing practice to be based on evidence.

Wong, Cummings, and DuCharme (2013) performed a systematic review focused on nursing leadership and patient outcomes. The research indicated that there is a negative correlation between relational leadership styles and patient mortality, medication errors, and adverse events

(p. 719). While not addressed specifically, this evidence may support the positive effect of nursing leadership, similar to the horizontal leadership displayed by CNLs. As the role of the CNL has spread to other small and large healthcare organizations, executives are continuing to see positive effects by implementing the role and having CNLs as horizontal leaders.

Lateral Integrator

In describing the evolution of the CNL role, Tornabeni (2006) defines *lateral integration* as "the integration of care provided by multiple interdependent, and independent disciplines across a continuum of patient admission or experience" (p. 6). The CNL lateral integrator role can be compared to that of the air traffic controller who has a balcony view of what is happening with the patient and healthcare team and system. The Magnet® model supports lateral integration of care by encouraging structural empowerment, whereby the flow of information and decision making is multidirectional between the nurse at the bedside, clinical leadership (i.e., the CNL), interprofessional teams, and nursing administration (American Nurses Credentialing Center, 2015). By providing lateral integration of care for the patient, the CNL breaks down barriers and proactively manages care across the care continuum. This role is further discussed in Chapter 9.

Use of Feedback

Effective communication is an important skill for all CNLs. As Antai-Otong (2014) discusses, communication involves numerous aspects. A few of these include verbal and nonverbal communication, active listening, assertiveness, conveying clear and simple messages, and being specific. Giving and receiving feedback are part of horizontal leadership. When giving feedback, (a) clearly state what you plan to say, (b) emphasize the positive, (c) focus on the behavior or problem rather than the person, (d) use "I" statements rather than "you" statements, (e) avoid giving advice, and (f) avoid generalizations (Antai-Otong, 2014).

Coaching and Mentoring

The CNL has been identified as a crucial link in creating an environment of improved quality of care, safety, and performance. The CNL acts as a coach and mentor to all members of the healthcare team. Coaching and mentoring are ways the CNL can help new graduate nurses as well as experienced nurses. *Mentoring* involves a long-term relationship oriented toward nurses who are focused on advancing clinically. Instead, coaching is an ongoing two-way process in which the CNL can share knowledge and experience to help other nurses achieve desired professional goals. It focuses on learning more complex ways of thinking and problem solving, rather than focusing on tasks (Clark, 2009). The CNL is perfectly positioned to *coach* new graduate nurses as they transition from education into practice. As the nurse gains skill and confidence, the CNL continues to act as a mentor in the design of care, as well as in the professional development of the individual nurse. When coaching, the CNL is evaluating team members and constructively criticizing team members' performance. Other team members can also be coached; for example, in the use of EBP to improve care.

Leading Teams

The CNL is the logical choice to lead teams to improve the quality of care in the microsystem. The process of designing quality improvement requires the CNL to develop and lead a team of like-minded individuals toward a common goal. Likewise, the care of patients in a complex healthcare system demands an integrated team approach to care in order to have optimal outcomes. With education in leadership, change, and EBP principles, the CNL has or develops the skills to lead teams to reach the desired goal (Clark, 2009; Dye, 2010; Thomas, 2014). Thomas (2014) describes team leader tools for success and team charters. Furthermore, she provides team agendas, meeting-minutes templates, as well as team ground rules for CNLs to use. Dye (2010) actually describes team structure, team effectiveness, team activities and objectives, and rules and norms. These are all helpful for CNLs, especially when they first begin to lead teams.

Promoting a Safe and Ethical Environment

The CNL collaborates with the administration or nurse manager to promote an environment of safety and ethical care. To promote a culture of safety, the CNL learns how to evaluate and assess risks to patient safety and then works within the team to design and implement systems that support safe patient care (AACN, 2007, p. 36). An example of promoting safety is when the CNL is involved in the rate of falls for complex patients and determining methods to decrease the number of patient falls. Falls, especially among older adults, are a large national problem. CNLs need access to in-depth information related to safety within their organization as well as regionally and nationally. When developing a plan of care for the individual or the microsystem, ethical principles are used in the design and delivery of the care. This is based on the fact that CNLs are well-informed of the traditional ethical principles of nonmalfeasance, beneficence, autonomy, and distributive justice. Additionally, the CNL must act in an ethical manner in providing safe, humanistic care (AACN, 2007, p. 15). Awareness of the many ethical dilemmas that are present for patients and families as well as for nursing staff is also an important part of the role of horizontal leadership for CNLs.

Horizontal Leadership Content on CNL® Exam

According to the *Clinical Nurse Leader Job Analysis Report* (Commission on Nurse Certification, 2011) and *The Clinical Nurse Leader (CNL®) Certification Exam Blueprint* (Commission on Nurse Certification, 2014), horizontal leadership questions represent 7% of the exam content. The content related to horizontal leadership covered on the exam is found in Table 5.1.

TABLE 5.1 Horizontal Leadership Content Outline for the CNL Exam

CATEGORY	WEIGHT
A. Horizontal Leadership	**7%**
1. Applies theories and models (e.g., nursing, leadership, complexity, change) to practice	
2. Applies evidence-based practice to make clinical decisions and assess outcomes	
3. Understands microsystem functions and assumes accountability for healthcare outcomes	
4. Designs, coordinates, and evaluates plans of care at an advanced level in conjunction with interdisciplinary team	
5. Utilizes peer feedback for evaluation of self and others	
6. Serves as a lateral integrator of the interdisciplinary health team	
7. Leads group processes to meet care objectives	
8. Coaches and mentors healthcare team serving as a role model	
9. Utilizes an evidence-based approach to meet specific needs of individuals, clinical populations, or communities within the microsystem	
10. Assumes responsibility for creating a culture of safe and ethical care	
11. Provides leadership for changing practice based on quality improvement methods and research findings	

Used with permission from the Commission on Nurse Certification (2011, 2014).

Conclusion

Leadership is essential in the current healthcare climate in order to have optimal patient outcomes, yet the traditional model of top-down vertical leadership may not be an effective strategy for the CNL working with interdisciplinary teams. CNL education provides the CNL with the skills not only to assume leadership in patient care, but also to mentor others in sharing horizontal leadership to improve patient outcomes.

Resources

American Association of Colleges of Nursing. (2007). *White paper on education and role of the clinical nurse leader.* Retrieved from http://www.aacn.nche.edu/publications/white-papers/ClinicalNurseLeader.pdf

American Nurses Credentialing Center. (2015). *Magnet model.* Retrieved from http://www.nursecredentialing.org/magnet/programoverview/new-magnet-model

Antai-Otong, D. (2014). Effective communication and team coordination. In J. L. Harris & L. Roussel (Eds.), *Initiating and sustaining the clinical nurse leader role: A practical guide* (2nd ed.). Sudbury, MA: Jones & Bartlett Publishers.

Cannon, S., & Boswell, C. (2010). The clinical nurse leader as a transformed leader. In J. L. Harris & L. Roussel (Eds.), *Initiating and sustaining the clinical nurse leader role: A practical guide.* Sudbury, MA: Jones & Bartlett Publishers.

Clark, C. C. (2009). Coaching and mentoring. *Creative nursing leadership & management.* Boston, MA: Jones & Bartlett Publishers.

Commission on Nurse Certification. (2011). *Clinical Nurse Leader job analysis report.* Retrieved from http://www.aacn.nche.edu/cnl/Job-Analysis-Report.pdf

Commission on Nurse Certification. (2014). *Clinical Nurse Leader (CNL®) certification exam blueprint.* Retrieved from http://www.aacn.nche.edu/leading-initiatives/cnl/cnl-certification/pdf/ExamContentOutline11.pdf

Dye, C. F. (2010). *Leadership in healthcare: Essential values and skills* (2nd ed.). Chicago, IL: Healthcare Administration Press.

Ott, K. M., Haddock, K. S., Fox, S. E., Shinn, J. K., Walters, S. E., Hardin, J. W., ... Harris, J. L. (2009). The clinical nurse leader: Impact on practice outcomes in the Veterans Health Administration. *Nursing Economics, 27*(6), 363–371.

Thomas, P. (2014). Quality care and risk management. In J. L. Harris & L. Roussel (Eds.), *Initiating and sustaining the clinical nurse leader role: A practical guide* (2nd ed.). Sudbury, MA: Jones & Bartlett Publishers.

Tornabeni, J. (2006). Evolution of a revolution. *Journal of Nursing Administration, 36*(1), 3–6.

Wong, C. A., Cummings, G. G., & Ducharme, L. (2013). The relationship between nursing leadership and patient outcomes: A systematic review update. *Journal of Nursing Management, 21*(5), 709–724. doi.org/10.1111/jonm.12116

6

Interprofessional Communication and Collaboration Skills

Denise M. Bourassa

Communication is an activity of conveying information and can be visualized in the form of a cycle. There is a sender of information, a receiver of information, and a method of sending information. In order for the communication cycle to be complete, the information must be received as it was intended by the sender to the receiver. Communication can be nonverbal, mainly through the use of body language; oral, as information that is shared face to face; and, finally, it can be written. Good communication skills are the cornerstone of interpersonal relationships; as a result, they are necessary for *collaboration* and interdisciplinary relationships among healthcare providers. These relationships become crucial when providing safe patient care that is also cost effective. How we communicate with each other plays a very important role in the overall patient experience.

Communication and Collaboration as a Cultural Foundation of Healthcare

Communication skills are acquired and learned through social interaction as we develop and mature. However, not everyone's experience with communication is the same; therefore, we all come to adulthood with different levels and types of communication skills. As healthcare providers, we are taught the essentials for communicating with patients, families, staff members, and other disciplines that are involved with the care of our patients. But do we understand the crucial importance of being able to communicate clearly and effectively? Do we know the inherent risk in poor communication? And how will we, as clinical nurse leaders (CNLs), lead the way to better interdisciplinary communication and collaboration skills?

Groundbreaking reports published by the Institute of Medicine (IOM) since 1999 have singled out communication and collaboration between healthcare workers and patients as leading causes of patient harm. The first of these, *To Err Is Human: Building a Safer Health System*, reports that an estimated 98,000 people die in hospitals every year as a result of medical errors. The specific types of errors outlined in this report include diagnostic errors, treatment errors, prevention, and failure of communication (Institute of Medicine [IOM], 1999). These errors often occur in a triangle of miscommunication between patients, providers, and other team members. Adding to the complexity of communication, healthcare providers are providing care among diverse individuals. As we become a more global society, our obligation as healthcare providers is to become aware of the diverse cultures for whom we are caring. There is a complex myriad of social customs, religious practices, language barriers, belief systems, and cultural barriers that are faced every day. These factors can enhance or complicate communication and collaboration depending on the approach. As a CNL working within a microsystem, there is a unique opportunity to bridge that communication gap Box 6.1 describes such a scenario.

In 2001, the publication of *Crossing the Quality Chasm: A New Health System for the 21st Century* addressed issues in healthcare such as decentralization, fragmentation of the healthcare system, and changing and nonintegrated technology systems. The report stated that medical science

BOX 6.1
Scenario

In a large tertiary hospital that delivers over 4,000 babies yearly, staff are accustomed to several different languages and cultures in their practices related to childbirth. At one point, however, a pattern emerged of patients coming from one particular clinic who had emigrated from a very small area of Burma, speaking a language called Karen. The nurses and other members of the healthcare team have been finding it difficult to find interpreters who speak anything close to Karen through the hospital language line, leaving a significant communication gap and posing a safety risk. This situation was brought to the CNL, who then researched the culture and spoke to key people at the clinic who were providing prenatal care for these patients. As it turns out, a large number of refugees were brought to the area by a religious organization protecting them from war in their country. Based on these facts, in-services were offered to educate staff about this culture, why they are here, how many people have recently immigrated, and approximately how many were receiving prenatal care. This information went a long way to help bridge the gap that seemed impossibly large. The hospital language line became aware of this need, and provided translations closer to the Karen language. A better cultural understanding and clear communication aided healthcare providers with the necessary tools to provide safe care that met the needs of the patient.

and technology have advanced at an unprecedented rate and healthcare is increasingly more complex, while public healthcare needs are changing. People are living longer and, as a result, healthcare providers are seeing a higher prevalence of chronic conditions. The quality chasm is also due to a healthcare delivery system that is poorly organized, often overly complex, and uncoordinated, and does not lend itself to easy communication between healthcare providers. In this report, "10 rules for redesign" are suggested in order to redesign a fragmented system and provide better quality and safety for our patients. Of particular importance is rule 10—"Cooperation among clinicians is a priority. Clinicians and institutions should actively collaborate and communicate to ensure an appropriate exchange of information and coordination of care" (IOM, 2001).

Communication Essentials

As outlined in the AACN *White Paper on the Education and Role of the Clinical Nurse Leader*, communication is complex, interactive, and ongoing, and forms the basis for building interpersonal relationships. These interpersonal relationships will include patients, healthcare providers, families, and other key stakeholders. Essential in good communication is critical listening, critical reading, and quantitative literacy, as well as oral, nonverbal, and written communication skills (American Association of College of Nursing [AACN], 2007). The white paper challenges CNLs "to establish and maintain effective working relationships within an interdisciplinary team, communicate confidently and effectively with healthcare workers both collegial and subordinate, produce clear, accurate, and relevant writing and communicate with diverse groups and disciplines using a variety of strategies" (AACN, 2007).

Critical Listening

The essentials of *critical listening* concepts originated 2000 years ago in Aristotle's treatise, *The Rhetoric* (www.rhetoric.eserver.org/aristotle/oneindex.html). Three major components of critical listening are ethos, or speaker credibility; logos, or logical arguments; and pathos, or psychological appeal.

Ethos—This refers to the credibility of the speaker. Two critical factors of speaker credibility are expertness and trustworthiness. As a CNL, you will need to listen critically while weighing decisions for practice and the implications they may have on staff and patients. On the other hand, your credibility as a CNL is rooted in your expert knowledge of your microsystem and the level of trustworthiness that you have earned with the people you interact with on a daily basis.

Logos—Does the speaker make errors in logic? By accident, carelessness, inattention to detail, or lack of analysis? Well-supported arguments from speakers are expected—these arguments contain both true propositions and valid inferences or conclusions. Ask the following: Are the statements true? Are the data supplied the best and most recent? Are the data known and respected by the listener? Are the data accurately presented? Is there evidence of logical thinking by the speaker? And, as a speaker, are you logical; do you support your arguments with well-founded, recent, evidence-based knowledge?

Pathos—This is the psychological or emotional element of communication that is often overlooked or misunderstood. Pathos is when the speaker appeals to one or several needs or values of the audience to which he or she is targeting. The critical listener asks himself or herself: Is the speaker attempting to manipulate rather than persuade? What is the speaker's intent? Does the speaker combine logos with pathos?

Effective critical listening depends on the listener keeping all three elements of the message in the analysis and in perspective (Kline, 1996). But what does all of this have to do with patients in healthcare and why is it so important to clinical outcomes and patient satisfaction?

Collaborative Partners

The white paper identifies *Ten Assumptions for Educating the Clinical Nurse Leader*, and it is no mistake that of those 10 assumptions, three of them directly relate to *interdisciplinary communication* of information related to patient care. Assumption 4 states that the CNL has the most comprehensive knowledge of the client and will be responsible for coordinating the variety of disciplines that will be participating in the plan of care. It goes on to caution that "lack of communication results in a discontinuous and frequently unsafe, uncoordinated, inappropriate care. Learning to advocate for clients by communicating effectively with other interdisciplinary team members is crucial, including nurses in other settings" (AACN, 2007). Accordingly, Assumption 5 states that information will maximize self-care and client decision making, and Assumption 9 states that communication technology will facilitate the continuity and comprehensiveness of care.

The CNL is expected to possess essential qualities that are the foundation of effective communication and *interdisciplinary collaboration*. These essential qualities are known as therapeutic use of self, genuineness, warmth, empathy, acceptance, maturity, and self-awareness. These essential qualities enable the CNL to quickly establish trust and foster cooperative behavior with patients, staff members, and other healthcare team members. In addition to the essential qualities, a strong professional value system is necessary to garner cooperation and effective communication with interdisciplinary teams and patients. These values include altruism, accountability and responsibility, human dignity, integrity, and ethical principles. Strong professional values will distinguish the CNL as a trusted leader and facilitator of communication and collaboration that is for the sole benefit of patient care (Harris & Roussel, 2010). Thus, the CNL is the conduit for communication that places the patient as the central focus (see Figure 6.1). The CNL communicates with patients, families, staff members at all levels, and providers of medical care.

Bedside nurses and CNLs are at the frontline caring for patients, assessing interventions, and listening to patient concerns, The CNL has the responsibility to make clinical decisions using a perspective that encompasses family/patient preferences while adhering to clinical specific protocols and institutional constraints. If there is a family concern because a patient is unable to communicate, it is up to the nurse (who is an advocate for that patient) to develop a therapeutic alliance to bridge the gap between patient and provider. A CNL may be instrumental in this process. This may be done in various ways, such as coaching by the CNL and supporting the nurse and the entire healthcare team to provide a plan of care for the patient that is respectful and safe. In November 2011, the U.S. Department of Health and Human Services Agency for Healthcare Research and Quality (AHRQ) began a new initiative "Questions Are the Answer." This initiative encourages healthcare providers and patients to engage in effective two-way communication to ensure safer care and better health outcomes (AHRQ, 2011). In a series of patient testimonies videographed for this initiative, it was revealed that good communication between patient and provider resulted in more accurate diagnosis, a reduction in medications, and increased education to patients regarding when to seek medical help. As an end result,

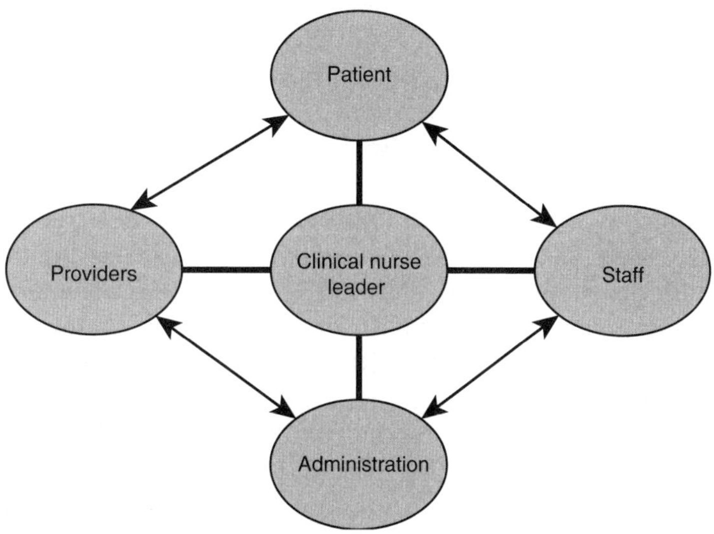

FIGURE 6.1 The CNL as a "conduit" of communication.

this led to better quality care for the patient and potential cost savings. It is very possible that The Joint Commission will be evaluating institutions to determine what work is being done to improve patient/provider communications (*Case Management Advisor*, 2012). As an advocate for the patient, bedside nurse, and lateral integrator, the CNL will be beneficial in facilitating communication and collaboration between patient and provider that will address this issue. If patient teaching is proving to be ineffective, it is important to investigate why. Is there a language or cultural barrier that has been overlooked by staff? Is staff communicating with patients in a way that will retain their attention? Are there more innovative ways to educate patients by computer? Has staff become stagnant and not grown with the technological changes that are facing us every day and our patients we serve? These questions can be asked by the CNL, and the discovery of the answers can be a joint effort between staff working with patients and CNLs.

Collaboration Among the Team of Care Providers

The consistent use of interdisciplinary communication and collaboration has been identified as not only important, but also crucial to the safety of patient care. Although the word *interdisciplinary* conveys many assumptions, for the purposes of this chapter, it refers to registered nurses, physicians, midlevel providers, and all others associated with the medical care of a patient. Without free-flowing, timely, and accurate communication of test/lab results and changes in patient status between disciplines, care is compromised. When disciplines disagree with the plan of care and do not discuss it, care is compromised. When there is a lack of respect and trust between disciplines, care can be compromised. The goal is interdisciplinary communication and collaboration. However, in order to achieve that goal, the CNL must be able to communicate in a way that is understood and respected by the intended audience, most of them healthcare providers working within the multidisciplinary network of people engaged in the patient's care.

Documented studies show the extent to which poor communication and lack of respect between physicians and nurses lead to harmful outcomes for patients, while good working relationships between physicians and nurses have been cited as a factor in improving the retention of nurses in hospitals. A study conducted in 2005 regarding the behavior outcomes of nurses and physicians sought to assess perceptions of the impact of disruptive behavior on nurse–physician relationships (Rosenstein & O'Daniel, 2005). The study specifically addressed the relationship among stress, concentration, frustration, team collaboration, information transfer, communication, and clinical outcomes, such as adverse events, errors, patient safety, quality of care mortality, and patient satisfaction. In the category of reduced communication, 94% of the nurses responded that disruptive behavior affected communication and 89% reported that information transfer was reduced (Rosenstein & O'Daniel, 2005). As delivery of care has become more complex, the need to coordinate care among multiple providers is necessary, putting the bedside nurse at the center of communication and the common denominator (IOM, 2011).

In 2004, the IOM publication *Keeping Patients Safe: Transforming the Work Environment of Nurses* suggested several recommendations to promote patient safety, in particular, fostering interdisciplinary collaboration. Bedside nurses interact with multiple levels of patient caregivers. In addition to the multiple levels, there are multiple changes from day to day and even shift to shift. It is not inconceivable that one nurse will interact with four different groups of healthcare providers for each patient he or she is assigned. As part of a study conducted by the IOM committee, a review of published research on team functioning and collaboration supports the effectiveness of teams and interdisciplinary collaboration in improving patient outcomes (IOM, 2004).

As the AACN has developed the CNL role with visions of better communication between healthcare workers, it is important to keep in mind the hallmarks of effective interdisciplinary collaboration: clinical competence, mutual trust, and respect. Clinical competence is crucial in gaining mutual trust and respect, implying that nurses and other disciplines are more likely to collaborate with each other when it is perceived that clinical knowledge is strong. Collaborative behaviors include shared goals and roles, effective communication, shared decision making, and conflict management strategies (IOM, 2004). Education goals of the CNL are aimed at addressing these issues to increase collaboration and communication between disciplines.

As a CNL who understands the importance of collaborative and interdisciplinary communication as it relates to patient safety, it is imperative that the CNL model communication that is clear, concise, and effective. This may be in the form of instituting bedside reporting, multidisciplinary rounding, intentional hourly rounding, interdisciplinary simulation, or the situation background assessment recommendation (SBAR) form of communicating with healthcare workers. Using SBAR is a prime example of bridging the way medical professionals communicate with each other. When there is a patient concern, communication that is clear, concise, and to the point when making a recommendation for action is valued and respected. Box 6.2 displays SBAR for CNLs.

As you can see in Box 6.2, this type of communication is direct, provides specifics about the current situation, and offers a bit of background information that may be essential. There was no hesitation on the nurse's part that she wanted further evaluation. Instead of hinting around the matter and suggesting an evaluation from the neonatal intensive care unit (NICU), she recommended it as the natural course of action. As a result, the infant was seen promptly by a neonatal cardiologist.

SBAR is a trend in healthcare communication that is being trialed by inpatient settings. The trend toward simulation learning has also been seen as a viable vehicle to address communication issues in healthcare. CNLs should place themselves in a position to participate in simulation exercises developed to increase communication skills for both nurses and other healthcare providers.

Introducing and implementing change is not easy, so it is not surprising that there has been significant resistance in the past from bedside nurses and others who do not understand (a) the need for better communication and (b) the significant research behind the success of these methods in creating a safer environment to deliver healthcare. This is where the CNL can blend his or her expert knowledge of the microsystem with the larger body of evidence that is guiding current practice. Although the concepts may change over time as healthcare continues to evolve, the CNL is the change agent that not only sees the need for change, but also seeks out literature to support best practice, relate it to staff at the bedside, and eventually track the progress of changes and make any necessary adjustments.

The CNL has been described as the lateral integrator of care; this role facilitates, coordinates, and oversees care provided by the healthcare team.

BOX 6.2
SBAR Reporting of Patient Data to a Physician

After assessing a 3-day-old neonate, you discover that the heart rate is irregular, from 60 to 90 beats per minute. The conversation to the attending pediatrician should sound like this:

- **Situation:** Hi, this is Mary. I am taking care of the baby Jones in room 620. She is a 3-day-old newborn and I am concerned about her assessment findings.
- **Background:** Mom is a 3-day post-c-section for a nonreassuring fetal heart rate during labor. APGAR scores were 8 to 8 at birth. The infant has not breastfed well, has lost over 10% of birth weight; mom is working with lactation, and just accomplished a good feeding using supplementation.
- **Assessment:** Infant's temperature is 97.7°F, respirations 33, and heart rate is irregular, difficult to determine, and bradycardic between 60s and 90s; O_2 saturation is 94% to 97%. Infant is sleepy, tone is good, and skin slightly pale.
- **Recommendation:** I would like you to call the NICU and have someone come to further evaluate the infant.

The goal of these actions is to meet care objectives by promoting a sense of shared responsibility for the patient between healthcare providers. Thus far, the discussion has been focused on patient/provider/bedside RN/CNL. Within that lateral integration of care, there is the relationship between the CNL, staff nurse, and nursing administration. There will be times when the CNL will need to address issues to administration on behalf of staff to indicate why a new protocol is problematic. On the other hand, staff may need to hear communication from the CNL that certain protocols are not up for debate; that it has been required by a governing body such as The Joint Commission. However, what the CNL can and should do is look for reasons why the staff does not think it will work, investigate the barriers that staff point out, and either advocate for staff or coach them on developing ways to make the new protocol fit into the present microsystem. The end result will be adherence to protocol and increased patient safety due to the implementation of best practice.

TABLE 6.1 Interdisciplinary Communication and Collaboration Skills

CATEGORY	WEIGHT
B. Interdisciplinary Communication and Collaboration Skills	**7%**
1. Establishes and maintains working relationships within an interdisciplinary team	
2. Bases clinical decisions on multiple perspectives including the client and/or family preferences	
3. Negotiates in group interactions, particularly in task-oriented, convergent, and divergent group situations	
4. Develops a therapeutic alliance with the client as an advanced generalist	
5. Communicates with diverse groups and disciplines using a variety of strategies	
6. Facilitates group processes to meet care objectives	
7. Integrates concepts from behavioral, biological, and natural sciences in order to understand self and others	
8. Interprets quantitative and qualitative data for the interdisciplinary team	
9. Uses a scientific process as a basis for developing, implementing, and evaluating nursing interventions	
10. Synthesizes information and knowledge as a key component of critical thinking and decision making	
11. Bridges cultural and linguistic barriers	
12. Understands clients' values and beliefs	
13. Completes documentation as it relates to client care	

(*continued*)

TABLE 6.1 Interdisciplinary Communication and Collaboration Skills *(continued)*

CATEGORY	WEIGHT
B. Interdisciplinary Communication and Collaboration Skills	**7%**
14. Understands the roles of interdisciplinary team members	
15. Participates in conflict resolution within the healthcare team	
16. Promotes a culture of accountability	

Used with permission from the Commission on Nurse Certification (2011, 2014).

BOX 6.3
Web Resources for Interdisciplinary Collaboration

Quality and Safety Education for Nurses—www.qsen.org
National League for Nursing—www.nln.org
Institute of Medicine—www.iom.edu
Institute for Healthcare Improvement—www.ihi.org

Conclusion

The effective CNL is respected, relied on as an advanced clinician, and serves as a mentor for strong interdisciplinary communication and collaboration skills. The CNL will translate advanced knowledge in communication principles and technologies to staff, patients, and interdisciplinary providers. The CNL® certification exam explores many areas of interdisciplinary communication and collaboration (Table 6.1). There are also many resources available from reputable online sources (Box 6.3). The CNL will model and facilitate collaboration, which will serve as a reminder that only with cooperation, collaboration, and clear communication will the patient's best interests be served.

Resources

Agency for Healthcare Research and Quality. (2011). *AHRQ initiative encourages better two-way communication between clinicians and patients.* Retrieved from http://ahrq.gov/research/nov11/1111RA19.htm

American Association of Colleges of Nursing. (2007). *White paper on the education and role of the clinical nurse leader.* Retrieved from http://www.aacn.nche.edu/cnl-certification

Case Management Advisor. (2012). Communication critical with patient, provider. *23*(2), 18–20.

Commission on Nurse Certification. (2011). *Clinical Nurse Leader job analysis report.* Retrieved from http://www.aacn.nche.edu/cnl/Job-Analysis-Report.pdf

Commission on Nurse Certification. (2014). *Clinical Nurse Leader (CNL®) certification exam blueprint.* Retrieved from http://www.aacn.nche.edu/leading-initiatives/cnl/cnl-certification/pdf/ExamContentOutline11.pdf

Harris, J. L., & Roussel, L. (2010). *Initiating and sustaining the clinical nurse leader role: A practical guide.* Sudbury, MA: Jones & Bartlett Publishers.

Institute of Medicine. (1999). *To err is human: Building a safer health system.* Retrieved from http://www.nap.edu/books/0309068371/html/

Institute of Medicine. (2001). *Crossing the quality chasm: A new health system for the 21st century.* Retrieved from http://www.nap.edu/books/0309068371/html

Institute of Medicine. (2004). *Keeping patients safe: Transforming the work environment of nurses.* Retrieved from http://www.nap.edu/catalog/10851.html

Institute of Medicine. (2011). *The future of nursing: Leading change, advancing health.* Retrieved from http://iom.nationalacademies.org/Reports/2010/The-Future-of-Nursing-Leading-Change-Advancing-Health.aspx

Kline, J. A. (1996). *Listening effectively-types of listening.* Maxwell, Alabama: Air University Press, Maxwell Air Force Base. Retrieved from http://www.au.af.mil/au/awc/awcgate/kline-listen/b10ch4.htm

Rosenstein, A. H., & O'Daniel, M. (2005). Disruptive behaviors & clinical outcomes: Perceptions of nurses and physicians. *American Journal of Nursing, 105*(1), 54–64.

7

Healthcare Advocacy

Jonathan P. Auld

Advocacy is the act of expressing or defending the rights or causes of another. Professional nursing standards and the *Code of Ethics for Nurses* by the American Nurses Association (2015) represent advocacy as an important characteristic of professional nursing. Advocacy plays a central role in professional nursing values, as well as serving as a core competency for the clinical nurse leader (CNL). The modern healthcare environment—with rapid advances in technology, increasing complexity, and a more critically ill and aging population—is an important reason advocacy is a prominent competency in the CNL role. Central principles of advocacy include the protection of patients' *autonomy*, acting on behalf of patients, advancement and protection of the profession, and *social justice*.

Protection of Patient Autonomy

A core nursing value is that patients or clients are autonomous beings who have the right to make their own decisions. The role of the CNL is to protect patients' rights to *self-determination* by working with the interdisciplinary team and the analysis of organizational structures and processes to ensure patient autonomy is maintained. The following are examples in which the CNL can protect patient autonomy:

- Ensure patients and families have information and understanding to facilitate informed decision making about their plan of care.
- Analyze systems in the organization to ensure informed consent is accessible and consistent.
- Participate in the analysis of benefits and burdens of the treatment plan with consideration of the patient's cultural background.
- Facilitate nurses' and the interdisciplinary team's communication of the treatment options to the patients and families, including the right to accept, refuse, or terminate treatment.

- Ensure patients have the opportunity to make decisions with their desired support network of family, caregivers, and health professionals.

Acting on Behalf of Patients

When patients are unable to make their own decisions, a foundational role of the nurse is to act on behalf of the patient. The CNL has the responsibility to work with the direct care nurses and the interdisciplinary team to uphold the patient's wishes to the extent that they are known. The following are ways in which the CNL can influence this aspect of advocacy:

- Assessing and analyzing organizational structures and processes that ensure advance directives are accessible to healthcare providers
- Facilitating communication with patient surrogates
- Providing guidance and support for patient surrogates in order for them to make informed decisions
- Performing policy or guideline evaluation and development to guide decision making when acting on behalf of patients
- Ensuring quality care through the development of evidence-based guidelines for care
- Coordinating care through referrals to other resources or services
- Utilizing chain of command policies to resolve conflicts in the identification of patient wishes or surrogacy, which may include an ethics consultation

Community Advocacy and Social Justice

Social justice is a guiding principle for the nursing profession. Through the analysis of the social, economic, and cultural environment in which healthcare is consumed and delivered, the CNL addresses the antecedents to poor health outcomes in communities and populations. The following are some examples of how CNLs incorporate social justice into the practice:

- Engaging policy makers and elected officials to influence health policy at institutional and governmental levels
- Engaging institutional leaders around health disparities and improving outcomes for populations and communities by
  - Talking with local, state, and federal lawmakers
  - Writing opinion articles for local or national newspapers
  - Lobbying elected officials to support programs that improve health outcomes for populations

- Examining legal and regulatory processes that influence patient outcomes and the healthcare system (AACN, 2013)
- Building partnerships with community organizations to identify and address health disparities and perceived discrimination in the healthcare system
- Applying knowledge of historical, social, and cultural contexts to address the needs of patient or community populations and to ensure nondiscriminatory practices
- Analyzing and developing evidence-based programs to ensure improved health outcomes for populations or communities, including home healthcare (Stocker Schneider, 2014).

Advocacy for the Professional

The CNL is a leader in the nursing profession. An important aspect of this leadership is protecting and advancing nursing as a profession. Advocacy for the nursing profession can take a number of forms.

- Assessing and developing nurse competency and the development of the nursing professional role
- Advocating for the CNL role and the value of the CNL role to an organization and the healthcare team (AACN, 2013)
- Establishing role clarity for nurses and the CNL in the interdisciplinary team and in an organization
- Developing and adhering to standards of practice for self and others to enhance quality outcomes
- Participating with professional organizations
- Participating in nursing education
- Influencing organizational and government policy that protects the rights of nurses in the workplace
- Engaging organizational and government leaders in establishing legislation that supports nurses practicing to the full extent of their licensure

Exam Content Outline and Advocacy

Advocacy is an important part of the CNL role. Additionally, it is a key topic on the CNL® certification exam. The CNL certification exam has changed slightly on the basis of recent job analysis. Thus, Table 7.1 displays the new detailed content outline for the advocacy portion of the certification exam. This section of the exam is worth 5% of the total points.

TABLE 7.1 Healthcare Advocacy

CATEGORY	WEIGHT
C. Healthcare Advocacy	**5%**
1. Interfaces between the client and the healthcare delivery system to protect the client's rights	
2. Ensures that clients, families, and communities are well informed and engaged in their plan of care	
3. Ensures that systems meet the needs of the populations served and are culturally relevant	
4. Articulates healthcare issues and concerns to officials and consumers	
5. Assists consumers in informed decision making by interpreting healthcare research	
6. Serves as a client advocate on health issues	
7. Utilizes chain of command to influence care	
8. Promotes fairness and nondiscrimination in the delivery of care	
9. Advocates for improvement in the healthcare system and the nursing profession	

Used with permission from the Commission on Nurse Certification (2011, 2014).

Conclusion

As can be seen in the Examination Content Outline, advocacy is a clear part of the CNL role. CNLs are leaders; through this role, they are responsible for advocacy in a variety of ways. For example, CNLs are involved in advocacy in the following ways: (a) establishing health goals for patients/families, (b) determining plan of care with patients/families rather than for them, (c) conducting evidence-based practice (EBP) and research, (d) promoting fairness, (e) using the chain of command, when needed, to advocate for clients, and (f) improving care for all patients and families. Advocacy has always been a part of the role of professional nurses, but it is also a critical role for CNLs as advanced generalists, role models, and leaders.

Resources

American Association of Colleges of Nursing. (2007). *White paper on the education and role of the clinical nurse leader*. Retrieved from http://www.aacn.nche.edu/publications/white-papers/ClinicalNurseLeader.pdf

American Association of Colleges of Nursing. (2013). *Competencies and curricular expectations for clinical nurse leader education and practice*. Retrieved from http://www.aacn.nche.edu/cnl/CNL-Competencies-October-2013.pdf

American Nurses Association. (2015). *Code of ethics for nurses with interpretive statement*. Silver Springs, MD: Author.

Bu, X., & Jezewski, M. A. (2006). Developing a mid-range theory of patient advocacy through concept analysis. *Journal of Advanced Nursing*, *57*(1), 101–110.

Commission on Nurse Certification. (2011). *Clinical Nurse Leader job analysis report*. Retrieved from http://www.aacn.nche.edu/cnl/Job-Analysis-Report.pdf

Commission on Nurse Certification. (2014). *Clinical Nurse Leader (CNL®) certification exam blueprint*. Retrieved from http://www.aacn.nche.edu/leading-initiatives/cnl/cnl-certification/pdf/ExamContentOutline11.pdf

Koizer, B. J., Erb, G., Berman, A. J., & Snyder, S. (2004). Values, ethics, and advocacy. In *Fundamentals of nursing: Concepts, process, and practice* (7th ed.). Upper Saddle River: New Jersey: Pearson/Prentice Hall.

Paquin, S. O. (2011). Social justice advocacy in nursing: What is it? How do we get there? *Creative Nursing*, *17*(2), 63–67.

Smith, A. P. (2004). Patient advocacy: Roles for nurses and leaders. *Nursing Economics*, *22*(2), 89–90.

Stocker Schneider, J. (2014). Clinical nurse leader. *Home Healthcare Nurse*, *32*(9), 563–564.

8

Implementation of the Clinical Nurse Leader Role

Cynthia R. King

It is difficult for any nurse to integrate a new role into practice (e.g., nurse manager, nurse practitioner, clinical nurse leader [CNL]). As of 2003, the CNL role was the first new role in nursing in about 35 years (AACN, 2013). Thus, transitioning into this role may be especially difficult for nurses. There are numerous nursing schools that now have CNL programs. The curriculum covers many of the key aspects that are the basis of the CNL role. However, not all programs help students learn to integrate their new role into practice. The CNL role, specifically, is aimed at managing a distinct population group through day-by-day management of clinical issues and decisions and focusing on patient outcomes. Moreover, the primary focus is on evaluating and supporting evidence-based decisions to ensure the best possible clinical outcomes (Thompson & Lulham, 2007). Educated at the master's degree level, the nurse leader possesses a higher level of clinical knowledge and leadership that creates positive patient outcomes (Hartranft, Garcia, & Adams, 2007). Because the CNL role is new and is different from other nursing roles, it is not always easy to implement the role in healthcare settings. There are expectations from nursing administration and many other disciplines, as well as each CNL's individual expectations. It is preferable that all of these expectations align; however, they may be in competition, which can create tension and anxiety. Poorly defined roles can lead to conflict in clinical teams and decrease effectiveness of care provided, communication, and collaboration (Brault et al., 2014). Additionally, not all employers know how to help new CNLs integrate their role in their specific setting.

Essential Aspects of the CNL's Role

The most critical period in the CNL's career will be the transition from staff nurse to CNL. The initial efforts as a CNL will set precedents and establish the individual's basic style, and may even cause the CNL to change some of his/her attitudes. Before integrating the CNL role into a particular setting, it is crucial that the CNL understand his or her broad areas of responsibility. These are outlined by the American Association of Colleges of Nurses and the broad areas are summarized as follows:

- **Clinician:** The CNL is designer/coordinator/integrator/evaluator of care to individuals, families, groups, communities, and populations. He or she is able to understand the rationale for care and competently deliver this care to complex and diverse populations. The CNL provides care at the point of care with particular emphasis on health promotion and risk reduction services.
- **Outcomes manager:** The CNL regularly synthesizes data, information, and knowledge to evaluate and achieve optimal client outcomes.
- **Client advocate:** The CNL becomes competent at ensuring that clients, families, and communities are well-informed and included in care planning. The CNL also serves as an informed leader for improving care and as an advocate for the profession and the interdisciplinary healthcare team.
- **Educator:** The CNL uses appropriate teaching principles and strategies as well as current information, materials, and technologies to teach clients, healthcare professionals, and communities.
- **Information manager:** The CNL is proficient in using information systems and technology to improve healthcare outcomes.
- **Systems analyst/risk anticipator:** The CNL participates in systems review to improve quality of nursing care delivered and at the individual level to critically evaluate and anticipate risks to client safety with the aim of preventing medical error.
- **Team manager:** The CNL properly delegates and manages the nursing team resources and serves as a leader in the interdisciplinary healthcare team.
- **Member of a profession:** The CNL remains accountable for the ongoing acquisition of knowledge and skills related to his or her profession and to effect change in healthcare practice and outcomes in the profession.
- **Lifelong learner:** The CNL recognizes the need for and actively pursues new knowledge and skills as one's role and needs of the healthcare system evolve.

All CNLs need to be able to integrate these areas of responsibility. They may also have their role as a professional staff nurse focused on self-performance (e.g., self-direction) to a leader helping oversee the work of staff nurses (e.g., selfless service). Moreover, they need to be able to articulate the significant aspects of the CNL role to other nurses and other disciplines.

Articulating the Significance of the CNL Role

Once a CNL moves into his or her role or position, it is crucial to be able to state the essential aspects of that role. One method to learn how to articulate the key aspects of the CNL role is to practice an "elevator speech" (2 to 5 minutes in length) during the CNL's residency. This simply means the CNL learns how to explain his or her role succinctly in 2 to 5 minutes. However, whatever the method, transitioning into a new role involves articulating newly acquired knowledge, skills, and abilities that differ from the ones used in the past role(s).

In order to articulate the significance of this new CNL role, individuals need to define the role for themselves, form expectations about the new role, describe to others, and encourage them to help make this role a success. However, there can be barriers to integrating and articulating the new CNL role. For example, there may be role conflict (when the role is different from what the new CNL expected) or isolation (e.g., if the CNL is the only one in the organization), or staff nurses and nurse managers do not perceive or embrace the new CNL role as being important.

In addition to being able to articulate what is involved in the CNL role to other disciplines, the CNL should be able to describe his or her role to patients and families. It is important to explain to patients/families that the CNL does not provide direct care for a particular group of patients, but instead is responsible for being a leader and guiding and influencing staff nurses with complex patient situations. Furthermore, CNLs should show a strong service orientation with a firm commitment to each patient/family.

Assuming Responsibility of One's Own Professional Identity and Practice

When CNLs begin their new role, and throughout their professional years in nursing, it is essential that they take responsibility for identifying their own professional practice and how that differs from other professional nurses. For example, CNLs must accept responsibility to demonstrate competence in their role and continually update their competencies, knowledge, and skills through professional education. Additionally, CNLs need to demonstrate they are competent leaders by (a) developing relationships with patients/families and many disciplines, (b) participating in and leading interdisciplinary teams, (c) being approachable and supportive, (d) appropriately delegating, (e) creating trust within relationships, (f) basing practice on evidence, and (g) effectively resolving conflict.

Networking is a vital strategy for CNLs, especially when beginning to integrate that role into practice. Some individuals appear to have an easy time networking (e.g., extroverts), whereas others might need a mentor. Networking can be learned. However, networking is not just simply meeting other individuals in your organization. It involves the cultivation of productive relationships for employment or business. The relationships developed become a supportive system of sharing information and services among individuals and groups having a common interest. For CNLs, networking is crucial both with staff on their unit (or setting) and with other disciplines. Developing a strong network early on will help CNLs with problems or issues they may face later.

Maintaining and Enhancing Professional Competencies and Lifelong Learning

As new CNLs learn to be responsible for professional development, it is important for these individuals to understand what it means to maintain professional competencies. This specifically encompasses a wide range of learning activities through which professionals (e.g., CNLs) maintain and develop through their career to ensure they continue to practice safely, effectively, and legally within their scope of practice. In order to maintain and enhance these initial competencies and lifelong learning, the CNLs will need to participate in a required number of hours of learning activities each year, maintain a personal professional profile of learning activities, and comply with any requests to audit how they have met the requirements.

As new CNLs, it is important to keep the supervisor informed of their career goals, as well as training and education needs. They should also express interest to their supervisor in succeeding in their new role and developing a plan for their professional development. In addition, CNLs should remember to learn from their colleagues (other CNLs) in their healthcare organization, at conferences, and through nursing organizations.

Understanding the Scope of Practice and Adhering to Licensure Law and Regulations

All professional nurses, including CNLs, are required to understand and abide by their scope of practice and follow all requirements and regulations needed to maintain their license. In order to accomplish this, CNLs should provide a high standard of practice and care at all times and model this for staff nurses. Moreover, CNLs need to:

- Use the best evidence possible to help oversee care provided.
- Keep skills and knowledge up to date.
- Follow regulations on delegation of care and tasks to other nurses.
- Maintain skills related to the eight roles outlined by the American Association of Colleges of Nursing.

Advocating for Professional Standards of Practice Using Organizational and Political Processes

As a CNL transitioning into this new position, it is important to advocate for professional standards, policies, and procedures, both inside the organization and in the political world outside. This is an even more urgent issue if the new graduate is the first CNL in the organization. He or she must blaze the trail for the other CNLs who will join the institution and the political arena. Some of the types of policies and standards to consider as a priority include (a) long-range goals, (b) immediate needs, (c) daily requirements, (d) organizational mandates, (e) quality issues, (f) safety issues, and (g) cost savings.

Politics is a process of finding solutions to universal concerns of humanity. This includes concern for public health. All nurses, including CNLs, advocate for the health of people and policies aimed at health promotion. Thus, it is imperative that CNLs become involved in making changes in public policy at the local, state, and national levels. Nurses are effective in the political process when they understand the sources of power and are willing to be involved and make a difference. Because the CNL role is the first new role in nursing in 45 years, it will be even more vital that CNLs become involved in the political process, as they will be able to speak most effectively to topics such as quality and safety issues related to patient care.

CNLs, and nurses in general, play a role in the development and implementation of policy. Ways in which nurses are involved in health policy are:

- Providing expertise
- Understanding consumer needs

- Assisting consumers in making healthcare decisions
- Providing a link to healthcare professionals and organizations
- Understanding the healthcare system
- Understanding interdisciplinary care

Articulating to the Public the Values of the Profession as They Relate to Client Welfare

When learning to integrate into their new role, CNLs need to be able to discuss both personal and professional values, which are individual and organizational expectations and ideas that help direct responsibilities, accountability, and proficiency. These values can influence decision making and communication, as well as judgment and daily routines. Professional values can include accountability, responsibility, and ethical principles.

As master's-prepared generalists, CNLs play a vital role in supporting and mentoring staff nurses at the bedside. Unfortunately, in some settings, staff have had little support from nursing.

Understanding and Supporting High-Quality, Cost-Effective, Safe Healthcare

The CNL role is the first new role in nursing in more than 45 years. Improving patient outcomes was one of the main reasons the role was developed. The Institute of Medicine (IOM) found in several studies that the healthcare system was fragmented and in need of improvement. Development of the CNL was a step in the right direction. Specifically, the CNL role can help improve the quality of care provided to patients in terms of structure, process, and outcomes. Other areas in which the CNL role helps issues raised by the IOM are cost-effectiveness and safe care. The IOM suggests six goals for improvement in patient care: (1) safe, (2) effective, (3) patient-centered, (4) timely, (5) efficient, and (6) equitable. Keeping these goals in mind, using the best evidence, and collecting data, CNLs can have an impact on quality, safety, and cost-effectiveness of care.

Publishing and Presenting CNL Impact and Outcomes

As evidence-based practice (EBP), research, or quality improvement (QI) projects come to an end, enthusiasm may tend to wane; however, dissemination is crucial to further nursing knowledge. Dissemination is actually part of the EBP/research/QI process and should not be an afterthought. Several motivations for CNLs to disseminate findings include the following:

- Improve health
- Do better research
- Change policy
- Develop career
- Help someone
- Use resources wisely
- Increase funding

There are a variety of options for dissemination both for CNLs and for staff nurses. A number of these may include the following:

- Journal publication
  - Full paper
  - Short report/letter
  - News item
  - Editorial
- Conference
  - Local/national/international
  - Poster
  - Oral presentation
- Report to funder
  - Publish as a report
- Set up conference or seminar
  - Within department
  - Area or regional meeting
  - National
- TV/lay press/media
  - Hospital newsletter
  - Newspapers
  - Radio
- Internet
  - Podcast
  - CD-ROM/DVD
- Teaching

Dissemination can be scary if an individual has not been a part of this process previously. That is why CNLs should be educated during their curriculum and encouraged to disseminate the results of their master's program. They may be mentored by their faculty advisor to submit an article for publication and give presentations. Once CNLs have participated in dissemination of a project, they can serve as excellent role models for staff nurses who have completed projects and do not know where or how to disseminate.

EBP and Nursing Research

EBP and nursing research are core competencies for the CNL and are connected to providing patient-centered care and to interdisciplinary teams. Increasing use of evidence helps the quality of care, safety of care, and avoidance of underuse, misuse, and overuse of care. CNLs understand the difference between nursing research (when there is a gap in knowledge) and EBP (when there are best outcomes that can be implemented in practice). In school, CNLs usually conduct an EBP or research project. This allows them to be role models for staff nurses when they transition into their CNL role. Equally important to the CNL role is the fact that each CNL learns in school how to search the literature for current evidence and research and apply it to clinical practice and potential patient outcomes.

It is also expected that CNLs will continue to be involved in EBP and nursing research once they have settled into their role. They may conduct nursing projects, serve on EBP/research shared governance councils, or work with other disciplines to conduct studies. The CNLs may also develop educational materials to help staff nurses better understand EBP and nursing research. In addition, CNLs may help staff nurses to plan, develop, and implement projects for clinical ladders.

Conclusion

Currently, the CNL role is being integrated in many different settings. There is potential for this role to be integrated in all areas of practice in all care settings (see Table 8.1). With the implementation of this new role comes the promise of streamlining coordination of care for all patients. For this role to be successful, it must be championed by executive leadership (e.g., the chief nursing officer) and understood by other nurses and disciplines as being a pivotal role at the point of care. The organizations that hire CNLs want to see them succeed just as much as the CNLs want to be successful. Furthermore, it is vital that CNLs implement the following roles: coordinate care for a specific microsystem (group of patients/families); oversee care across the continuum (lateral integration); and provide leadership to, and serve as a role model for, other professional nurses (Ott et al., 2009).

TABLE 8.1 Integration of the CNL Role

CATEGORY	WEIGHT
D. Integration of CNL Role	**8%**
1. Articulates the significance of the CNL role	
2. Advocates for the CNL role	
3. Assumes responsibility of own professional identity and practice	
4. Maintains and enhances professional competencies	
5. Assumes responsibility for lifelong learning and accountability for current practice and healthcare information and skills	
6. Advocates for professional standards of practice using organizational and political processes	
7. Understands the history, philosophy, and responsibilities of the nursing profession as it relates to the CNL	
8. Understands scope of practice and adheres to licensure law and regulations	
9. Articulates to the public the values of the profession as they relate to client welfare	
10. Negotiates and advocates for the role of the professional nurse as a member of the interdisciplinary healthcare team	
11. Develops personal goals for professional development and continuing education	
12. Understands and supports agendas that enhance both high-quality, cost-effective healthcare and the advancement of the profession	
13. Supports and mentors individuals entering into and training for professional nursing practice	
14. Publishes and presents CNL impact and outcomes	
15. Generates nursing research	

Used with permission from the Commission on Nurse Certification (2011, 2014).

Resources

American Association of Colleges of Nursing. (2007). *White paper on the education and role of the clinical nurse leader*. Retrieved from http://www.aacn.nche.edu/publications/white-papers/ClinicalNurseLeader.pdf

American Association of Colleges of Nursing (2013). *Competencies and curricular expectations for clinical nurse leader education and practice*. Washington, DC. Retrieved from http://www.aacn.nche.edu/cnl/CNL-Competencies-October-2013.pdf

Brault, I., Kilpatrick, K., D'Amour, D., Contandriopoulos, D., Chouinard, V., Dubois, C.A., … Beaulieu, M.D. (2014). Role clarification processes for better integration of nurse practitioners into primary healthcare teams: A multiple-case study. *Nursing Research and Practice.* doi:10.1155/2014/170514.

Burton, R., & Ormrod, G. (2011). *Nursing: Transition to professional practice.* Oxford, UK: Oxford University Press.

Clark, C. C. (2009). *Creative nursing leadership & management.* Boston, MA: Jones & Bartlett Publishers.

Commission on Nurse Certification. (2011). *Clinical Nurse Leader job analysis report.* Retrieved from http://www.aacn.nche.edu/cnl/Job-Analysis-Report.pdf

Commission on Nurse Certification. (2014). *Clinical Nurse Leader (CNL®) certification exam blueprint.* Retrieved from http://www.aacn.nche.edu/leading-initiatives/cnl/cnl-certification/pdf/ExamContentOutline11.pdf

Dye, C. F. (2010). *Leadership in healthcare: Essential values and skills* (2nd ed.). Chicago, IL: Healthcare Administration Press.

Finkelman, A., & Kenner, C. (2014). *Professional nursing concepts: Competencies for quality leadership* (3rd ed.). Boston, MA: Jones & Bartlett Publishers.

Hartranft, S. R., Garica, T., & Adams, N. (2007). Realizing the anticipated effects of the clinical nurse leader. *Journal of Nursing Administration, 37*(6), 261–263.

Kearney-Nunnery, R. (2012). *Advancing your career: Concepts of professional nursing* (5th ed.). Philadelphia, PA: F. A. Davis.

Ott, K. M., Haddock, K. S., Fox, S. E., Shinn, J. K., Walters, S. E., Hardin, J. W., …, Harris, J. L. (2009). The clinical nurse leader: Impact on practice outcomes in the Veterans Health Administration. *Nursing Economics, 27*(6), 363–383.

Thompson, P., & Lulham, K. (2007). Clinical nurse leader and clinical nurse specialist role delineation in the acute care setting. *Journal of Nursing Administration, 37*(10), 429–431.

9

Lateral Integration of Care Services

September T. Nelson

The *White Paper on the Education and Role of the Clinical Nurse Leader* states, "the CNL provides lateral integration of care services within a microsystem of care to effect quality, client care outcomes" (American Association of Colleges of Nursing [AACN], 2007, p. 6). Tornabeni defines *lateral integration* as "the integration of care provided by multiple, interdependent, and independent disciplines across a continuum of patient admission or experience" (2006, p. 6). This means not just in the acute care setting, but also in areas such as home care and hospice. Integration also means involving potential key stakeholders in addition to healthcare providers (healthcare administrators, financial representatives, and ombudsmen) in order to improve the quality and value of healthcare. The combination of multiple contributors into a unified whole is the crux of integration. This unification is necessary to remove the walls created by individual silos of fragmented care that impede communication and collaboration, thus contributing to errors and poor outcomes (Begun, Tornabeni, & White, 2006). A fundamental function of the clinical nurse leader (CNL) is to intentionally and proactively manage patient care services across professional boundaries to implement best practice (Begun et al., 2006; Bender, Connelly, & Brown, 2013). In order for the CNL to successfully design and implement a holistic plan of care, all members of the team should be included. Therefore, communication with all the stakeholders is a crucial part of providing high quality, safe care (Hartranft, Garcia, & Adams, 2007). According to Begun and associates (2006), the role of lateral integration of care is what has been missing in the care of patients with complex needs. There has been no nursing role that oversees care laterally and over time and that can then intervene and coordinate a holistic plan of care. With the implementation of the 2010 Patient Protection and Affordable Care Act, increased focus has been placed on integrated care to improve the quality and value of care (Jeffers & Astroth, 2013). The CNL is poised to play an instrumental role through coordination of patient care provided by an interprofessional team across care settings.

Components of Lateral Integration

Understanding the interdependency of all disciplines in providing care is an essential part of the CNL role and lateral integration. Once the CNL understands the roles and expertise of the interdisciplinary team members, he or she can laterally integrate the team to deliver patient-centered care. Stanley (2010) described lateral integration as one of the defining aspects of CNL practice. Effective lateral integration requires multiple ongoing components:

- Communication
- Collaboration
- Coordination
- Evaluation

These components are not effective on their own, but require a coordinated flow between them. The CNL is integral to this process. These components will be described further.

Communication

The CNL serves as a liaison between the members of the healthcare team, fostering the flow of information and serving as a translator (Stanley et al., 2008). As a lateral integrator, effective communication skills are essential in order to disseminate healthcare information to all members of the healthcare team, across disciplines. The quality of all relationships stems from effective communication and the rights and respect for others. Communication occurs in all situations. It involves the transmission of feelings, attitudes, and ideas between people. This is an essential tool for the CNL, regardless of the setting. To foster this effective communication, Akper et al. (2006) suggest that the professional nurse should:

- Actively solicit input from all players
- Foster open rapport across professional boundaries
- Disseminate healthcare information with other disciplines
- Share clear goals, messages, and plans with all players
- Keep team members informed

Additionally, the CNL needs to be aware of both verbal and nonverbal communication. A crucial skill for CNLs to be successful communicators is active listening (Antai-Otong, 2010). These strategies ensure that all participants have the needed healthcare-related information and are engaged in the discussion. If the verbal and nonverbal messages are conflicting, meaning and trust can be lost. Asking for clarification and restating what is heard will improve understanding among the participants and help bring them together. This intentional, thoughtful communication provides a foundation for collaboration.

Collaboration

Collaboration is defined by McKay and Crippen as an "interdisciplinary process of problem solving that involves shared responsibility for decision making as well as the execution of specific plans of care while working toward a common goal" (2008, p. 110). In the context of healthcare, the role of the CNL is to develop an effective holistic plan of care across settings in collaboration with all disciplines, professions, and stakeholders—including the patient (Begun et al., 2006).

To promote collaboration, the CNL:

- Seeks collaboration and consultation with all contributors to the healthcare delivery process, including the patient and family
- Synthesizes gathered input and information to find common goals
- Translates discipline-specific language to a common message, so that everyone has a clear understanding of the goals
- Evaluates information for relevance and appropriateness
- Not only communicates with members of the team, but also facilitates communication between members of the team
- Engages in and fosters shared decision making within the healthcare team

The CNL understands that the knowledge and perspective of just one discipline are limited and biased. Therefore, collaboration is essential to optimal outcomes and to provide a more complete, richer picture by incorporating multiple viewpoints into patient care.

Coordination

Coordination requires intentional planning and direction. The CNL is responsible for coordinating the flow of communication, activities of the team members, and the services provided to the patients.

The CNL coordinates care by:

- Organizing team members toward a common goal
- Creating and fostering systems that encourage communication, teamwork, and collaboration
- Performing risk analysis to ensure client safety

- Coordinating care of patients and groups of patients using appropriate technology and information systems that are accessible to team members
- Managing the care of clients through transitions across settings and episodes of care
- Clearly delegating tasks and responsibilities
- Ensuring each member of the team has a clear understanding of each member's role and work flow

Within large healthcare systems such as the Veterans Administration, the CNL role is implemented in all practice areas to provide streamlined, coordinated care across the spectrum, from acute care to ambulatory and long-term care (Ott et al., 2009). In other healthcare organizations, the CNL is implemented in the most critical areas first (e.g., medical–surgical units and units with the most acute patients). Then, as more nurses graduate from CNL programs, the role is added to other units. Additionally, the CNL role is used in settings outside of acute care, including public health, home-based care, long-term facilities, and schools (Lammon, Stanton, & Blakney, 2010).

Ongoing Evaluation

Ongoing evaluation of care delivery systems and processes is an important component of lateral integration. The CNL continually monitors not only the final outcomes of care, but also the implementation and progression of care delivery strategies along the way. Evaluation of healthcare delivery teams and processes must be concurrent and ongoing. By seeing what is working as well as what is not, adjustments can be made to improve the overall outcomes.

Specific areas the CNL should monitor and evaluate include:

- The plan of care for specific patients and populations of patients
- Analysis of risk to promote client safety
- Perspectives of all team members
- Communication strategies and processes used by the team members
- Efficacy of coordination of services
- Use of technology and information systems
- Appropriateness and relevancy of current and newly emerging healthcare information
- Environment and system to optimize healthcare quality and outcomes
- Design and delivery of interventions and team processes

Through intentional, ongoing assessment of processes and systems, the CNL is able to identify areas of needed improvement and implement changes to improve the efficiency, efficacy, safety, and quality of care as well as improve the satisfaction of those involved in the process (Baernholdt & Cottingham, 2011; Hix, McKeon, & Walters, 2009).

Lateral Integration Content on the CNL® Exam

According to the *Clinical Nurse Leader Job Analysis Report* (Commission on Nurse Certification, 2011) and the *Clinical Nurse Leader* (CNL®) *Certification Exam Blueprint* (Commission on Nurse Certification, 2014), lateral integration of care questions represent 6% of the exam content. The content related to lateral integration covered on the exam is found in Table 9.1 and Appendix A.

For example, the CNL will generally need to involve multiple disciplines in the plan for discharge to home or transition to a different level of care. Other disciplines may be needed for assistance in financial, social, and transportation issues if the patient has no active family or social support. Lateral integration may appear to be similar to client advocacy. However, client and family advocacy involves the CNL participating with other disciplines along with the patient and family to decide current healthcare issues. One of the original four articles by *The Joint Commission Journal on Quality and Patient Safety* (Watson et al., 2008) describes the important role of the CNL in facilitating interdisciplinary team care. This function can help overcome the difficulty of implementing change via CNL-led lateral integration.

TABLE 9.1 Lateral Integration

CATEGORY	WEIGHT
E. Lateral Integration of Care Services	**6%**
1. Delivers and coordinates care using current technology	
2. Coordinates the healthcare of clients across settings	
3. Develops and monitors holistic plans of care	
4. Fosters a multidisciplinary approach to attain health and maintain wellness	
5. Performs risk analysis for client safety	
6. Collaborates and consults with other healthcare professionals in the design, coordination, and evaluation of client care outcomes	
7. Disseminates healthcare information with healthcare providers to other disciplines	

Used with permission from the Commission on Nurse Certification (2011, 2014).

Conclusion

Healthcare delivery is an extremely complex process involving numerous disciplines, practitioners, and services. Each member of this healthcare team is at risk for practicing within the silo of one specific perspective. Through lateral integration, the CNL intentionally and proactively brings this team together to improve not only the healthcare delivery process but also patient outcomes. An important role of the CNL is to support and facilitate ongoing and evolving communication, collaboration, coordination, and evaluation among the multidisciplinary team, patient, and family.

Resources

American Association of Colleges of Nursing. (2007). *White paper on education and role of the clinical nurse leader.* Retrieved from http://www.aacn.nche.edu/publications/white-papers/ClinicalNurseLeader.pdf

Antai-Otong, D. (2010). Introducing the clinical nurse leader: A catalyst for quality care. In J. L. Harris & L. Roussel (Eds.), *Initiating and sustaining the clinical nurse leader role: A practical guide.* Boston, MA: Jones & Bartlett.

Apker, J., Propp, K., Ford, W., & Hofmeister, N. (2006). Collaboration, credibility, compassion, and coordination: Professional nurse communication skill sets in health care team interactions. *Journal of Professional Nursing, 22*(3), 180–189.

Baernholdt, M., & Cottingham, S. (2011). The clinical nurse leader—New nursing role with global implications. *International Nursing Review, 58*, 74–78.

Begun, J. W., Tornabeni, J., & White, K. R. (2006). Opportunities for improving patient care through lateral integration: The clinical nurse leader. *Journal of Healthcare Management, 51*(1), 19–25.

Bender, M., Connelly, C. D., & Brown, C. (2013). Interdisciplinary collaboration: The role of the clinical nurse leader. *Journal of Nursing Management, 21*, 165–174.

Commission on Nurse Certification. (2011). *Clinical Nurse Leader job analysis report.* Retrieved from http://www.aacn.nche.edu/cnl/Job-Analysis-Report.pdf

Commission on Nurse Certification. (2014). *Clinical Nurse Leader (CNL®) certification exam blueprint.* Retrieved from http://www.aacn.nche.edu/leading-initiatives/cnl/cnl-certification/pdf/ExamContentOutline11.pdf

Commission on Nurse Certification and Schroeder Measurement Technologies, Inc. (2011). *Exam content outline.* Washington, DC: Author.

Hartranft, S. R., Garcia, T., & Adams, N. (2007). Realizing the anticipated effects of the clinical nurse leader. *Journal of Nursing Administration, 37*(6), 261–263.

Hix, C., McKeon, L., & Walters, S. (2009). Clinical nurse leader impact on clinical microsystems outcomes. *The Journal of Nursing Administration, 39*(2), 71–76.

Jeffers, B. R., & Astroth, K. S. (2013). The clinical nurse leader: Prepared for an era of healthcare reform. *Nursing Forum, 48*(3), 223–229.

Lammon, C. B., Stanton, M. P., & Blakney, J. L. (2010). Innovative partnerships: The clinical nurse leader role in diverse clinical settings. *Journal of Professional Nursing, 26*(5), 258–263. doi:10.1016/j.profnurs.2010.06.004.

McKay, C. A., & Crippen, L. (2008). Collaboration through clinical integration. *Nursing Administration Quarterly, 32*(2), 109–116.

Ott, K. M., Haddock, K. S., Fox, S. E., Shinn, J. K., Walters, S. E., Hardin, J. W., ... Harris, J. L. (2009). The clinical nurse leader: Impact on practice outcomes in the Veterans Health Administration. *Nursing Economics, 27*(6), 363–370, 383.

Stanley, J. M. (2010). Introducing the clinical nurse leader: A catalyst for quality care. In J. L. Harris & L. Roussel (Eds.), *Initiating and sustaining the clinical nurse leader role: A practical guide*. Boston, MA: Jones & Bartlett.

Stanley, J. M., Gannon, J., Gabaut, J. Hartranft, S., Adams, N., Mayes, C., ... Burch, D. (2008). The clinical nurse leader: A catalyst for improving quality and patient safety. *Journal of Nursing Management, 16*, 614–622.

Tornabeni, J. (2006). Evolution of a revolution. *Journal of Nursing Administration, 36*(1), 3–6.

Watson, J. H., Anders, S. G., Moore, L. G., Ho, L., Nelson, E. C., Godfrey, M. M., & Batalden, P. B. (2008). Clinical microsystems, part 2. Learning from micro practices about providing patients the care they want and need. *The Joint Commission Journal on Quality and Patient Safety, 34*(8), 443–452.

III

Key Certification Topics: Clinical Outcomes Management

10

Illness/Disease Management

Audrey Marie Beauvais

Chronic illnesses, such as diabetes, cancer, and cardiovascular disease, are some of the most common and expensive of all global health issues (Schulman-Green, et al., 2012; World Health Organization, 2011a). Chronic illnesses are the main reason that adults obtain healthcare and are the principal cause of disability and death in the United States (Schulman-Green et al. 2012; Centers for Disease Control and Prevention, 2011). Approximately half (117 million) of the adults in the United States have at least one chronic condition (Ward, Schiller, & Goodman, 2014). One in every four adults has two or more chronic health conditions (Ward et al., 2014). Seven of the leading 10 causes of death were chronic diseases. Two of those chronic diseases, cancer and heart disease, combined are responsible for approximately 48% of all deaths (Centers for Disease Control and Prevention, 2015). Chronic illnesses are long term and interfere with the person's everyday life (Schulman-Green et al., 2012). Management of these chronic illnesses is an essential component of healthcare that clinical nurse leaders can perform to make a valuable difference.

Chronic Illness

Improving healthcare for people with chronic illnesses is one of the most significant challenges confronting the U.S. healthcare system (Trehearne, Fishman, & Lin, 2014). Chronic conditions are quite costly. In fact, 86% of healthcare spending is for people with one or more chronic medical conditions (Gerteis et al., 2014). The cost of heart disease and stroke are over $300 billion (Go et al., 2014). Cancer care costs are over $150 billion (National Cancer Institute, 2014). Costs associated with diabetes are over $240 billion (American Diabetes Association, 2014). Costs associated with obesity are over $140 billion. The good news is that these conditions are often preventable, as they are attributed to lifestyle and environmental factors such as lack of physical activity, poor nutrition, tobacco use, chronic stress, excessive alcohol use, and environmental toxins (Chambers & Grolman, 2011; Hyman et al., 2009).

Individuals with chronic conditions are complicated and need someone to screen and address any physical, psychological, or social issues (Chambers & Grolman, 2011). Clinical nurse leaders (CNLs) can take an active role in illness and disease management, as they are knowledgeable about chronic diseases, able to assess and manage physical and psychological symptoms related to disease and treatment, able to recommend preventive measures, and able to engage in patient and family teaching (Chambers & Grolman, 2011; Fuller, 2013).

When assessing and screening patients, CNLs need to be cognizant of both the *nonmodifiable and modifiable risk factors* for chronic diseases. Table 10.1 identifies some nonmodifiable risk factors using the example of diabetes. CNLs should assist in the development of individual interventions based on modifiable risk factors. Table 10.2 identifies some modifiable risk factors and potential interventions using the example of diabetes.

TABLE 10.1 Nonmodifiable Risk Factors for Diabetes

Age	As age increases, so does the risk for developing diabetes.
Race/ethnicity	The risk of diabetes is greater in certain ethnic groups such as African Americans and Mexican Americans.
Family history/genetics	An individual's chances of developing diabetes are greater if someone in his or her family has the disease.

TABLE 10.2 Modifiable Risk Factors for Diabetes

	POTENTIAL INTERVENTIONS
Obesity	Provide nutritional education (such as portion control and food choices), increase physical activity, decrease calorie intake, modify lifestyle, modify behavior
High-blood glucose	Follow dietary guidelines, perform regular home glucose testing, treat blood glucose as ordered by APRN or physician, pursue medication education
Sedentary lifestyle	Help patients discover a way to put physical activity into their daily life. For example, the CNL may suggest that the patient take the stairs rather than the elevator, park farther away from his or her destination to encourage walking, wear a pedometer, join a walking group, join a gym, etc.
Smoking	Offer education regarding smoking cessation
Excessive alcohol intake	Offer alcohol counseling

CNLs will be most effective when part of a collaborative team of nurses, physicians, dietitians, social workers, and behavior health specialists (Chambers & Grolman, 2011; Hegney, Patterson, Eley, Mohomed, & Young,, 2013). In addition, CNLs will want to develop community partnerships, which will enable them to connect their patients to programs that provide exercise, nutrition, and disease management education. CNLs should advocate for their patients to help them navigate the healthcare system as well as identify resources that will assist with healthcare and social needs (Chambers & Grolman, 2011).

CNLs, with their skills, abilities, and knowledge of research and outcomes, are an asset for individuals with chronic illness, as they can assist with the creation of treatment plans and self-management approaches while anticipating and managing complications of disease progression (Schulman-Green et al., 2012). In creating treatment plans, CNLs should make certain that patients are partners in healthcare decisions. CNLs can help individuals with chronic illness by providing support, guidance, and education about the benefits of implementing a healthy lifestyle (Chambers & Grolman, 2011). Not only do CNLs play a vital role with developing plans and goals in partnership with patients as well as following up with ongoing healthcare needs, but they also play an essential role in evaluating and modifying the care that is received.

CNLs will need to be aware that focusing solely on the individual and his or her lifestyle will not be addressing the entire issue. Society as a whole has contributed largely to this problem by promoting such behavior as increasing portion sizes, consuming soft drinks, eating processed foods, and sitting for extended periods of time playing video games and watching television. As a result, disease management and prevention need to be addressed at two levels within *primary prevention* (Centers for Disease Control and Prevention, n.d.). The first is the *individual level*, which includes healthcare interventions (Centers for Disease Control and Prevention, n.d.). The second level is at the *population level*, which includes policies and environments that promote health (Centers for Disease Control and Prevention, n.d.). CNLs can play an active role by advocating for social change that addresses these unhealthy lifestyle choices (Chambers & Grolman, 2011; Centers for Disease Control and Prevention, n.d.).

Disease Management

Disease management typically has the following goals: to prevent chronic disease, reduce rates of death and disability, improve quality of life, and reduce costs. To reach these goals, CNLs can implement primary and *secondary prevention* strategies as described in Table 10.3.

CNLs should incorporate primary and secondary prevention techniques into their practice. Concentrating on secondary prevention will not yield favorable long-term outcomes with regard to better health conditions or decreased cost (Delaware Health Care Commission [DHCC], 2004).

CNLs need to be aware of some key factors impacting chronic disease management. Table 10.4 highlights some of the important concepts in disease management. Additional information can be found at the Centers for Disease Control and Prevention website under "Chronic Disease Prevention and Health Promotion" (www.cdc.gov/chronicdisease/index.htm). The website offers information on chronic diseases and health promotion, statistics and tracking, tools and resources, state profiles, and health equity.

TABLE 10.3 Disease Management Strategies

Primary prevention strategies	Purpose	Prevent the onset of chronic illness
	Focus	On a healthy lifestyle
		Healthy habits and behaviors
	Intention	To result in long-term positive outcomes
		(*Note*: It is difficult to determine actual long-term cost savings)
	Examples	Healthy eating habits, maintaining a healthy weight, increased physical activity, smoking cessation
Secondary prevention strategies	Purpose	Lessen the effect of chronic disease once it has occurred
		Evade needless complications
		Avoid serious illness or disease advancement
	Focus	Assure that individuals with chronic illness receive the needed medical treatment and tests to manage their disease
	Intention	To produce faster outcomes
		Easier to measure improvement in health and cost-saving outcomes
	Examples	Blood sugar testing and altering the diet of an individual diagnosed with diabetes

Source: DHCC (2004).

TABLE 10.4 Important Concepts in Disease Management

Patient-centered care/partnering	Patient-centered care is care that is grounded in a mutually beneficial partnership between the patient, family, and healthcare team. It involves the following: dignity, respect, information sharing, participation, and collaboration. CNLs should develop their partnering skills in order to enhance shared decision making with patients and the healthcare team (Saxe et al., 2007).

(*continued*)

TABLE 10.4 Important Concepts in Disease Management *(continued)*

	CNLs should focus on individual assessment and needs of the patients, in part with effective interviewing and communication skills (Saxe et al., 2007). CNLs should focus on self-care behaviors (e.g., taking medications correctly), emphasize patient choice, and encourage shared decision making (Forbes & While, 2009), as well as assist individuals to make informed choices, develop a joint crisis plan, and create a wellness recovery action plan (Kemp, 2011).
Education	CNLs should ensure that education is provided for patients, families, caregivers, employers, insurers, and legislators. Outside agencies such as state health departments and national organizations may be able to provide educational materials on managing chronic diseases. Accurate information about chronic illness and disease management is necessary for effective plans, policies, and programs to be developed and implemented (DHCC, 2004).
Data collection and analysis	CNLs will need to evaluate interventions by gathering and analyzing data to ensure they are obtaining positive outcomes. Accurate and current data regarding effective and efficient treatment guidelines will be needed as evidence to support and improve practice (Saxe et al., 2007). Data collection and analysis can be utilized to: • Identify and monitor the most common chronic illnesses • Identify effective strategies to manage chronic illnesses • Identify effective treatment protocols (Saxe et al., 2007).
Information and communication technology	CNLs should utilize technology to help monitor care and outcomes of individuals with chronic diseases. This technology can be used to share information with patients and health care professionals (AHRQ, 2009; Saxe et al., 2007).
Motivation	Changing behavior and habits is difficult. As a result, it may be necessary to offer some incentives for individuals to make positive changes to their lifestyle and to embrace healthy behaviors. Incentives will need to be individualized to the person's interest. For example, incentives can be such things as saving money on medication and healthcare bills, improving the quality of life, and having the ability to enjoy time with children or grandchildren.
Health literacy	According to the Institute of Medicine Report on Health Literacy, almost half of all Americans have trouble comprehending the health information that is provided to them. CNLs can play a valuable role to help ensure that patients are educated as well as engaged and included in their healthcare decisions (DHCC, 2004).

(continued)

TABLE 10.4 Important Concepts in Disease Management *(continued)*

Identifying key population	CNLs need to remain cognizant of the public health perspective. Some groups are at increased risk for chronic illness relative to other groups. In addition, certain strategies are more effective with particular diseases and populations. As a result, CNLs will need to identify target populations. Also, they will need to complete a needs assessment and develop strategies that work for that population, as there is no single set of strategies that will work for the needs of all individuals (DHCC, 2004; Saxe et al., 2007).
Determining resources	Operating a disease/illness management program will require financial and physical resources. As such, CNLs will need to identify approaches that are feasible, given the cost and availability of resources.
Identifying responsible parties	Operating a disease/illness management program will require that roles and responsibilities are assigned. In addition, it is essential to determine who will lead this effort and will be accountable for its success.
Key stakeholders	Key stakeholders are individuals or groups of people who have a vested interest in the disease/illness management program. They can prevent a project from reaching its goals as well as help a project be successful. Key stakeholders that may be involved with disease/illness management include employers, government agencies, healthcare providers, insurers, patients themselves, and family caregivers (DHCC, 2004; Jamison, 1998).
Clinical practice guidelines	CNLs should play an active role in developing and revising clinical practice guidelines for specific diseases/illnesses (Jamison, 1998). This involves monitoring the effectiveness of the guidelines as well as making modifications to the guideline based on the analysis of the data with the team. As mentioned above, information technology will help with the evaluation process (Jamison, 1998).

Source: DHCC (2004).

Transitions Between Levels of Care and Readiness for Discharge

The Joint Commission, a group focused on improving healthcare and patient outcomes, dedicates a great deal of resources to the topic of Transitions of Care (www.jointcommision.org). In every area of the healthcare spectrum, this time of change sets up the potential for miscommunication, medication errors, oversight of key patient issues, lapses in patient safety, and increased patient/family stress. CNLs will need to remain aware that transitions between levels of care are a critical time for patients (Weiss, Yakusheva, & Bobay, 2010). A patient who returns to the emergency department or is readmitted to an acute care facility within a month after hospital discharge may not have been ready to leave, may not have been adequately prepared, may not have had a well-coordinated aftercare plan, or may not have been able to deal with the demands of self-management at the next level of care (Weiss et al., 2010). A return to the hospital may result in outcomes that are adverse, potentially avoidable, and costly (Weiss et al., 2010).

The Joint Commission (2013) notes some common approaches to successful transitions. For example, one successful approach is to address sender/receiver concerns with partner organizations. Another successful strategy is to provide a screening process to identify those individuals at greater risk for healthcare problems that could potentially lead to readmission. Individuals such as CNLs should complete an assessment of needs and work collaboratively with the healthcare team to coordinate the transition to the next setting. Such an assessment should include the following factors, which can increase the risk of readmission:

- Patients who have diagnoses that are associated with readmissions
- Patients who have comorbidities
- Patients who are receiving numerous medications
- Patients with a history of readmissions
- Patients who have psychosocial and/or emotional factors (e.g., mental health issues, interpersonal relationship concerns, family conflict)
- Patients who have a lack of family members, friends, or other caretakers who could offer support
- Patients who are older in age
- Patients with financial concerns
- Patients who do not have adequate housing (The Joint Commission, 2013)

When a patient transitions to another level of care, the CNLs need to support patient safety. This can be accomplished by focusing on self-management of medication and medication reconciliation, follow-up with the primary care provider and specialists, and patient understanding regarding key clinical signs about his or her condition, as well as ensuring that support systems and sufficient services are arranged (Agency for Healthcare Research and Quality [AHRQ], 2010). CNLs should look to key healthcare organizations for resources and research regarding this important patient issue. Without a doubt the true value of a CNL in coordination of care can be operationalized at this critical time for patients.

Pain Management, Palliative Care, and End-of-Life Issues

If CNLs are going to play a role in managing diseases, they will most certainly be involved with managing pain, palliative care, and end-of-life issues. The following sections briefly cover pain management, palliative care, and end-of-life issues.

Pain

According to the Institute of Medicine (IOM, 2011), approximately 116 million adult Americans are affected by chronic pain. Medical treatment and lost productivity attributed to chronic pain are said to cost our nation approximately $635 billion annually (IOM, 2011). In light of this information, CNLs will need to find ways to improve pain assessment and management. CNLs will need to assess, design, and provide interventions for moderation of pain and suffering and try to maintain, restore, and optimize patients' level of functioning. CNLs need to complete pain assessments to help ascertain the cause, understand how it influences the individual, specify suitable pain strategies, and evaluate the helpfulness of these strategies (Briggs, 2010). Table 10.5 provides some key aspects regarding pain assessment. The websites listed in Box 10.1 provide additional resources for pain assessment.

Palliative Care

Palliative care focuses on improving the symptoms, dignity, and quality of life for individuals who are suffering with a serious illness or disease (World Health Organization, 2011b). Palliative care concentrates on pain and symptom management, communication, and coordinated care. It can be provided from the time of diagnosis and can be provided along with curative treatment. Palliative care does not accelerate or delay death. Rather, it offers respite from pain and other symptoms, incorporates the psychological and spiritual components of care, and provides assistance for patients to actively participate in life until they die. In addition, it offers support to families through the patient's illness and death, as well as throughout the family's grieving process (World Health Organization, 2011a).

BOX 10.1
Web Resources for Pain Assessment

- American Pain Foundation: www.painfoundation.org
- American Pain Society: www.ampainsoc.org
- Institute of Medicine: http://iom.nationalacademies.org/reports/2011/relieving-pain-in-america-a-blueprint-for-transforming-prevention-care-education-research.aspx

TABLE 10.5 Key Aspects of Pain Assessment

Site	Identify the location of the pain. Where does it hurt?
Amount/severity	How intense is the pain? How bad is the pain? Pain is an individual experience, so the CNL will need to have the patient rate it. Ask patients to rate their pain during movement and at rest. There are a variety of pain assessment tools available.
Characteristics/ description of pain	What is the quality and type of pain? Describe the pain. Does the pain radiate/spread anywhere? Is the pain throbbing, burning, aching, tender, dull, sharp, crushing, gnawing, stabbing, cramping, sore, discomfort, etc.? There are several kinds of physical causes of pain. Nociceptive pain: Typically localized, constant, aching, throbbing. Typically time limited and responds well to treatment. Neuropathic pain: Often described as burning, shooting, and pins and needles. The pain can also result from light touch. Typically chronic. Mixed category of pain: A combination of the above two.
Onset and timespan	When did it begin? Was it sudden or gradual? How long did it continue? Is there a pattern to the pain? Does the pain vary during the day? Is it sporadic? Is it constant? What started the pain? What things make it hurt more (e.g., activity)?
Prior pain management techniques used and relief from pain	What medications and nonmedication approaches have been tried? Were they successful? What makes the pain better or worse?
Related symptoms and effect on level of functioning/activity	Do you have any other symptoms associated with the pain (nausea, photosensitivity, stiff neck, etc.)? What effects has the pain had on you and your family? Has the pain affected your mood, your dietary intake, your functioning, and your sleep?

Source: Briggs (2010).

Hospice and End-of-Life Care

Palliative care differs from end-of-life care and hospice care. *Hospice/end-of-life care* provides quality care to people in the last months of their life who have decided to stop curative treatments. CNLs should help ensure that individuals in the last phase of life get the dignity and respect they deserve. Every person should be afforded the chance to discuss how he or she would like to be treated. Each person should be given an opportunity to formulate a "living will" and determine a healthcare proxy. CNLs can play an important role by making certain that physical and psychological suffering will be attended to and by taking measures to ensure comfort will be sought out. For additional information, CNLs can access the National Hospice and Palliative Care Organization (NHPCO) website (www.nhpco.org/templates/1/homepage.cfm).

Common Geriatric Problems

Given the aging population, CNLs will need to be knowledgeable about common geriatric problems. There are 13 principal clinical issues for geriatric care:

- Cognitive impairment
- Depression
- Behavioral issues
- Gait/mobility
- Incontinence
- Nutrition
- Sleep
- Vision
- Hearing
- Caregiver issues (social support/isolation)
- Home safety
- Driving safety
- Health and financial planning (Bogardus, Richardson, Maciejewski, Gahbauer, & Inouye, 2002)

CNLs will need to bear in mind these common issues as they consider the plan of care most appropriate for the geriatric population. In addition, the CNL should recognize that there are certain patterns of problem occurrences in the population as a whole, such as:

- Several acute-care admissions
- Two or more visits to the emergency department during a 6-month period
- Discharge from a hospital or skilled nursing facility
- Inadequate nutrition
- Medication nonadherence
- Lack of psychosocial support necessary to sustain wellness
- Expected increased use of medical services following hospital discharge
- Asthma in children, which is chronic and severe (AHRQ, 2010)

Being aware of the data and outcomes around these issues will help CNLs anticipate needed interventions, develop risk reduction strategies, and implement holistic care of the patient and family. As CNLs continue to move out of the acute care setting across the spectrum of healthcare services, an understanding of the larger healthcare system will be imperative.

Assessing Health Literacy

CNLs will need to be able to identify whether patients have issues with health literacy (Cornett, 2009). Patients will frequently hide their deficits due to feelings of embarrassment and shame. They develop coping skills that help them conceal their limited literacy, and that may lead healthcare providers to misjudge their ability to comprehend patient teaching. A recent article by Cornett provides some practical ways to identify behavioral clues for low health literacy. For example, patients who provide incomplete forms, make excuses such as they forgot their glasses, or state that they will complete the paperwork at home may be trying to hide low literacy. Low-literacy skills can be uncovered when CNLs ask certain nonthreatening assessment questions (Cornett, 2009). Cornett provides some useful sample questions. For example, a CNL could say the following to a patient: Many people have trouble understanding the healthcare information given to them. Do you ever have (or would you like to have) someone help you with your forms, your insurance information, and your medication labels?

The previous information can be supplemented with additional useful resources:

- The U.S. Department of Health and Human Services (Office of Disease Prevention and Health Promotion) *Quick Guide to Health Literacy* can be accessed at the following website: www.health.gov/communication/literacy/quickguide/quickguide.pdf
- The Council of State Governments *Health Literacy Tool Kit* can be accessed at the following website: www.csg.org/knowledgecenter/docs/ToolKit03HealthLiteracy.pdf

Cultural Competence

CNLs will be expected to offer illness and disease management while also providing culturally competent care. Culturally competent care requires that the CNL is sensitive to matters related to culture, race, gender, and sexual orientation. Cultural competence can be viewed as an extension of patient-centered care. Cultural competence can be conceptualized as the process in which CNLs continuously strive to achieve the skills, knowledge, and ability to work effectively within the cultural context of the patient. There is evidence to support a relationship between patient outcomes and nurses' cultural competence (Boyer, 2006). In order to become culturally competent, Boyer suggests that there are several stages through which CNLs will need to progress:

- **Cultural awareness:** CNLs need to recognize their own individual values, beliefs, and prejudices. CNLs should reflect on their own cultural practices.
- **Cultural knowledge:** CNLs should stay unbiased and find information concerning other cultures to establish educational underpinnings.
- **Cultural skills:** CNLs need to demonstrate the ability to communicate efficiently. Additionally, they should have the ability to identify, assess, and incorporate the values, beliefs, and cultural customs of the person under their care.
- **Cultural interaction:** CNLs will need to work with individuals from various cultural backgrounds to expand their understanding and become more at ease and self-assured.
- **Cultural sensitivity**: CNLs will need to understand and accept the individual's values and beliefs. The CNL will need to show presence, support, empathy, flexibility, and tolerance (Boyer, 2006).

TABLE 10.6 Illness and Disease Management

CATEGORY	WEIGHT
A. Illness and Disease Management	**7%**
1. Assumes responsibility for the provision and management of care at the point of care in and across all environments	
2. Coordinates care at the point of service to individuals across the life span, with particular emphasis on health promotion and risk reduction services	
3. Identifies client problems that require intervention, with special focus on those problems amenable to nursing intervention	
4. Designs and redesigns client care based on analysis of outcomes and evidence-based knowledge	
5. Completes holistic assessments and directs care based on assessments	
6. Applies theories of chronic illness care to clients and families	
7. Integrates community resources, social networks, and decision support mechanisms into care management	

(continued)

TABLE 10.6 Illness and Disease Management *(continued)*

CATEGORY	WEIGHT
A. Illness and Disease Management	**7%**
8. Identifies patterns of illness symptoms and effects on clients' compliance and ongoing care	
9. Educates clients, families, and caregivers to monitor symptoms and take action	
10. Utilizes advanced knowledge of pathophysiology and pharmacology to anticipate illness progression and response to therapy, and to educate clients and families regarding care	
11. Applies knowledge of reimbursement issues in planning care across the life span	
12. Makes recommendations regarding readiness for discharge, having accurately assessed the client's level of health literacy and self-management	
13. Applies research-based knowledge from nursing and the sciences as the foundation for evidence-based practice	
14. Develops and facilitates evidence-based protocols and disseminates these among the multidisciplinary team	
15. Understands the role of palliative care and hospice as a disease management tool	
16. Understands cultural relevance as it relates to healthcare	
17. Educates clients about healthcare technologies using client-centered strategies	
18. Synthesizes literature and research findings to design interventions for select problems	
19. Monitors client satisfaction with disease action plans	
20. Evaluates factors contributing to disease, including genetics	
21. Designs and implements education and community programs for clients and health professionals	
22. Applies principles of infection control, assessment of rates, and inclusion of infection control in plan of care	
23. Integrates advanced clinical assessment	

Used with permission from the Commission on Nurse Certification (2011, 2014).

Conclusion

CNLs can play a vital role in disease and illness management given their ability to assess and manage symptoms related to disease and treatment, ability to recommend interventions, and ability to provide education to patients, families, and communities (Chambers & Grolman, 2011). In order for CNLs to manage diseases and illnesses appropriately, they will need to consider certain key factors. For example, CNLs will need to be aware that transitions in level of care are a critical time for patients and will thus need to ensure that patients are assessed for their readiness for discharge. Given the nature of disease management, CNLs will also need to be involved in managing pain, palliative care, and end-of-life issues. In addition, as our population ages, CNLs will need to be well versed in issues that affect our geriatric population. Finally, CNLs will need to be cognizant of their patient's health literacy as well as cultural considerations. The concepts of illness and disease management included in the CNL® exam are broad and challenging for CNL students (Table 10.6).

Resources

Agency for Healthcare Research and Quality. (2009). Innovations in using health IT for chronic disease management. Retrieved from http://healthit.ahrq.gov/sites/default/files/docs/page/09-0029-EF_cdm_1.pdf

Agency for Healthcare Research and Quality. (2010). *Chronic care and disease management improves health, reduces cost for patients with multiple chronic conditions in an integrated health system*. Retrieved from http://www.innovations.ahrq.gov/content.aspx?id=1696

American Diabetes Association. (2014). The cost of diabetes. Retrieved from http://www.diabetes.org/advocate/resources/cost-of-diabetes.html.

Bogardus, S. T., Richardson, E., Maciejewski, P. K., Gahbauer, E., & Inouye, S. K. (2002). Evaluation of a guided protocol for quality improvement identifying common geriatric problems. *Journal of the American Geriatrics Society*, *50*(2), 328–335.

Boyer, D. (2006). Cultural competence at the bedside. *Pennsylvania Nurse*, *61*(4), 18–19.

Briggs, E. (2010). Assessment and expression of pain. *Nursing Standard*, *25*(2), 35–38.

Centers for Disease Control and Prevention. (2011). *Chronic disease overview*. Retrieved from http://www.cdc.gov/nccdphp/overview.htm

Centers for Disease Control and Prevention. (2015). *Death and mortality*. NCHS FastStats website. Retrieved from http://www.cdc.gov/nchs/fastats/deaths.htm

Centers for Disease Control and Prevention. (n.d.). *The four domains of chronic disease prevention*. Retrieved from http://www.cdc.gov/chronicdisease/pdf/four-domains-factsheet-2015.pdf

Chambers, P., & Grolman, C. (2011). The emerging role of disease management nurses for chronic disease care. *Viewpoint*, January/February, 4–6.

Commission on Nurse Certification. (2011). *Clinical Nurse Leader job analysis report*. Retrieved from http://www.aacn.nche.edu/cnl/Job-Analysis-Report.pdf

Commission on Nurse Certification. (2014). *Clinical Nurse Leader (CNL®) certification exam blueprint*. Retrieved from http://www.aacn.nche.edu/leading-initiatives/cnl/cnl-certification/pdf/ExamContentOutline11.pdf

Cornett, S. (2009). Assessing and addressing health literacy. *Online Journal of Issues in Nursing*, *14*(3), 1.

Council of State Governments. (n.d.). *State officials guide chronic illness*. Retrieved from http://www.csg.org/knowledgecenter/docs/SOG03ChronicIllness.pdf

Delaware Healthcare Commission. (2004). *Chronic illness and disease management: House joint resolution 10 task force key findings and recommendations*. Retrieved from http://dhss.delaware.gov/dhss/dhcc/files/chronicillnessreportfinal0804.pdf

Forbes, A., & While, A. (2009). The nursing contribution to chronic disease management: A discussion paper. *International Journal of Nursing Studies*, *46*, 120–131.

Fuller, J. (2013). Nurses key to effective chronic disease management in primary care. *Australian Nursing Journal*, *20*(11), 53.

Gerteis, J., Izrael, D., Deitz, D., LeRoy, L., Ricciardi, R., Miller, T., & Basu, J. (2014). *Multiple chronic conditions chartbook.* AHRQ Publications No, Q14-0038. Rockville, MD: Agency for Healthcare Research and Quality. Retrieved from http://www.ahrq.gov/sites/default/files/wysiwyg/professionals/prevention-chronic-care/decision/mcc/mccchartbook.pdf

Go, A. S., Mozaffarian, D., Roger, V. L., Benjamin, E. J., Berry, J. D., Blaha, M. J., ... American Heart Association Statistics Committee and Stroke Statistics Subcommittee. (2014). Heart disease and stroke statistics—2014 update: A report from the American Heart Association. *Circulation, 129*(3), e28–e292.

Hegney, D. H., Patterson, E., Eley, D. S., Mohomed, R., & Young, J. (2013). The feasibility, acceptability and sustainability of nurse-led chronic disease management in Australian general practice: The perspective of key stakeholders. *International Journal of Nursing Practice, 19*, 54–59.

Hyman, M., Ornish, D., & Roisen, M. (2009). Lifestyle medicine: Treating the causes of diseases. *Alternative Therapies, 15*(6), 12–14.

Institute of Medicine. (2011). *Relieving pain in America: A blueprint for transforming prevention, care, education, and research.* Washington, DC: The National Academies Press.

Jamison, M. (1998). Chronic illness management in the year 2005. *Nursing Economics, 16*(5), 246–253.

The Joint Commission. (2013). *Transitions of care: The need for collaboration across entire care continuum.* http://www.jointcommission.org/assets/1/6/TOC_Hot_Topics.pdf

Kemp, V. (2011). Use of "chronic disease self-management strategies" mental healthcare. *Current Opinion in Psychiatry, 24*, 144–148.

National Cancer Institute. (2014). *Cancer prevalence and cost of care projections.* Retrieved from http://costprojections.cancer.gov/.

Saxe, J., Janson, S. L., Dennehy, P. M., Stringari-Murray, S. S., Hirsch, J. E., & Waters, C. M. (2007). Meeting a primary care challenge in the United States: Chronic illness care. *Contemporary Nurse, 26*(1), 94–103.

Schulman-Green, D., Jaser, S., Martin, F., Alonzo, A., Grey, M., McCorkle, R., ... Whittemore, R. (2012). Processes of self-management in chronic illness. *Journal of Nursing Scholarship, 44*(2), 136–144.

Trehearne, B., Fishman, P., & Lin, E. (2014). Role of the nurse in chronic illness management: Making the medical home more effective. *Nursing Economics, 32*(4), 178–182.

Ward, B. W., Schiller, J. S., & Goodman, R. A. (2014). Multiple chronic conditions among U.S. adults: A 2012 update. *Preventing Chronic Disease, 11*, E62. doi:10.5888/pcd11.130389.

Weiss, M., Yakusheva, O., & Bobay, K. (2010). Nurse and patient perceptions of discharge readiness in relation to post discharge utilization. *Medical Care, 48*(5), 482–486.

World Health Organization. (2011a). *Scaling up action against noncommunicable diseases: How much will it cost?* Retrieved from http://whqlibdoc.who.int/publications/2011/9789241502313_eng.pdf

World Health Organization. (2011b). *Palliative care for older people: Better practices.* Retrieved from http://www.euro.who.int/__data/assets/pdf_file/0017/143153/e95052.pdf

11

Knowledge Management

Deborah C. Jackson and Katherine A'Hearn

The clinical nurse leader (CNL) white paper dictates that the CNL is an outcomes manager who synthesizes data, information, and knowledge to evaluate and achieve optimal client outcomes (American Association of Colleges of Nursing [AACN], 2007). The CNL has the ability to acquire a wealth of data from multiple sources within the microsystem and throughout the mesosystem. Beginning with listening to shift-to-shift reports at the start of her day, to multidisciplinary rounds, physical assessments of patients, lab reports, hourly rounding, and reviewing electronic medical record (EMR) documentation, there is no lack of topics upon which the CNL might focus to evaluate for potential outcome improvement.

Driving Forces and Outcomes

Since October 2012, hospitals have been trying to adjust to the latest wrinkle in the world of healthcare: the impact of linking patient-satisfaction scores to Medicare payments. Formerly, in the fee-for-service payment system, the Centers for Medicare & Medicaid Services (CMS) paid all healthcare providers without discriminating on the basis of quality of care (Fenter & Lewis, 2008). Ascertaining that this method is no real incentive to improve outcomes, CMS changed its payment strategy to a pay for performance (P4P) reimbursement that links payment to the quality of care provided by clinicians, offering financial incentives for improvements in care, as well as disincentives for care that does not achieve adequate outcomes. The standardized tool being utilized that measures patient perception of the quality of care received is the Hospital Consumer Assessment of Healthcare Providers and Systems (HCAHPS). Since 2007, CMS has required most hospitals to submit HCAHPS; failure to do so has resulted in payment reductions (Dunn, 2011). Although HCAHPS measures patients' perception of quality, the results are also directly connected to quality, such as medication information, preprocedural education, and discharge instructions (Dunn, 2011).

As a result of these changes, the role of the CNL regarding knowledge management has been expanded. Figure 11.1 depicts the cycle of knowledge management. Data from nurse-sensitive indicators, quality improvement initiatives, patient satisfaction, advancing technology, and competent clinical care are even more critical in the age of the P4P, owing to the transparency of data. The CNL synthesizes all microsystem data, including information obtained from HCAHPS scores, and strives to achieve improvement outcomes, which favor improving patient outcomes. The P4P indicators are another defining, justifying feature of the CNL role—to promote cost-effectiveness.

AACN (2007) has challenged nursing educators and professionals to accept the "unparalleled opportunity and capability to address the critical issues that face the nation's current health care system." The nursing profession can have an impact on changing our current healthcare system by reshaping nursing practice. Nursing has been, and continues to be, described as an art and a science. Science is based on facts and evidence. Going forward, nursing practice must be established by the same method, which is the most recent evidence. The CNL, practicing within a microsystem, has the ability to, and is obligated to, obtain this evidence by a variety of methods: literature search using electronic search engines such as the Cumulative Index of Nursing and Allied Health Literature (CINAHL) or Cochrane Database of Systematic Reviews, as well as online software programs such as Mosby's Nursing Consult. In addition, the CNL utilizes access to EMR documentation of patient care and medication administration, multidisciplinary rounds on the microsystem, nursing grand rounds, and first-hand observation of the problems and challenges presented at the bedside with the ability to obtain quantitative and qualitative data. The transformation of nursing practice should have evidence-based research (EBR) as the prototype for changing all aspects of practice such as

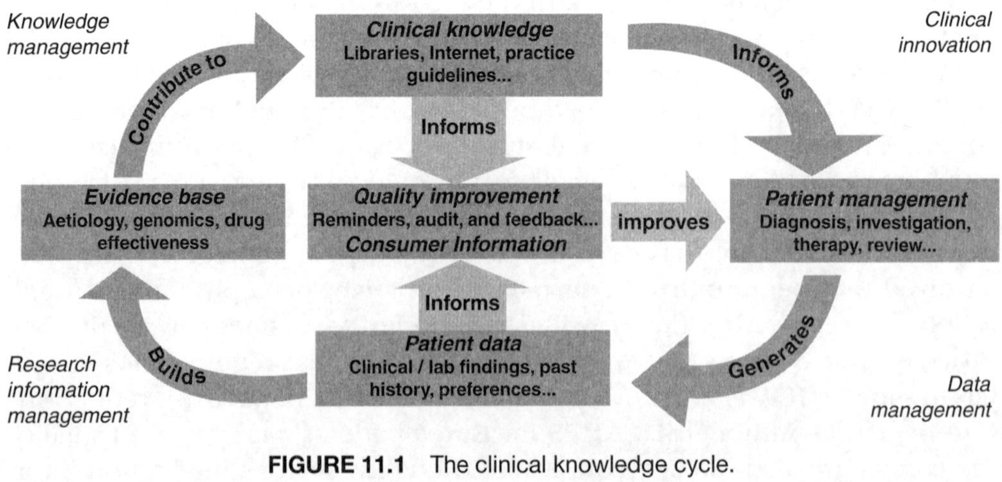

FIGURE 11.1 The clinical knowledge cycle.

Source: World Health Organization (2015).

policies, procedures, guidelines, and standards of care. "The credibility of health professions will be judged by practices based on the latest and the best evidence from sound scientific studies in combination with clinical expertise, astute assessment, and respect for patient values and preferences" (Melnyk & Fineout-Overholt, 2015).

The value of a clinical nurse leader will be measured by the high-quality outcomes in individuals and groups of clients, as well as the ability to manage waste and control costs within a microsystem. The CNL compares desired effect outcomes with national benchmarks against like institutions. Going along with the goals of the CMS, the CNL strives to identify quality measures that need improvement, incorporates new evidence into practice, implements new guidelines for patient care, tracks data on these projects, and is able to show improved clinical outcomes that are cost effective within the microsystem. The CNL needs to understand economies of scale, how to read a balance sheet, the difference between fixed and incremental costs, how to establish per unit costs, and some basic marketing strategies (Boxes 11.1 and 11.2). Basic business skills and organizational theory must become accepted components of CNL education (AACN, 2007).

BOX 11.1
Examples of Outcomes Tracked in Acute Care

- Falls
- Falls with injuries
- Pressure ulcers
- Central line catheter infections
- Catheter-related urinary tract infections
- Ventilator-acquired pneumonias (VAPs)
- Use of restraints
- Hospital readmission rates

BOX 11.2
HCAHPS Categories of Data

- Care from nurses
- Care from doctors
- Experience in the hospital
- Preparation for discharge
- Overall rating of hospital

The CNL's Role in Epidemiology

As the CNL is accountable for designing and implementing measures that modify risk factors within the microsystem, it is also an expectation that data will be collected in an effort to predict expected health problems and healthcare–associated infections (HAIs). Knowledge of the epidemiological triad is essential as the starting point, prior to the collection of data, for the identification and prevention of present and future diseases and infections within the microsystem.

The epidemiological triad, a model explaining the spread of disease, consists of an agent, a host, and an environment; the agent being the organism, such as a virus or bacterium, that infects the host (person or animal) in an environment or place with the appropriate conditions that allow for the host to be infected. Epidemiology provides the CNL with a method or direct approach to uncovering the cause of a sudden increase in infections within the microsystem, such as multiple methicillin-resistant *Staphylococcus aureus* (MRSA). Of course, this applies to a variety of hospital-acquired infections that are a significant challenge in today's healthcare. Epidemiology allows for the development of and testing for hypotheses pertaining to occurrence and prevention of serious infections that increase morbidity and mortality. By collecting specific data related to each patient affected, discovery of either the agent or the environment will allow for future prevention of the disease.

Epidemiology has been described as the sum of factors that influence the incidence and distribution of disease (Morath & Turnbull, 2005). The evolution surrounding current thinking related to poor outcomes and errors has shifted around this "sum of factors." Medical errors and poor outcomes are now ascribed to faulty systems, not to an individual. "The focus on error in the research was a reflection of the medical culture's flawed, entrenched belief that the actions of individuals, 'bad apples,' were responsible for harm to patients" (Leape, 2001). By working closely with the professional disease professionals in nursing and medicine, the CNL can support this more productive approach to improvement by using knowledge of epidemiologic data in the microsystem to enact change.

The CNL on any microsystem would do well to focus on the two guiding principles that have emerged: (a) error is best viewed as a broken healthcare system and (b) errors will always exist and should be viewed as a data source, which can help to avoid harm (Leape, 2001). Research demonstrates that accidents and near misses are a result of faulty systems, culture- and system-based failures in teamwork, communications, and transitions (Morath & Turnbull, 2005). Data and errors of the microsystem must be made transparent, allowing the CNL to understand the epidemiology of the error, to learn from it, to alleviate it, and to prevent future mistakes in the care delivery system. Also, not to be dismissed is the public's outcry related to being held financially accountable for the cost of these medical errors. Consumers of healthcare are demanding that action be taken to reduce harm to patients. What better incentive to reduce and prevent these adverse events than to have the consumers demand that healthcare providers account for their erroneous actions?

In accordance with the information regarding epidemiology of the microsystem, the CNL will develop a disease surveillance plan, if one has not already been created. Knowing which resources within the microsystem are available and can be targeted for use, the CNL will begin by collecting EBR and best practice guidelines on the specific disease identified. EBR can help identify probable causes within the specific microsystem (acute care facility, extended care facility, community clinic, physician's office, etc.) as well as recommended treatments and prevention of future outbreaks. The Agency for Healthcare Research and Quality states that HAIs are one of the top 10 leading causes of death in the United States (AHRQ, 2010). Knowing this, the CNL incorporates infection control as a fundamental aspect of preventing disease on the microsystem, where the patient population already has a compromised immune system.

In addition, the CNL must be aware of surveillance compliance with state and local infection control agencies. Some diseases must be reported. Most hospitals are enrolled in the National Healthcare Safety Network (NHSN), an Internet-based surveillance system that integrates and expands a facility's own surveillance program to a national level. One purpose of NHSN is to conduct collaborative research studies with NHSN member facilities to describe the epidemiology of emerging HAIs, assess the importance of potential risk factors, further characterize HAI pathogens and their mechanisms of resistance, and evaluate alternative surveillance and prevention strategies (NHSN, 2011). The CNL should have a working knowledge of the data collected within the organization, who is responsible for what data, and to what data registries the organization is reporting.

Risk Anticipation and Evaluation

Individuals seeking healthcare can be at risk in a variety of settings. Since October 2008, when CMS refused to reimburse hospitals for *hospital acquired conditions* (HACs) such as falls, pressure ulcers, central line infections, and deep vein thrombosis, it has become fiscally prudent for each hospital to identify which patients may be at risk for such conditions during the admission process. Assessments initiated in the emergency department (ED), on admission to the microsystem, and then again on a daily basis (sometimes each shift), are utilized in an attempt to prevent such occurrences. Millions of dollars are spent annually on items used to prevent falls (bed alarms, safety slippers, etc.), pressure ulcers (skin creams, specialty beds, constant repositioning of the patient), and central line infections. Resources have been utilized in many environments for the Institute for Healthcare Improvement (IHI)'s use of bundles—order sets specific to prevent different HAIs and safety hazards. Hourly rounding by staff on units is meant specifically to prevent such conditions. Each hour, the nurse or another member of the healthcare team must enter the patient's room and address patient needs, such as pain assessment, elimination, and physical positioning. This level of risk identification and risk reduction is a significant shift in healthcare. Often it is the CNL who is leading the development or implementation of these changes.

For adequate treatment and risk reduction to be provided, all of the patient's conditions and health needs must be addressed upon admission to the hospital. Previous medical records and treatments for conditions such as diabetes, hypertension, congestive heart failure, chronic kidney disease, and chronic obstructive pulmonary disease must be carefully considered when treating the present condition. Failure to do so might result in a lengthier hospital stay or readmission. It is essential to review current hospital medications and treatments and how they interact with the list of comorbid conditions, developing an integrated, evidence-based treatment plan that considers primary diagnosis and comorbidities (Institute for Healthcare Improvement, 2012; Box 11.3).

Example: The STOPP and START criteria were developed in 2007 to serve as a screening tool for comprehensive assessment of safety and quality of prescription in patients 65 years and older (Topinková, Mádlová, Fialová, & Klán, 2009). Using STOPP criteria, potentially inappropriate drugs are identified in drug regimens, which could be stopped altogether

BOX 11.3
Medication Management

Medication management is a significant challenge in healthcare, and that challenge must be addressed by all members caring for individuals across systems. Issues for the CNL include:

- What tool is currently being used to address medication management/reconciliation?
- What are the most common high-risk medications patients are prescribed at discharge?
- How is the process of medication review, education, and intervention incorporated into the routine practices of the microsystem?
- What resources are available to support this issue?

or replaced by a safer drug alternative. Both screening tools represent a new method for improving quality of geriatric prescribing in clinical practice (Topinková et al., 2009).

Risk anticipation, the ability to critically evaluate and anticipate risks to client safety, is a critical component of the CNL role. The CNL also uses risk analysis tools and quality improvement methodologies at the systems level to anticipate risk to any client and intervenes to decrease the risk (AACN, 2013). *Root cause analysis* (RCA) is a structured method used to analyze serious adverse events. It is now widely deployed as an error analysis tool in healthcare (AHRQ, 2014).

The major concept of RCA involves identifying underlying problems related to the system, rather than concentrating on the mistakes made by an individual. If one should occur on the microsystem, the CNL would follow a "prescribed protocol that begins with data collection and reconstruction of the event through record review and participant interviews" (AHRQ, 2014). A multidisciplinary team should then analyze the sequence of events leading to the error, with the goals of identifying how and why the event occurred. The ultimate goal of RCA, of course, is to prevent future harm by eliminating the latent errors (the hidden problems within the systems that contribute to adverse events) that so often underlie adverse events (AHRQ, 2014).

Another tool for risk analysis in healthcare is failure mode effect and analysis (FMEA). As stated in Wilcox (2012), "A healthcare failure mode and effect analysis process is conducted in an effort to help identify weak points in a process, to prevent failures of a process/system and to reduce or prevent medical errors, before these processes have the chance to occur." Reporting of "near misses" in many organizations is a key opportunity to conduct a FMEA and analyze the components of the system that could allow for errors. Reports by nurses of medication "near misses" are a wonderful opportunity for this process. Suppose a CNL observes a nurse draw up a dose of insulin that seems much greater than the dose the patient normally requires. The staff nurse reports that the computerized medication administration record indicates the patient is due for the large dose when, in fact, the CNL realizes that the nurse has misread the insulin coverage. This near miss with a high-risk medication is an opportunity to analyze the factors involved, because if one nurse made the mistake, it can certainly happen again.

Electronic Medical Record

Modern technology has created an explosion in the world of healthcare related to new equipment designed to prevent medical errors and keep the patients' medical records safe. The EMR was implemented to prevent medical errors and plays a significant role in reducing the cost of healthcare, reducing complications, and achieving better outcomes (Harris & Roussel, 2013). With the implementation of the EMR, healthcare workers have the ability to access patient records nationwide. This process, now supported (and being made mandatory by 2015) by the federal government, is in the form of a health information exchange (HIE). It refers to the sharing of clinical and administrative data across the boundaries of healthcare institutions and other health data repositories (Harris & Roussel, 2013).

The CNL performs a critical part in developing, training, and auditing all documentation into the EMR. Order sets may be created at the request of physicians or staff in order to provide consistency in disease management and prevent variations in care when able. Clinical support systems can be put into place to share information with nurses at critical times to avoid or reduce the risk of error. The EMR affords greater access to data collection, facilitates communication across microsystems, and addresses some areas of safety. Physicians and CNLs may have the potential to communicate electronically with their patients after discharge, checking that patients are doing well, taking medications as instructed, and knowing when to call if not feeling well, all in an attempt to prevent readmissions. The complexity, functionality, and compatibility of EMRs vary greatly by institution and healthcare system. The CNL will be instrumental in supporting the development and integration of an EMR system that will continue to be developed in the coming decades.

Lastly, an important aspect for electronic communication is patient privacy. The CNL must do everything possible to ensure that patient records are not viewed inappropriately by anyone who is not directly caring for the patient. Enforcement of safety measures for the CNL as well as the staff on the microsystem, such as closing EMRs when completed, not leaving any paperwork for others to view, or giving passwords to fellow employees, is mandatory to protect privacy. Issues related to ethics and privacy in the EMR are discussed further in this book.

Benchmarking Data

On any given microsystem, the CNL continually strives to improve the quality of care for the patient population. Since good performance reflects good quality practice, it is essential that performance be measured both against other microsystems within the institution and against like microsystems on a national level. Competition can be healthy among these like microsystems, the goal being to strive for continually better outcomes and practices. The progress of quality improvement initiatives can be tracked by using measures of quality and safety. There is always a need to improve the quality of care or the safety of practice for a microsystem. The use of external benchmarks allows the CNL to determine whether or not improvement has truly been made. *Benchmarking* in healthcare has been defined as the continual and collaborative discipline of measuring and comparing the results of key work processes with those of the best performers in evaluating organizational performance (Hughes, 2008).

Benchmarking in healthcare allows the organization to improve the efficiency, cost-effectiveness, and quality of services performed in a meaningful manner. On the microsystem level, data collected by the CNL on each of the quality indicators can be compared to like microsystems nationwide and gauged on the effectiveness of protocols used. If falling below the national benchmark, the CNL reflects on practice used, researches best practices, and seeks out knowledge on what is used by like systems whose achievement levels are excellent. Likewise, if the microsystem is well above the benchmark (considering this the expectation), the CNL reflects on the methodology in place for this indicator and analyzes whether or not the same can be used elsewhere.

Designing Care to Optimize Outcomes

On a weekly, monthly, and quarterly basis, nursing administration, nursing management, and CNLs seriously evaluate the results of quality indicators for the individual microsystems, as well as the mesosystem as a whole. Comparisons are made against national benchmarks with like microsystems. Since the 2013 implementation of the CMS value-based incentive programs such as the Value-Based Purchasing, Hospital-Acquired Condition Reduction Program, and Hospital Readmissions Reduction Program, financial incentives and penalties have been linked to benchmarked performance and affect reimbursement (CMS, 2013). For those indicators whose rates lie below (or above, as the case may be) the benchmarks, it is necessary to determine where the variations lie and implement plans to improve the measures to meet or exceed the benchmarks. In addition to the most commonly thought attribution to variation in the work of the practitioners, the CNL must consider variability in the methodology of the system, which can produce variations in access and outcomes, as well as other significant results (Box 11.4). Specific variations must be dissected separately for true determination of causes. Each variation should have the following addressed: Is there a need to identify it? How will it be measured? Does it necessitate improvement? Can improvement occur?

BOX 11.4
Methods to Support Knowledge Sharing to Optimize Outcomes

- Electronic medical record
- Informational hurdles at the microsystem and mesosystem levels
- Shared governance council
- Unit practice councils
- Journal clubs
- Unit practice councils
- Data boards with benchmarks
- Staff involvement in RCA

Optimal client outcomes best occur when the healthcare team has the patient's *total* history: physical, social, and psychological. Without this being complete, the CNL begins with a handicap when trying to establish goals for this patient. Collaboration with the nursing staff, especially the primary nurse, and the entire interdisciplinary team is advantageous to the CNL in developing a specific, individualized plan of care that allows for optimal outcomes. Each of these healthcare workers is an expert in his or her field, and their suggestions are taken seriously. The AACN's Synergy Model stresses that responsibility and accountability for outcomes is a shared responsibility between the patient and the healthcare provider (Curley, 1998).

Keeping in mind that the patient's perception of what is an "optimal patient outcome" is most important in today's world of patient satisfaction scores, HCAHPS, and future reimbursement from CMS, it is imperative that the CNL educate the staff on the importance of developing a comprehensive plan, assessing risk, and individualizing care on admission to the microsystem. A proactive, evidence-based approach by the entire team will best support outcomes related to the patient's disease state.

Accountability for Knowledge Management

The American Nurses Association (ANA) *Code of Ethics for Nurses* (4.2) states, "Accountability means to be answerable to oneself and others for one's actions. In order to be accountable, nurses act under a code of ethical conduct that is grounded in moral principles of fidelity and respect for the dignity, worth, and self-determination of patients. Nurses are accountable for judgments made and actions taken in the course of nursing practice, irrespective of healthcare organizations' policies or providers' directives" (ANA, 2011).

Harris and Roussel (2013) further address accountability for the CNL by emphasizing that responsible people account for what they do and how well they perform, work effectively with others, complete tasks, and achieve outcomes. Accountability includes developing trust, being known to follow through on problems, keeping promises, and being persistent on problem resolution even when anticipated outcomes are not obtained.

These statements relate to the CNL even more than to the staff nurse, as the CNL plans, evaluates, and revises plans of care; develops and provides staff and patient education; and has input on many of the decisions made for the microsystem. The CNL on the microsystem assumes responsibility for the total care of the patients and families on a fair and equitable basis, advocating that all patients receive continuity of care without bias or unfair judgment. Being accountable, this leader asks for and offers feedback in an attempt to create desired improvements. Skills needed for accountability include remaining engaged when a situation continues to be problematic, persistence in seeking new and creative solutions, asking for advice of the experts and superiors when needed, and thinking outside the box to accomplish new pathways for accomplishment of goals. Continually striving to achieve the best results, the CNL does not give up when outcomes are under par; revision of strategies and further EBR demonstrate a determination that outcomes will be of the best quality possible.

Also taken into consideration, here is the cultural diversity of the patient population within the microsystem. Sensitivity and cultural competency must be displayed for each and every individual plan of care. It is the judgment of the CNL, usually through EBR, that formulates many of these decisions. If the patient's plan of care is less than adequate, or contains misinformation, harm may come to the patient. Utilizing input from patients and families, the CNL can support optimal care for diverse populations on the microsystem. The CNL assumes accountability for outcomes through the collection and application of research-based information to design, implement, and evaluate client plans of care (AACN, 2007). If there are errors in judgment made, the CNL is ethically accountable, and must correct, reevaluate decisions made, and develop new strategies. As stated earlier, the value of the CNL position is judged by the patient outcomes and cost efficiency that result from decisions made for the microsystem. The business case for the CNL role is intricately involved in the outcomes of a microsystem and the associated cost savings for the organization.

Knowledge of Complementary Therapy

Along with the standardized and common medical treatments, *complementary and alternative medicine* (CAM) has again made a place for itself in medicine in the 21st century. Long before doctors and hospitals were commonplace, there were individuals who practiced medicine utilizing what was on hand: plants, herbs, spices, and prayers. The shaman in China, the medicine man in America, and those who practiced witchcraft and voodoo were all familiar in towns and villages when one was sick or hurt. Yoga has been practiced for more than 5,000 years and improves flexibility, increases strength, develops better concentration, improves posture, and promotes breathing. Reiki healing promotes overall balance to feel and function well, is safe, and supports any medical treatment plan. Acupuncture and chiropractic medicine are other examples of CAM.

Over the past 20 years, many patients are turning to and adding CAM to the treatment plans prescribed by their doctors. Some avoid prescribed medicines at any cost, hoping that CAM will be sufficient. The CNL on any microsystem would be wise to impress upon the staff that it is prudent to consistently ask the patients upon admission if they take any vitamins, minerals, herbs, or supplements. Many of these CAMs potentiate, decrease, or negate the medicinal effects of traditional medications being taken. The CNL must educate the staff to be aware of such interactions. For example, garlic and ginko can increase the effect of some anticoagulants, while goldenseal can decrease the effectiveness; women who are on oral contraceptives may be surprised if also taking St. John's wort to fight depression, as it may also render the contraceptives ineffective (Ehrlich, 2011).

Herbs are unregulated and there are no standard doses, so it becomes imperative for the admission nurse to deliberately ask if the patient takes any vitamins or herbs, since many people do not think of them as medicine. On the other hand, when traditional treatment plans are not working or are not fully effective, the CNL might suggest CAM to the staff as well as the interdisciplinary team. This can be especially true for patients with refractory pain, such as cancer patients or those with migraine headaches. Together the staff nurse and the CNL might evaluate the success or failure of combined treatment care plans. If it proves that the CAM is unsuccessful, exploration of other CAMs is deemed necessary.

In addition to the traditional route of using EBR, today's nurse needs to also inquire about the possibility of CAM for patients. The CNL might be wise to include educational programs on this topic, so that staff will be prepared for this additional inclusion in medicine in today's world.

Conclusion

The CNL® certification exam covers a broad range of content related to knowledge management (Table 11.1). Clinical instructors and nurse educators continually educate and impart knowledge to students, nurses, and administration. The dilemma lies in having them retain and store this knowledge. Knowledge management promotes learning, the acquisition of new knowledge, and a systematic way of retaining this resource for future use. Acknowledging that explicit knowledge is easily retained and documented, we give credence to tacit knowledge within the minds of the most experienced nurses and seek ways to keep their knowledge and experience if they leave the institution. If we do not retain what we have discovered and learned, we will forever be reinventing the wheel.

Having discussed the various methodologies for obtaining data, the CNL synthesizes these data and applies it to developing improvement on the microsystem. Knowledge management permits quality improvement throughout the unit, strengthening practice and protocols, utilizing the latest in technology, and creating and strengthening a professional staff capable

TABLE 11.1 Knowledge Management

CATEGORY	WEIGHT
B. Knowledge Management	**5%**
1. Applies research-based information	
2. Improves clinical and cost outcomes	
3. Utilizes epidemiological methodology to collect data	
4. Participates in disease surveillance	
5. Evaluates and anticipates risks to client safety (e.g., new technology, medications, treatment regimens)	
6. Applies tools for risk analysis	
7. Uses institutional and unit data to compare against national benchmarks	
8. Designs and implements measures to modify risks	
9. Addresses variations in clinical outcomes	
10. Synthesizes data, information, and knowledge to evaluate and achieve optimal client outcomes	
11. Demonstrates accountability for processes for improvement of client outcomes	
12. Evaluates effect of complementary therapies on health outcomes	

Used with permission from the Commission on Nurse Certification (2011, 2014).

of continuing to acquire assets of knowledge. The CNL is continuously accountable for patient safety, HCAHPS results, and the discretionary use of CAMs on the microsystem. The future success of all of these depends on how the acquisition of knowledge is stored and retained. Well-managed knowledge will serve to strengthen both the microsystem and the organization, enable both to avoid repetition of problems, and store valuable evidence from research, which is readily accessible for practice when needed.

Resources

Agency for Healthcare Research and Quality. (2010, November 2). *AHRQ awards $34 million to expand fight against healthcare-associated infections*. U.S. Department of Health and Human Services. Press Release. Retrieved from http://archive.ahrq.gov/news/newsroom/press-releases/2011/haify11.html

Agency for Healthcare Research and Quality. (2014). *Patient safety primers—Root cause analysis*. Retrieved from http://psnet.ahrq.gov/primer.aspx?primerID=10

American Association of Colleges of Nursing. (2007). *White paper on the role of the clinical nurse leader*. Washington, DC. Retrieved from http://www.aacn.nche.edu/cnl-certification

American Association of Colleges of Nursing. (2013). *Competencies and curricular expectations for clinical nurse leader education and practice*. Retrieved from http://www.aacn.nche.edu/cnl/CNL-Competencies-October-2013.pdf

American Nurses Association. (2011). *Code of ethics for nurses with interpretative statement*. Retrieved from http://ana.nursingworld.org/MainMenuCategories/EthicsStandards/CodeofEthicsforNurses/Code-of-Ethics.aspx

Centers for Medicare & Medicaid Services. (2013). *Hospital quality initiatives*. Retrieved from https://www.cms.gov/Medicare/Quality-Initiatives-Patient-Assessment-Instruments/HospitalQualityInits/index.html

Commission on Nurse Certification. (2011). *Clinical Nurse Leader job analysis report*. Retrieved from http://www.aacn.nche.edu/cnl/Job-Analysis-Report.pdf

Commission on Nurse Certification. (2014). *Clinical Nurse Leader (CNL®) certification exam blueprint*. Retrieved from http://www.aacn.nche.edu/leading-initiatives/cnl/cnl-certification/pdf/ExamContentOutline11.pdf

Curley, M. (1998). Patient–nurse synergy: Optimizing patient outcomes. *American Journal of Critical Care*, *7*(1), 64–72.

Dunn, L. (2011). Quint Studer: Raising HCAHPS is about more than better service. *Becker's Hospital Review*. Retrieved from http://www.beckershospitalreview.com/hospital-management-administration/quint-studer-raising-hcahps-is-about-more-than-better-serviceits-about-better-quality.html

Ehrlich, J. (2011). *Herbal medicine. University of Maryland medical center*. Retrieved from http://www.umm.edu/altmed/articles/herbal-medicine-000351.htm

Fenter, T., & Lewis, S. (2008). Pay-for-performance initiatives. *Supplement to Journal of Managed Care Pharmacy*, *14*(6, Suppl. C), S12–S15.

Harris, J. L., & Roussel, L. (2013). *Initiating and sustaining the clinical nurse leader role* (2nd ed.). *A practical guide*. Sudbury, MA: Jones & Bartlett Publishers.

Hughes, R. (2008, April). *Patient safety and quality: An evidence-based handbook for nurses: Vol. 3*. AHRQ publication no. 08-0043.

Institute for Healthcare Improvement. (2012, January 20). *Disease specific care for common comorbidities*. Retrieved from http://www.ihi.org/search/pages/results.aspx?sq=1&k=Risk%20Assessment%20Tool%20For%20CHF

Leape, L. (2001). Foreword: Preventing medical accidents: Is systems analysis the answer? *American Journal of Law and Medicine, 27*, 145–148.

Melnyk, B., & Fineout-Overholt, E. (2015). *Evidence-based practice in nursing & healthcare. A guide to best practice* (3rd ed.). Philadelphia, PA: Lippincott Williams & Wilkins.

Morath, J., & Turnbull, J. (2005). *To do no harm. Ensuring patient safety in health care organization*. Foreward by Lucian L. Leape. San Francisco, CA: John Wiley & Sons.

National Health Care Safety Network. (2011). *About NHSN*. Home page. Centers for Disease Control and Prevention.

Topinková, E., Mádlová, P., Fialová, D., & Klán, J. (2009). New evidence-based criteria for evaluating the appropriateness for drug regimen in seniors. Criteria STOPP (screening tool of older person's prescriptions) and START (screening tool to alert doctors to right treatment). *Vnitr ˇníe lékarˇství, 54*(12), 1161–1169.

Wilcox, J. (2012). Failure mode effect and analysis—Nursing. *Phillips Learning Center*. Retrieved from http://www.theonlinelearningcenter.com/Catalog/product.aspx?mid=6357

World Health Organization. (2015). The clinical knowledge cycle. *Image Source Page*. Retrieved from http://www.who.int/management/general/knowledge/en/index.html

12

Health Promotion and Disease Prevention and Injury Reduction/ Prevention Management

Sally O'Toole Gerard

The stage is set for an unprecedented chapter in the history of nursing, as factors impacting health promotion and disease prevention come together in a time of great need. Healthcare has begun a new era of reform with an emphasis on prevention of illness, rather than treating existing diseases as they occur. The need for this change in ideology is apparent in the explosion of preventable conditions and associated illnesses. Obesity, for example, illustrates the impact of a preventable condition with a ripple effect that will greatly impact the healthcare resources of the future. The clinical nurse leader (CNL) stands poised to encompass health promotion and risk reduction in diverse settings to support individuals, families, and the American healthcare system.

Health promotion and risk reduction take on a variety of diverse scenarios for the master's-prepared generalist. Today's CNLs have expanded beyond the original vision of acute care and include community/public health, home health, outpatient settings, long-term care, hospice, and more (Stanley, 2010). Considering the variety of settings, CNLs can be involved in primary, secondary, and tertiary disease prevention in an array of clinical situations. The needs of the population being served in the CNL's particular microsystem will drive the specific approach to ensure positive patient outcomes. The CNL assumes the responsibility for those patient-centered outcomes through the assimilation and application of evidence-based information to design, implement, and evaluate appropriate health promotion interventions for individuals (American Association of Colleges of Nursing [AACN], 2007).

The complexity and fragmentation of the current healthcare system supports the role of the CNL as an advocate in the arena of health promotion and risk reduction. Integrating research, technology, best practice models, and individualized family care within a fast-moving, outcome-driven healthcare environment requires the CNL to practice to the fullest extent of the role. This chapter will review significant themes of health promotion and provide examples of CNL activities related to health promotion, risk reduction, resource management, and the common challenges of maintaining optimal health.

Health Promotion and Healthy People 2020

The impact of health promotion efforts by healthcare members is supported by the identification of national health issues. Key resources for healthcare providers include the U.S. Department of Health and Human Services (USDHHS) publication of *Healthy People: National Health Promotion and Disease Prevention Objectives* for health promotion programs. The Healthy People initiative provides science-based, 10-year national objectives for improving the health of all Americans. The program has established benchmarks for three decades and monitored progress over time to encourage collaboration across sectors, guide individuals in health decisions, and measure the impact of prevention activities (Healthy People, 2011). The vision of this work is to establish a society in which people live long and healthy lives (see Table 12.1 for additional details of the latest report, Healthy People 2020 [HP 2020]).

The HP 2020 initiative empowers CNLs, in all settings, to be aligned with the nation's healthcare priorities, focus areas, and goals. This most recent report continues to support all aspects of health promotion and gives specific guidance to the nurse's role. Undoubtedly, the CNL's academic preparation

TABLE 12.1 Healthy People 2020 Summary

HEALTHY PEOPLE 2020	RELEASED IN DECEMBER 2010
Mission: Healthy People strives to	• Identify nationwide health improvement priorities • Increase public awareness and understanding of determinants of health, disease, and disability and opportunities for progress • Provide measurable objectives and goals that are applicable at the national, state, and local levels • Engage multiple sectors to take action to strengthen policies and improve practices that are driven by the best available evidence and knowledge • Identify critical research, evaluation, and data collection needs

(*continued*)

TABLE 12.1 Healthy People 2020 Summary *(continued)*

HEALTHY PEOPLE 2020	RELEASED IN DECEMBER 2010
Overarching goals	• Attain high-quality, longer lives free of preventable disease, disability, injury, and premature death • Achieve health equality, eliminate disparities, and improve the health of all groups • Create social and physical environments that promote good health for all • Promote quality of life, healthy development, and healthy behaviors across all life stages
Health measures: Four categories will serve as indicators of progress toward the HP 2020 goals	• General health status • Health-related quality of life and well-being • Determinants of health • Disparities

Source: Healthy People (2011).

has introduced the Healthy People data as a valuable resource. These professionals can incorporate the mission, vision, and goals of HP 2020 into their own approach to health promotion as appropriate to their population. Data from the HP 2020 site can be analyzed and utilized to develop holistic health promotion initiatives. The CNL is strategically positioned to partner with individuals to initiate and maintain healthier lifestyles focusing on the human response to symptoms and diagnoses (Carranti, 2010). This collaboration of a national vision with a CNL who can individualize care, utilize resources, and support the uniqueness of the human response to health is invaluable to the challenge of attaining the HP 2020 goals.

The CNL Role in Health Promotion, Risk Reduction, and Disease Prevention

Regardless of the microsystem for which the CNL is responsible, the work of health promotion requires a multitude of skills. The CNL must have a strong theoretical foundation in health promotion. Not only does the master's curriculum introduce course content in health promotion, but the CNL also integrates the curriculum of epidemiology, health policy, research, health assessment, pathophysiology, and pharmacology to be a clinical expert in designing care. The goal of this care is to allow for an optimal level of wellness. The application of this knowledge is supported through practicum experience, which specifically involves health promotion activities and patient/family education. Effective health promotion, risk reduction, and disease prevention also require effective teaching and evaluation skills and knowledge, including knowledge of available resources, teaching, and communication methods and learning principles (AACN, 2007). A patient scenario is introduced and discussed through the chapter to help illustrate how relatively common patient situations can benefit from a CNL's approach to health promotion (Box 12.1).

BOX 12.1
Patient Scenario: Mrs. Louise

Mrs. Louise, a 56-year-old Haitian woman, is admitted to the emergency department with a chief complaint of severe headache.

Clinical data of note:

Blood pressure: 220/118 mmHg

Pulse: 90 bpm

Respirations: 22/min

Temperature: 97.9°F

ECG: normal

Routine lab work unremarkable with the exception of a random glucose of 245 mg/dL

Body mass index: 32

Other client information: Patient is non–English speaking, works full time as a maintenance worker for a large hotel, and lives with multiple family members, including a spouse and children of varied ages. Her father died of a heart attack, age unknown, and her mother died of unspecified causes at the age of 79. She has medical insurance through her employer. She has no private physician in the community.

Treatment: The patient is monitored for a number of hours. She is started on an antihypertensive and given a prescription to continue the medication after discharge. Prior to discharge, the patient is informed that she had high blood sugar and was prescribed a medication to treat this as well. She is told to follow up with a physician in the community in 1 week. Her teenage son acts as the interpreter for the patient. She is given written instructions for discharge from the emergency department regarding her medications and instructions for follow-up treatment. No appointment was made with a primary care provider (PCP) for her follow-up.

Patient Follow-Up: The patient filled the two prescriptions, believing both were to treat the cause of her headache, which she vaguely understood to be high blood pressure. She took the medications daily until the bottle was

(*continued*)

BOX 12.1 *(continued)*

finished, at which time her headaches had ceased. She had no understanding of her new diagnosis of diabetes.

Keep this patient scenario in mind as more commentary follows, including her readmission to the emergency department (ED) 2 years later.

Levels of Prevention

Primary prevention involves measures to prevent illness or disease from occurring. For a CNL in the public health or occupational health arena, this could include exercise programs, nutrition programs, weight loss initiatives, smoking cessation, stress reduction activities, and increased awareness of the body's well-being. The HP 2020 data continue to cite exercise as a top goal for our country. In examining Mrs. Louise, we see that the adoption of regular exercise could have supported decreased weight, decreased blood pressure, stress reduction, and improved insulin utilization. This type of primary prevention can occur at the workplace, through churches, or in other community organizations or healthcare–sponsored outreach programs. As CNLs continue to establish roles outside of acute care, the careful planning of culturally appropriate community programming and resource utilization is critical.

Secondary prevention refers to methods and procedures to detect the presence of disease in the early stages, so that the effective treatment can be initiated and complications decreased (Greiner & Edelman, 2010). Screenings of all types play a key role in secondary prevention. Cancer, cardiovascular, and diabetes screens are some of the most common. Heart disease is the leading cause of death in the United States, resulting in the death of 2,200 Americans daily, many of whom were unaware of their condition (American Heart Association, 2011). A screening program for Mrs. Louise could have alerted her to the presence of hypertension, hyperglycemia, or possibly both. A referral to a healthcare provider for management of her health could have prevented the emergency department visit and facilitated more appropriate use of resources.

The insidious nature of these often asymptomatic diseases allows for microvascular and macrovascular damage, leading to poorer outcomes. Initiation of health-promoting behavior can have a great impact on the course of a disease. Categories of prehypertension and prediabetes offer evidence-based research on the impact of behavior modification. Studies on prediabetes indicate that lifestyle interventions can reduce the rate of conversion to type 2 diabetes from 43% to 30% (Ackerman & Marrero, 2007). As the incidence of these types of diseases increases, CNLs in all areas of healthcare can be instrumental in developing age-appropriate, culturally appropriate, and accessible programs that promote health, reduce disease burden, and improve outcomes.

Tertiary prevention refers to prevention strategies needed after a disease or condition has been diagnosed in an attempt to return the client to an optimum state of health (Kazer & Grossman, 2011). This type of prevention can also occur in a variety of CNL settings. Acute care of the patient with coronary artery bypass graft (CABG), stroke, asthma, and cancer treatment are just a few of the many types of tertiary care. Often this type of care includes a team of professionals such as physical therapists, dietitians, occupational therapy, social workers, case managers, and more. The CNL has a vital role in the coordination of care within the interdisciplinary group.

Barriers to Health Promotion/Risk Reduction

The Healthy People documents have some overarching goals, one of which is to increase the quality and years of healthy life for an individual. Members of the healthcare team can support this goal in a variety of ways, but the ultimate determination for adopting positive health behaviors or lifestyle changes is ultimately up to the individual. The best possible scenario is that members of society are raised with healthy lifestyle choices, such as a healthy diet, tobacco-free environment, adherence to personal safety standards, and high levels of exercise. Unfortunately, many individuals have lifestyle indicators that are inconsistent with health and risk reduction. For this reason, it is commonly necessary for healthcare professionals to educate and support individuals and families in the adoption of behavior changes. CNLs may have studied a variety of theoretical models of behavior change, such as the health belief model and Pender's health promotion model.

A classic model of examining how people intentionally change their behaviors is described in Prochaska's work on behavior change, which is based on the study of addictions. It may be referred to as the *transtheoretical model of change*. The concepts and phenomenon of intentional change within an individual were studied to support professionals in their appreciation of successful change (Prochaska, DiClemente, & Norcross, 1992). This research produced a theory of stages in the process of change: precontemplation, contemplation, preparation, action, and maintenance (see Table 12.2). These stages are not linear, but spiral in nature, in which an individual may vacillate, moving forward and back with a varying degree of success toward change. The concepts of this model can be associated with other theoretical models of behavior change, all of which support an evolving and individualized approach to change.

TABLE 12.2 Stages of Change

STAGE OF CHANGE	DESCRIPTION
Precontemplation	Individuals are not considering change within the next 6 months. They may be resistant, have a lack of knowledge, or be overwhelmed by the problem.
Contemplation	Individuals are seriously thinking about changing within the next 6 months, but because of ambivalence, they may remain in this stage for years.
Preparation	Individuals are seriously planning to change within the next month and have already taken some steps toward action.
Action	This stage involves overt modification of the problem behavior; can last from 3 to 6 months.
Maintenance	This period begins after 6 months of continuous successful behavior change. Individuals can remain in maintenance from 3 to 5 years and still experience temptations to relapse and often do revert to the behavior.

Source: Prochaska et al. (1992).

The concept of modifiable versus nonmodifiable risk factors guides much of the work in health promotion. Let us take, for example, the CNL's role in adoption of healthy lifestyles regarding use of tobacco products. A CNL involved in public health or community health may assess the population/microsystem being served and provide educational interventions to deter individuals from trying tobacco products. Programming would be individualized to the target group, age appropriate, culturally appropriate, and may involve some type of incentive program. This primary prevention is the preferred situation, in which a person does not adopt a lifestyle that is inconsistent with health. For those in the community who do use tobacco, a series of cessation initiatives would also be individualized and deemed appropriate to the active smokers. In most cases, a CNL would have a diverse team of professionals to plan, implement, and evaluate program efforts. This team should analyze available data related to national, state, and local smoking trends, effectiveness of previous interventions, and available evidence for optimal outcomes related to tobacco use. For those smokers who are not ready to enter the action phase, the interventions can fuel the contemplative stage, as they understand the consequences of their actions, although they are not ready to change.

In the acute care setting, a tobacco user who had been in the precontemplative stage, in which there is no intention of changing behavior, may be catapulted into the action phase by an acute health issue. A heavy smoker, who is admitted to the hospital with shortness of breath and diagnosed with pneumonia, may be strongly motivated to take action, quit smoking, and commit to a smoke-free life. The concerns of serious health issues, cancer, and death that were present in the precontemplative phase may now be actualized into a readiness to take action. Although the person may truly be committed to quit, the maintenance phase often requires work to prevent relapse. Because many health-related behaviors truly stem from a physical and psychological addiction, relapse is the rule rather than the exception (Prochaska et al., 1992). The CNL can maximize success in the maintenance phase through patient education, preparing the client for the struggles of maintenance and offering strategies to promote success. Again, utilizing the resources of an interdisciplinary team in the acute care environment and in the community supports health promotion.

Healthcare Literacy

The issue of healthcare literacy challenges all aspects of health promotion and risk reduction. On a national level, this issue is gaining traction through a variety of sources. The Healthy People initiative, the Institute of Medicine (IOM), and the Centers for Disease Control are some of the national leaders in highlighting the importance of this central health issue, which goes beyond the ability to read. *Healthcare literacy* is the capacity to obtain, process, and understand basic health information and services to make appropriate health decisions (Baur, 2011). The Office of Disease Prevention and Health Promotion (ODPHP), U.S. Department of Health and Human Services, launched a National Action Plan to Improve Health Literacy (the "Action Plan") to draw attention to limited health literacy as a major public health issue (Baur, 2011). This collaborative work from a multitude of public and private sector organizations provides a framework to identify the most important actions to take to improve the society-wide problem of limited health literacy. The Action Plan outlines strategies for all disciplines to address this widespread problem and work to support a more health-literate society.

Nurses in all settings have a vital role in improving healthcare literacy, and CNLs in particular can be leaders in this initiative. In the complex setting of our current healthcare system—namely polypharmacy, ambiguous health recommendations, unclear medication instructions, insurance forms, multiple medical specialists, and medical terminology—navigating the healthcare system is challenging in the best of situations. Add to that an individual's illness, comprehension of medical issues, varied cognitive abilities, fears, cultural conditioning, vision, and hearing loss, and you have a vastly difficult situation for most people. Clearly communicated information to support health issues would seem to be a foundation for navigating this maze toward good health. CNLs should utilize research and resources to promote healthcare literacy in all settings.

As the vision of the CNL is to have direct contact with individuals receiving care, the comprehensive assessment of knowledge, literacy issues, cultural circumstances, and spiritual and socioeconomic factors are essential to support health. Through discussions with patients, families, members of the healthcare team, and community services, the CNL can support individualized care of complex patients. Through increased awareness of literacy issues and utilization of the Action Plan's resources, CNLs and all team members can support the vision of this work. The vision has been summarized in three points: A health-literate society is one that (a) provides everyone with access to accurate and actionable health information, (b) delivers person-centered health information and services, and (c) supports lifelong learning and skills to promote good health (Baur, 2011). The specific goals of the Action Plan are broad and lend support to CNLs in all settings. You may access these goals at www.health.gov/communication/literacy.

Health Promotion Disease Prevention Complexity

Admission Scenario

We return to the case of Mrs. Louise. Two years after her ED visit described previously, Mrs. Louise is admitted back to the ED. She had not been feeling well for a few days and began to have chest pain on a Friday night while working at her housekeeping job in the local hotel. A family member in attendance helps to communicate this information to the ED staff and shares the patient's medical history of being treated for headaches due to high-blood pressure. She is admitted for a cardiac workup and to rule out a myocardial infarction (MI). She is admitted to the cardiac telemetry unit at 3 a.m. on Saturday morning. The nursing report from the ED gives a medical history of hypertension, but notes that the patient's blood sugar is 536 mg/dL, and a new diagnosis of type 2 diabetes is assumed to be present.

Arrival at Inpatient Unit

The patient arrives at the unit sleepy with no family members present. The English-speaking nurse orients the patient to the room and tries to elicit some basic information for the admission process in addition to the objective data about her patient such as vital signs, weight, and physical assessment data.

Day 1: On Saturday at 8 a.m., the hospitalist assigned to this patient obtains her medical records from her previous ED visit 2 years earlier and notes that the type 2 diabetes was diagnosed at that time. The communication regarding this patient now changes from "new onset diabetes" to "a 2-year history of diabetes in which the patient was noncompliant in follow-up as instructed by the ED staff."

Family members were updated on the status of the cardiac testing and also told that the patient had indeed done the right thing by being evaluated for chest pain, but that it was most likely caused by her high blood sugars. The family stated they did not know she had blood sugar problems. In response to this conversation, the nurse gave the family information on diabetes, which was written in English.

Day 2: On Sunday, Mrs. Louise has a new nurse. This nurse received the following information about Mrs. Louise:

- Testing for MI was negative.
- She had a 2-year history of hypertension and diabetes.
- The patient was being treated with an antihypertensive, and blood pressure was now within acceptable limits.
- Blood glucose was still high, measuring in the high 300 range, and was being treated with oral medicines and insulin.
- The patient was scheduled for a stress test, and pending the results of that test she may be discharged.
- This nurse was also told that the family had been given information on care for people with diabetes.

The Critical Role of Discharge Planning

Later in the day, when the charge nurse, who was in a CNL program, received an overview of the patient, she questioned the nurse caring for Mrs. Louise regarding discharge planning. The primary nurse responded by saying she had just met the patient, but that the patient was negative for an MI and had a 2-year history of her medical issues but was noncompliant. In addition, the patient did not seem to speak English and the family was not present at this time, but that it was reported to her that patient education had been done the previous day. The nurse in charge of the unit then brought up the following questions to the more novice nurse:

- Have you spoken directly to the patient to assess what she may or may not know about her diabetes? (As a result of poor communication, the patient did not know she had diabetes at all and did not know that the high blood pressure for which she was previously treated was a lifelong condition.)

- What language does the patient speak? (Creole.)
- Have you checked the hospital's education database to provide the patient with information in her own language? (It was not available but was retrieved from the reputable government website.)
- Did you utilize the telephone interpreter system to communicate with the patient rather than using a family member to interpret? (No.)
- Does the patient know how to check blood sugar and have the equipment to do so at home? (No, she did not know she had diabetes.)
- Have you discussed with the physician what medications the patient will go home on and how the team can best educate her about this plan? (No.)
- Will she go home on insulin and does she know how to administer the medication? (Subsequent findings: The doctor would discharge her on insulin and no teaching had been started.)
- What outpatient and community resources can we connect her with to develop within her a deeper understanding about caring for herself and managing her two chronic conditions? (The hospital has a comprehensive outpatient diabetes management program at a nearby location, which the staff nurse knew little about.)
- Did you know there are social workers and nursing care managers who are available by request on weekends to support our safe discharge of this patient? (The novice nurse did not know this.)
- Have you notified the dietary department to come and speak regarding the dietary implications of both diabetes and hypertension? (Requesting a dietary consultation for a patient is an independent nursing function.)
- What risk factors for heart disease can you identify in this patient and how can you address them? (Patient has many modifiable risk factors for heart disease.)

Proper Assessment of Patient Needs for Discharge

On the basis of collaboration with her nursing peers, the primary nurse provided the patient with appropriate educational materials regarding diabetes, hypertension, and risk factors for related cardiovascular disease. After providing this information in the patient's language and asking her to review it, the nurse utilized a telephone interpreter system to communicate more effectively regarding these complicated issues. It became clear to this nurse that the patient clearly did not understand the information provided by the ED about her conditions and follow-up care on her last admission. The nurse also assessed that the patient seemed to be illiterate even in her own language. In discussing discharge with the healthcare team, the physician shared that the patient would be discharged on insulin and a variety of oral medications; would need to check blood sugar regularly; and should be advised to follow a low-salt, calorie-restricted diet and exercise regularly to promote weight loss. The physician made no reference to the healthcare organization's comprehensive outpatient diabetes education center, but did make the referral for when it was requested by the primary nurse.

When the nurse had accurate knowledge of the discharge plan and a more accurate assessment of the patient's needs, she worked with the various members of the team to properly prepare the patient for discharge, including connecting the patient with the outpatient diabetes office, where the patient would be seen the following day. Prior to discharge, the nurse worked with the patient and family on the procedures needed to check blood sugar and safely administer insulin. Knowing that insulin is a high-risk medication, and in light of this individual's situation, the nurse advocated that social services provide visiting nurse services to support the transition of the patient to her home environment. The nurse had previously been told that the patient did not qualify for home services because she was not homebound. This patient was discharged Sunday evening with a plan that addressed her immediate safety needs, her limited comprehension of her complex conditions, basic technical skills on necessary procedures, and outpatient resources to bridge the continuum of care and support long-term behavior changes to decrease the risk of associated illnesses.

Promoting Health Through Care Coordination

The situation described for Mrs. Louise is based on actual facts of a particular patient; these scenarios present themselves in varied settings every day. Without an assessment of individualized needs, including knowledge levels and healthcare literacy components, the system that works to treat and heal can go very much off course. The complexity of the healthcare system coupled with the complexity of a diverse population of consumers requires insightful and open-minded nurse leaders to improve care. In this scenario, Mrs. Louise could have been discharged with a longer list of instructions that she did not understand, leading to future admission for stroke, uncontrolled diabetes, or hypertension. The healthcare community could once again seek to blame Mrs. Louise for being noncompliant rather than examining their own system. The opportunities for health promotion and risk reduction with Mrs. Louise are vast, but they are not simple. Managing chronic illness, adopting health-promoting lifestyle changes, and eliminating risks such as smoking, sedentary lifestyle, and obesity are challenging in the best of situations. Often these situations are more complicated by low literacy, language barriers, cultural considerations, finances, family dynamics, and a lack of desire. These difficult situations are best optimized by nurses who welcome the challenges presented and collaborate with patients, families, and healthcare team members to provide care.

Health Promotion and the Affordable Care Act

A key principle of the Affordable Care Act (ACA) is to refocus the healthcare system from the treatment of disease to prevention of illness. Since the passage of the radically new laws governing healthcare, much has changed in the area of health promotion. Key provisions of the law require health insurance plans to include the following: preventive and wellness visit with no copay; maternity and newborn care, which is considered preventative and provided at no cost; mental and behavioral health treatment; lab work for issues considered preventive; pediatric, dental, and vision care; and prescription drug coverage (useconomy.about.com). As millions of previously uninsured Americans become eligible for benefits, there is much confusion and educational need in this area. CNLs should be well acquainted with provisions of the ACA and opportunities for health promotion support. Individuals in all settings may need counseling regarding plan selection and navigation of changing healthcare systems.

The CNL's Role in Risk Reduction and Patient Safety

Measures of healthcare quality and outcomes have become an integral part of the nursing profession from the bedside to the boardroom. Measures of patient outcomes, financial outcomes, and transparency of organizational quality measures have forever changed the healthcare playing field. Much of this change can be attributed to landmark reports from the IOM and the work of The Joint Commission regarding patient safety (IOM, 2009). The work of these organizations has been part of the impetus for the AACN to bring the vision of the CNL to reality. For this reason, it is logical that patient safety is at the core of the CNL role. Concepts of health promotion and disease prevention are aligned with patient safety to maximize the most positive patient outcomes in any healthcare setting.

The Joint Commission is dedicated to a safe healthcare environment and is a valuable resource for practicing CNLs. Annual patient safety goals for acute care and ambulatory care help all healthcare leaders to prioritize initiatives to improve the environment, which seeks to care for, help, and heal people of infinite diversity. Some of the very public reports regarding healthcare mistakes that have resulted in injuries and death have spurred a new level of awareness from the public regarding risks of seeking care. Media reports of wrong-site surgeries, fatal and near-fatal medication errors, and lethal hospital-acquired infections are plentiful, not to mention Internet access to credible or less credible information. Nonetheless, these factors all add up to a new era of public awareness of safety issues in healthcare settings. CNLs should be very knowledgeable of The Joint Commission's annual goals, which can be found at www.jointcommission.org.

The influence of patient safety metrics cannot be minimized in the role of today's healthcare settings, and the CNL must possess not only an understanding of these metrics but also an ability to share that understanding with direct care providers in all settings. Nurses have traditionally been a profession of caregivers who were not educated in data measures, run charts, control charts, and histograms. These types of data may be involved in the "dashboard" measures of their care area. These are the areas that have been chosen for a particular unit to measure the quality of care in that area. Patient satisfaction, fall rates, infection rates, and so on, may be posted on a monthly or quarterly basis for staff to evaluate. For many, the direct link between the care they provide every day and those metrics of quality are not well connected. The CNL and others, who are often accountable to those measures, have a vested interest in a staff of professionals and ancillary caregivers who can provide safe, high-quality care and can understand the metrics surrounding that care in a measurable way. Dashboard indicators should also be aligned with the strategic mission of the organization, so that the direct link can be made from the bedside to the boardroom.

The running scenario of Mrs. Louise in this chapter is a very familiar and relatively uncomplicated situation considering the complex conditions encountered in all areas of healthcare. Our population of healthcare consumers is aging rapidly and living longer. Multiple chronic diseases, polypharmacy, complex social issues, lack of adequate healthcare coverage, and spiritual needs can complicate the care of persons in all settings. The relatively new role of the CNL originated in the current and future need to have someone directly involved in care, who can see the big picture.

TABLE 12.3 Health Promotion and Disease Prevention Management

CATEGORY	WEIGHT
C. Health Promotion and Disease Prevention Management	**5%**
1. Teaches direct care providers how to assist clients, families, and communities to be health literate and manage their own care	
2. Applies research to resolve clinical problems and disseminate results	
3. Engages clients in therapeutic partnerships with multidisciplinary team members	

(continued)

TABLE 12.3 Health Promotion and Disease Prevention Management *(continued)*

CATEGORY	WEIGHT
C. Health Promotion and Disease Prevention Management	**5%**
4. Applies evidence and data to identify and modify interventions to meet specific client needs	
5. Counsels clients and families regarding behavior changes to achieve healthy lifestyles	
6. Engages in culturally sensitive health promotion/disease prevention intervention to reduce healthcare risks in clients	
7. Develops clinical and health promotion programs for individuals and groups	
8. Designs and implements measures to modify risk factors and promote engagement in healthy lifestyles	
9. Assesses protective and predictive (e.g., lifestyle, genetic) factors that influence the health of clients	
10. Develops and monitors holistic plans of care that address the health promotion and disease prevention needs of client populations	
11. Incorporates theories and research in generating teaching and support strategies to promote and preserve health and healthy lifestyles in client populations	
12. Identifies strategies to optimize client's level of functioning	

Used with permission from the Commission on Nurse Certification (2011, 2014).

Conclusion

The conditions of society are ever changing as are the needs of that society. Nurses have always been at the forefront of health promotion and continue to be strengthened in that role with the CNL. The liberal education for the master's prepared generalist supports the vast array of settings for the CNL throughout the healthcare continuum. Through research, application of evidence, and the study of populations CNLs utilize science in the application of improved care. The CNL® certification exam covers many of the concepts of health promotion that are applied in a variety of clinical situations (Table 12.3). The practicum experience of CNL students allows for practical application of the multiple and diverse roles described. As we stand on the edge of healthcare reform, all citizens have a vested interest in how healthcare can be safer, more cost effective, less fragmented, and focused on health promotion rather than on disease treatment. Our current resources are being burdened with many preventable illnesses, and primary prevention is critical to the health of our nation. Achievement of improved outcomes must take into account issues of health literacy.

As CNLs are establishing practice in a number of healthcare settings, national resources can help to recognize and focus care based on patient safety goals, healthcare indicators, and best-practice publications. From public health, school settings, acute care, outpatient facilities, and long-term care, the CNL has vast opportunities to make improvements. The skill set acquired through a liberal education at a graduate level prepares these expert clinicians for the challenge.

Resources

Ackerman, R., & Marvero, D. (2007). Adapting the Diabetes Prevention Program Lifestyle intervention for delivery in the community. *The Diabetes Educator, 33*(1), 68–78.

American Association of Colleges of Nursing. (2007). *White paper on the education and role of the clinical nurse leader*. Washington, DC. Retrieved from http://www.aacn.nche.edu/cnl-certification

American Heart Association. (2011). *Heart disease and stroke statistics—2011 update: A report from the American Heart Association*. Retrieved from http://circ.ahajournals.org/content/123/4/e18.full.pdf

Baur, C. (2011). Calling the nation to act: Implementing the national action plan to improve health literacy. *Nursing Outlook, 59*, 63–69.

Carranti, B. (2010). CNL role in health promotion and disease prevention. In J. Harris & L. Roussel (Eds.), *Initiating and sustaining the clinical nurse leader role: A practical guide* (pp. 197–218). Sudbury, MA: Jones & Bartlett Publishers.

Commission on Nurse Certification. (2011). *Clinical Nurse Leader job analysis report*. Retrieved from http://www.aacn.nche.edu/cnl/Job-Analysis-Report.pdf

Commission on Nurse Certification. (2014). *Clinical Nurse Leader (CNL®) certification exam blueprint*. Retrieved from http://www.aacn.nche.edu/leading-initiatives/cnl/cnl-certification/pdf/ExamContentOutline11.pdf

Greiner, P., & Edelman, C. (2010). Health defined: Objectives for promotion and prevention. In C. Edelman & C. Mandle (Eds.), *Health promotion throughout the life span* (pp. 3–21). St. Louis, MO: Elsevier.

Healthy People. (2011). *About Healthy People*. Retrieved from http://www.healthypeople.gov/2020/about/default.aspx

Institute of Medicine. (2009). *Informing the future—Critical issues in health*. Retrieved from http://www.iom.edu/~/media/Files/About%20the%20IOM/ITF2009.pdf

Kazer, M. K., & Grossman, S. C. (2011). *Gerontological nurse practitioner. Certification review*. New York, NY: Springer Publishing.

Prochaska, J., DiClemente, C., & Norcross, J. (1992). In search of how people change. Applications to addictive behaviors. *American Psychologist, 47*(9), 1102–1114.

Stanley, J. (2010). Introducing the clinical nurse leader: A catalyst for quality care. In J. Harris & L. Roussel (Eds.), *Initiation and sustaining the clinical nurse leader role. A practical guide*. Sudbury, MA: Jones & Bartlett Publishers.

The 10 essential health benefits of Obamacare. Accessed from Useconomy.about.com/od/healthcarereform

13

Evidence-Based Practice

Cynthia R. King

Evidence-based practice (EBP) has been clearly defined in general and for nursing. However, there continues to be confusion about what EBP is and how nurses should utilize this important concept in clinical practice. It is important that clinical nurse leaders (CNLs) and other healthcare providers not confuse the term *research utilization* (RU) with EBP. RU refers to the review and critique of scientific research and then the application of the findings to clinical practice. EBP is a broader concept that includes using the best and current evidence, the patient's preferences, and the clinician's expertise or judgment. Thus, the three key components in EBP are:

- Use of evidence
- Patient preferences and values
- Clinical or professional judgment based on clinical expertise

It is also important to remember the difference between research and EBP. Research is conducted when there is a gap in knowledge, whereas EBP is conducted when there are one or more best practices that can be applied to clinical practice.

The American Association of Colleges of Nursing (AACN; 2007) established a number of assumptions about the CNL role. EBP is threaded throughout a variety of assumptions, such as the following:

- Assumption 2: Client care outcomes are the measure of quality practice.
- Assumption 3: Practice guidelines are based on evidence.
- Assumption 5: Information will maximize self-care and client decision making.

- Assumption 6: Nursing assessment is the basis for theory and knowledge development.
- Basing nursing care on the best evidence is characteristic of clinical leadership. This is the expectation of CNLs as leaders.

The more recent AACN document on CNL competencies (AACN, 2013) clearly outlines the design and implementation of EBP as a fundamental aspect of the CNL role. Rankin also cites EBP as a key aspect of the CNL role and even cites EBP projects at her institution that have had a significant effect on patient outcomes (Rankin, 2015).

The Evidence-Based Process

Once a CNL clearly understands the definition of EBP, it is crucial to understand the steps in the process. Most professional nurses have learned the research process during nursing school, but it is only in recent years that faculty have spent much time describing the EBP process and the difference between that and the research process. Table 13.1 displays the steps in the EBP process and the research process.

As is shown in Table 13.1, both the EBP and the research process start the same way. The key to both processes is identifying a clinical question or issue. From there, the CNL must review the literature and obtain evidence (e.g., data from admissions or human resources). Only after the literature is reviewed can an individual decide if he or she needs to conduct an EBP project or conduct research. The decision is based on whether there is a gap in knowledge (then the CNL designs research) or whether there are one or more best practices in the literature (then the CNL can conduct an EBP project). Although some of the middle steps are different, the final step should be the same in each process—disseminate findings via presentations or publications.

TABLE 13.1 EBP Process Versus Research Process

EBP PROCESS	RESEARCH PROCESS
Identify clinical problem	Identify clinical problem
Review literature/search for evidence	Review literature/search for evidence
Critique evidence	Design study
Synthesize evidence and patient view	Write research proposal
Implement evidence-based change	Obtain IRB approval
Evaluate outcomes	Collect and analyze data
Present or publish findings	Present or publish findings

EPB, evidence-based practice; IRB, Institutional Review Board.

The Clinical Question or Issue

As seen in Table 13.1, both EBP and research start with a clinical question or issue. Therefore, a well-designed clinical question is crucial. Once CNLs learn how to design thorough clinical questions, they can easily design the remainder of the EBP (or research) project. Although most research and EBP books briefly describe the importance of the clinical question, Melnyk and Fineout-Overholt's (2014) seminal book on EBP provides an excellent chapter on developing the clinical question or issue. Not only do the authors describe the most common method for developing a clinical question (called PICOT), but also they provide a variety of examples of well-designed questions.

The most common way to develop the clinical question is using the PICOT method. By carefully developing each of the five components of the question, it helps to clearly articulate the question, which then drives the remainder of the steps of the EBP process. Table 13.2 helps to describe the various components of the PICOT method.

While Melnyk and Fineout-Overholt (2014) provide an excellent description of PICOT, they also give a template to use for practice and many excellent examples. The more CNLs and professional nurses practice writing clinical questions, the easier it will become.

Where and How to Locate Evidence

Once the clinical question has been refined, the next step is to locate appropriate evidence in the literature. In general, CNLs and other disciplines will find the most current evidence in academic journals and by utilizing databases such as CINAHL, PubMed, and MEDLINE. Other ways to access journals are via (a) the journal website, (b) a search engine (e.g., Google Scholar), (c) an electronic library, (d) the Cochrane Databases (e.g., they contain systematic reviews), or (e) the *British Medical Journal of Clinical Evidence* (e.g., it provides summaries of evidence with recommendations).

TABLE 13.2 The PICOT Method for Developing Clinical Questions

LETTER AND DESCRIPTION	EXAMPLE(S)
P = Patient population/disease	Elderly with congestive heart failure; obese adolescents
I = Intervention or issue of interest	A specific therapy or educational intervention
C = Comparison intervention	An alternative therapy, placebo, disease vs. no disease
O = Outcome	Outcome expected from therapy, patient outcome
T = Time	The time it takes for intervention

Sometimes evidence or data is also found in other departments (e.g., admissions, physical therapy, human resources). Searching for evidence can be overwhelming. In order to increase the chances that CNLs and other disciplines access the right information, some of the following strategies can be implemented:

- Be familiar with and practice different methods for searching for evidence and data
- Search for literature reviews and meta-analyses
- Set up e-mail alerts to receive content lists of the most relevant journals
- Attend EBP workshops and conferences
- Set up a journal club

Melnyk and Fineout-Overholt (2014) provide detailed descriptions regarding how to search for evidence. They also provide specific websites for specific EBP databases and screenshots of how the databases and websites will look. Furthermore, they provide descriptions on specialized search functions. Because nursing schools often do not provide thorough lectures on searching literature, the information contained in the EBP book by Melnyk and Fineout-Overholt (2014) is even more valuable to CNLs conducting EBP projects.

Critically Appraising the Literature and Determining the Strength of the Evidence

Once the literature is obtained, it has to be synthesized and critically appraised. The literature may be quantitative or qualitative or both (e.g., mixed methods). There are many sources that list questions to ask when critically appraising the literature. Many of these questions are used in EBP projects but also in journal clubs. When appraising the literature, CNLs must also evaluate the literature for the strength of evidence or credibility.

There are different methods for CNLs to use to select the most credible evidence. The competencies developed by AACN for CNLs include a role to make point-of-care decisions on the basis of best possible evidence (AACN, 2007; Herrin & Spears, 2007). There are a variety of hierarchies that can be used to determine how credible the collected evidence is. Each of these hierarchies has different levels. Some are designated by letters (A–D or A–F) and some are designated by numbers (e.g., Level 1–Level 4 or Level 1–Level 7). Melnyk and Fineout-Overholt (2014) recommend using a hierarchy with seven levels based on the design as follows:

- Level 1: Systematic review or meta-analysis of randomized controlled trials (RCTs) and evidence-based clinical practice guidelines.
- Level 2: One well-designed RCT.

- Level 3: Quasi-experimental studies documented without randomization.
- Level 4: Well-designed case-control and cohort studies.
- Level 5: Systematic reviews of descriptive and/or qualitative studies.
- Level 6: Single descriptive and/or qualitative studies.
- Level 7: Expert opinion and/or expert committee reports.

As described, CNLs must have the skills to critically appraise the literature gathered for the EBP project. Critical appraisal involves the structured process of examining research in order to determine its strengths and limitations, and therefore, the relevance it should have in addressing the clinical question. Moreover, CNLs need to understand the difference between quantitative and qualitative articles and data. *Quantitative studies* investigate clinical questions that involve the collection of data in numeric form, whereas *qualitative studies* involve the collection of data in nonnumeric form (e.g., using words in forms such as personal interviews, observation). Although the terminology used to describe whether evidence is quantitative or qualitative is slightly different, it is still important that CNLs learn to critically appraise both quantitative and qualitative evidence.

CNLs are not only expected to develop and implement EBP projects, but they are also required to partner with patients/families and other disciplines to improve patient outcomes within their microsystem (AACN, 2013). There are many different ways to use evidence to improve patient outcomes. For example, CNLs may use evidence to (a) start journal clubs, (b) start nursing grand rounds, (c) develop or update policies and procedures, or (d) create care pathways or protocols.

Use of Measurement Tools During the Implementation of the EBP

As CNLs are accountable for healthcare outcomes in a particular microsystem, unit, or setting, it is crucial they accept responsibility for the assimilation and application of evidence to design, implement, and evaluate client plans of care with staff nurses. When working with staff nurses on plans of care for patients, it is important to teach staff nurses how to locate current practices and evidence as well as measurement tools to apply to plans of care. Frequently in practice settings, assessment tools are used for clinical decisions, because they have been used in that microsystem or setting for many years. This does not mean the tool is the most appropriate for that patient population or acuity of patients. Thus, one key skill that CNLs may need to teach staff nurses is how to locate measurement tools for assessment that are reliable and valid and are based on solid evidence. It may be that while searching, reviewing, implementing, and evaluating a new assessment tool for a specific microsystem, the staff nurses and CNLs discover that the new measurement tool may actually be best applied in multiple microsystems, the mesosystem, or throughout the entire organization.

Putting Evidence Into Practice

Once the literature has been critically appraised and one or more of the best practices have been identified, it is time to put the evidence or best practice into the clinical practice. However, there continue to be barriers for staff nurses and CNLs in implementing EBP in the practice setting. Some of these barriers include:

- Lack of staff understanding about EBP and research
- Failure to understand the importance of EBP and research in the clinical setting
- Difficulty in determining a clinical question or issue
- Lack of time and/or competing priorities
- Lack of knowledge and skills related to searching current literature
- Lack of access to library and/or computers
- Lack of support from administration (e.g., director of nursing, chief nursing officer)
- Lack of money for EBP and research projects

Despite potential barriers, there are many different types of interventions or best practices that can be implemented as part of EBP. It seems simple to say that CNLs should apply the "best evidence" in a clinical decision. However, it is crucial to remember that the EBP involves considering the patient's concerns and preferences. Thus, CNLs need to use their good clinical judgment as well as the current evidence and the way in which it is most relevant to a specific patient's concerns.

There are definite advantages to CNLs overcoming barriers and creating a culture where patient care is based on evidence. Some of the more global advantages include (a) increased professionalism, (b) increased collaboration, (c) decreases in length of stay and costs, and (d) increased patient safety and quality of care. Besides conducting a specific EBP or nursing research project, there are specific strategies that CNLs can use to create a culture where patient care is based on evidence. Some of these strategies include

- Ensure all policies and procedures are based on the latest research-based literature.
- Start a journal club on the unit for staff nurses.
- Post a summary of research studies on a topic of interest to staff.

- Update staff on the latest evidence in short staff gatherings (e.g., 15 minutes).
- Link quality indicators to EBP.
- Invite nursing faculty members to unit meetings or to help with a project.
- Mentor staff nurses who have to complete EBP activities for school or a clinical ladder.

Results of Intervention and Evaluation

After implementing a change based on the critical appraisal of the literature for a specific period, the CNL needs to analyze the results and evaluate the implemented change. The CNL may be analyzing a wide array of important outcomes. Some of these may include patient health outcomes, provider and patient satisfaction, efficacy, and economic analysis. The question is, how does a CNL apply the results of the project to patient care? For instance, are there patient differences (e.g., biological, socioeconomic) that may diminish the response to the intervention? Based on the evaluation, the CNL may need to alter the intervention slightly, expand the intervention to other settings, or decide the intervention is not appropriate for this clinical setting.

Communication of Results in a Collaborative Manner

Although any nurse with the appropriate knowledge and skills can implement EBP in a clinical setting, most staff nurses are not taught these skills. However, if they do learn how to search for best practices and evidence (e.g., finding reliable and valid measurement tools for assessment), rarely are staff nurses taught how to disseminate and communicate their findings to other nurses and disciplines. CNLs, however, learn how to use leadership skills as well as interdisciplinary collaboration and communication skills to successfully help staff communicate important EBP and research results within the microsystem, clinical setting, and, specifically, to other disciplines. There are a variety of options for dissemination both for CNLs and staff nurses. A number of these may include the following:

- Journal publication
  - Full paper
  - Short report/letter
  - News item
  - Editorial

- Conference
  - Local/national/international
  - Poster
  - Oral presentation
- Report to funder
  - Publish as a report
- Set up conference or seminar
  - Within department
  - Area or regional meeting
  - National
- TV/lay press/media
  - Hospital newsletter
  - Newspapers
  - Radio
- Internet
  - Podcast
  - CD-ROM/DVD
- Teaching

TABLE 13.3 Evidence-Based Practice

CATEGORY	WEIGHT
D. Evidence-Based Practice	**8%**
1. Communicates results in a collaborative manner with client and healthcare team	
2. Uses measurement tools as foundation for assessments and clinical decisions	
3. Applies clinical judgment and decision-making skills in designing, coordinating, implementing, and evaluating client-focused care	
4. Selects sources of evidence to meet specific needs of individuals, clinical groups, or communities	
5. Applies epidemiological, social, and environmental data	
6. Reviews datasets to anticipate risk and evaluate care outcomes	

(continued)

TABLE 13.3 Evidence-Based Practice *(continued)*

CATEGORY	WEIGHT
D. Evidence-Based Practice	**8%**
7. Evaluates and applies information from various sources to guide client through the healthcare system	
8. Interprets and applies quantitative and qualitative data	
9. Utilizes current healthcare research to improve client care	
10. Accesses, critiques, and analyzes information sources	
11. Provides leadership for changing practice based on quality improvement methods and research findings	
12. Identifies relevant outcomes and measurement strategies that will improve patient outcomes and promote cost-effective care	
13. Synthesizes data, information, and knowledge to evaluate and achieve optimal client outcomes	

Used with permission from the Commission on Nurse Certification (2011, 2014).

What is most important is to disseminate findings in some manner. If nurses do not disseminate the results of EBP and research projects, nursing knowledge will not advance. Additionally, other staff and CNLs will not have access to best practices that have been developed at other institutions. Thus, the last step of the EBP project is not analysis of the results, but dissemination of the findings.

Conclusion

Understanding and using EBP is a part of the leadership role of CNLs (Table 13.3). It is imperative that CNLs understand the EBP and research processes and are able to describe them to staff nurses. It is part of the CNL's role to be sure that he or she creates a culture of evidence. The steps in the EBP process have been described here as well as other strategies that can be used to assist CNLs in creating a working environment based on evidence.

Resources

American Association of Colleges of Nursing. (2007). *White paper on the education and role of the clinical nurse leader*. Washington, DC: Author.

American Association of Colleges of Nursing. (2013). *Competencies and curricular expectations for clinical nurse leader education and practice.* Washington, DC. Retrieved from http://www.aacn.nche.edu/cnl/CNL-Competencies-October-2013.pdf

Aveyard, H., & Sharp, S. (2011). *A beginner's guide to evidence based practice in health and social care professions.* New York, NY: Open University Press.

Commission on Nurse Certification. (2011). *Clinical Nurse Leader job analysis report.* Retrieved from http://www.aacn.nche.edu/cnl/Job-Analysis-Report.pdf

Commission on Nurse Certification. (2014). *Clinical Nurse Leader (CNL®) certification exam blueprint.* Retrieved from http://www.aacn.nche.edu/leading-initiatives/cnl/cnl-certification/pdf/ExamContentOutline11.pdf

DiCenso, A., Guystt, G., & Ciliska, D. (2014). *Evidence-based nursing: A guide to clinical practice.* St. Louis, MO: Elsevier.

Herrin, D., & Spears, P. (2007). Using nurse leader development to improve nurse retention and patient outcomes: A framework. *Nursing Administration Quarterly, 31*(3), 231–243.

LoBiondo-Wood, G., & Haber, J. (2014). *Nursing research: Methods and critical appraisal for evidence-based-practice.* St. Louis, MO: Elsevier.

Malloch, K., & Porter-O'Grady, T. (2006). *Introduction to evidence-based practice in nursing and health care.* Boston, MA: Jones & Bartlett.

Melnyk, B., & Fineout-Overholt, E. (2014). *Evidence-based practice in nursing & healthcare* (3nd ed.). Philadelphia, PA: Wolters Kluwer: Lippincott Williams & Wilkins.

Powers, B. A., & Knapp, T. R. (2010). *Dictionary of nursing theory and research* (4th ed.). New York, NY: Springer Publishing Company.

Rankin, V. (2015). Clinical nurse leader: A role for the 21st century. *MedSurg Nursing, 24*(3), 199–201.

Schmidt, N. A., & Brown, J. M. (2012). *Evidence-based practice for nurses: Appraisal and application of research.* Boston, MA: Jones & Bartlett.

14

Patient Assessment

Grace O. Buttriss

The skills of advanced clinical assessment are essential for the clinical nurse leader (CNL) to master, comprehend, and perform on clients within their individual microsystems. The information acquired from the clinical assessment will provide the CNL with the data needed to continuously monitor client care and enhance the quality of ongoing care. Client assessments should be evidence based and require competent observation techniques, clinical reasoning skills, and individual consideration of all cultural aspects related to their care. Assessments should also incorporate concepts of pathophysiology and pharmacology to support decisions and care.

Linguistically appropriate services must be provided, and religious beliefs and genetics should be considered in planning client care. These specific components will provide the CNL with the foundation to collect and differentiate, verify and organize the collected data, and initiate the client plan of care and provide support for electronic documentation of client data and care.

Advanced clinical assessment skills also include the collection of data related to an individual's past and current health status as well as his or her health promotion, risk reduction, and disease prevention strategies. The condition and consideration of the whole person is considered to be the essence of holistic health. *Holistic health* views the total mind, body, and spirit as interdependent and functioning as a unit. A client's health status depends on all areas operating together to promote an individual's optimal health (Jarvis, 2016).

The client's advanced clinical assessment should also be considered from a life cycle view and attainment for age-appropriate *development tasks* should be evaluated. The reinforcement of positive health behaviors provides encouragement to clients and helps to establish a provider-client relationship and support of client health goals (Jarvis, 2016).

Designing, Coordinating, and Evaluating Plans of Care

The advanced clinical assessment commences with the collection of data related to an individual's current and past healthcare condition. This process involves the initial client survey and the collection and analysis of both subjective and objective data. The information obtained in conjunction with the client's healthcare record and diagnostic information will be utilized to formulate an individual client database and plan. The database will provide a baseline for client care and an ongoing assessment and plan for the client response to all medical and nursing interventions that are executed.

The database also provides the CNL with the foundation for formulating both clinical judgments and diagnoses through the process of diagnostic reasoning. These components are essential for client care planning with the advanced clinical assessment serving as the foundation for this process.

Additionally, the CNL will coordinate the process of risk reduction for assigned clients and will refer to the "Guide to Clinical Preventive Services," which is updated annually for the evidence-based, gold-standard recommendations used for populations. This include recommendations for screening, counseling, and using preventative medications, and is a source for decision making about preventative services and is associated with specific, proven screening, counseling, and preventive strategies (Jarvis, 2016; USPSTF, 2014).

The CNL will also use the Healthy People 2020 *Leading Health Indicators* (LHIs) to coordinate client care. LHIs are science-based, 10-year national objectives to improve health and communicate the high-priority health issues for individuals living within the United States. They can be utilized to guide clients to identify health improvement priorities; identify critical research, evaluation, and data collection needs; and support the promotion of health and avoidance of preventable illness. These indicators are a guide to empower individuals to initiate and sustain informed health choices (http://www.healthypeople.gov/2020/Leading-Health-Indicators).

These 12 leading health indicators have associated actions that can be taken by individuals and communities to address the importance of promoting health improvement to support the maintenance of a healthy lifestyle (Box 14.1).

BOX 14.1
Healthy People 2020 Leading Health Indicators

- Access to health services
- Clinical preventive services
- Environmental quality

(*continued*)

BOX 14.1 (*continued*)

- Injury and violence
- Maternal, infant, and child health
- Mental health
- Nutrition, physical activity, and obesity
- Oral health
- Reproductive and sexual health
- Social determinants
- Substance abuse
- Tobacco

Source: 2020 Healthy People Leading Indicators (2015).

Developing a Therapeutic Alliance With the Client

The CNL begins the clinical assessment by developing a *therapeutic relationship* with his or her assigned clients. This relationship begins with the first client encounter and continues throughout his or her affiliation. The client is always considered to be the principal source for personal data and this is identified as primary data. Additional data obtained about the client from family members, support persons, members of the healthcare team, diagnostics, or the utilization of current research are considered to be secondary or indirect sources of data. These secondary sources are important, but should always be validated for accuracy.

The exchange of healthcare information between the CNL and the client can be achieved by many techniques, including observation, one-on-one client interviews, and physical assessment techniques. The client interview is a structured form of communication that provides the basis for acquiring specific client information related to his or her current needs and symptoms. The procedure is conducted to obtain a confidential, comprehensive health history and should be held in a private and comfortable setting, if possible, for both the CNL and the client. The comprehensive health history should include those items found in Box 14.2.

The present health or history of present illness is the reason the client is currently seeking care. This relates to the client's description of what he or she is experiencing and the signs and symptoms related to his or her decision to seek medical attention at this time. There are eight critical characteristics used to summarize the client's presenting symptoms (see Box 14.3). The mnemonic PQRST can also be used to organize the client's symptoms (see Box 14.4).

BOX 14.2
Comprehensive Health History

- Biographic data
- Reason for seeking care
- Present health or history of present illness
- Medications/allergies
- Medical/surgical history
- Family history/genogram
- Review of systems
- Psychosocial history
- Diagnostic results

Source: Jarvis, 2016.

BOX 14.3
Characteristics to Describe Symptoms

- Location
- Character or quality
- Quantity or severity
- Timing
- Setting
- Aggravating or relieving factors
- Associated factors
- Client's perception

BOX 14.4
Mnemonic for Symptoms

- P: Provocative or palliation
- Q: Quality or quantity
- R: Region or radiation
- S: Severity scale
- T: Timing

Source: Jarvis, 2016.

Current medications (including over-the-counter herbs and any supplements), along with dosages and frequency, should also be recorded for the client. Allergies and symptoms to medications are also important and should be included. The specific type of allergic reaction is important to clarify and record during the data collection. An immunization history should also be determined and documented for any client seeking care.

The client's past medical and surgical history are significant because of the potential effect on his or her current health. This history includes childhood illnesses; accidents or injuries; serious or chronic conditions; any hospitalizations, surgeries, or obstetric history; last physical exam; and dental, vision, hearing, or applicable screenings. The client's family history is essential to obtain and relate to his or her ongoing care and risk factors. A genogram is an important tool for the CNL to create for organizing and tracking a client's family history for a minimum of three generations (Jarvis, 2016).

A review of systems is performed on each client to evaluate the health condition of systems and to assess the effectiveness of his or her individual health promotion practices. According to Jarvis (2016), the review of systems should include subjective and objective data areas (see Box 14.5).

A mental status exam that includes cognitive functioning data should be included with all advanced clinical assessments and should evaluate those areas listed in Box 14.6.

Substance use and abuse should be a component of the assessment based on the negative effects on many body systems. The most commonly used questionnaires include the CAGE, which takes less than a minute

BOX 14.5
Review of Symptoms

- General health status
- Skin
- Hair
- Head
- Eyes
- Ears
- Nose and sinus
- Mouth and throat
- Neck
- Breast

(*continued*)

BOX 14.5 (*continued*)

- Axilla
- Respiratory
- Cardiovascular
- Peripheral vascular
- Gastrointestinal
- Urinary
- Male and female genital
- Musculoskeletal
- Neurological
- Hematological
- Endocrine
- Pain
- Nutrition

BOX 14.6
Mental Status Exam

- Consciousness
- Language
- Mood and affect
- Orientation
- Attention
- Memory
- Abstract reasoning
- Thought process
- Thought content
- Perceptions
- Mini mental exam includes A, B, C, T: appearance, behavior, cognition, and thought process

Source: Jarvis, 2016.

to complete, but is less effective in women and minorities. The TWEAK questionnaire helps to identify at-risk women who drink, particularly pregnant women. This tool measures the client's tolerance to alcohol consumption (see Boxes 14.7 and 14.8).

BOX 14.7
CAGE Questionnaire

- Have you ever felt you should *cut down* on your drinking?
- Have people *annoyed* you by criticizing your drinking?
- Have you ever felt bad or *guilty* about your drinking?
- Have you ever had a drink first thing in the morning to steady your nerves or get rid of a hangover (*eye-opener*)?

BOX 14.8
TWEAK Questionnaire

- **Tolerance**—Number of drinks tolerated or how many drinks it takes to feel "high."
- **Worry**—Do you have close friends or relatives worried about your drinking in the past year?
- **Eye-opener**—Do you sometimes take a drink in the morning when you get up?
- **Amnesia**—Has a friend or family member ever told you things you said that you could not remember saying?
- **Kut Down**—Do you sometimes feel the need to cut down on your drinking?

Score 2 points for Tolerance and Worry

Score 1 point for the others.

>2 points = a drinking problem, and further assessment is needed

Source: Jarvis, 2016.

Intimate partner violence, child abuse, and elder abuse are health problems that the CNL must recognize and assess. These assessments include both physical and sexual violence, psychological and emotional abuse or neglect, or financial abuse. There are multiple tools and questionnaires available for use in all clinical settings. The key is recognition and documentation, including photography and the use of forensic terminology, for legal purposes.

A sleep assessment should be conducted on every client due to the detrimental cumulative effects of sleep loss and disorders on the body systems. The assessment should consider the quality of sleep and factors associated with sleep loss, including napping, insomnia caused by age, medications, psychological factors, gender, and lifestyle. Pain, sleep apnea, shortness of breath, and restless leg syndrome interfere with sleep. An assessment of sleep apnea should also be included to help in determining the cause of the sleep loss (Wilson & Giddens, 2013).

A *functional assessment* is an additional important assessment tool and should be completed on each client to evaluate his or her activities of daily living. This information will provide the CNL with the information to evaluate the client's self-care abilities, current and past relationships, and his or her individual coping techniques. A functional assessment is performed during the interview phase and should include those areas listed in Box 14.9.

Identifying Client Problems That Require Intervention

The advanced clinical assessment is a systematic data collection method that utilizes the techniques of:

- Inspection
- Auscultation
- Palpation
- Percussion

These techniques are organized according to the CNL's preference for the head-to-toe (cephalocaudal) or the body system approach. These techniques are also prioritized on the basis of the client's current diagnosis and symptoms. The primary focus will be on the individual physiological

BOX 14.9
Functional Assessment

- Self-esteem/self-concept
- Activity level/exercise
- Sleep/rest
- Nutrition/elimination
- Interpersonal relationships/resources
- Spiritual resources
- Coping/stress management
- Use of tobacco, alcohol, illegal substances
- Environment/exposures
- Sexual history
- Abuse

(Jarvis, 2016)

system that correlates with the client's current symptoms and diagnosis (Smith, Duell, & Martin, 2013). The immediacy of the symptoms can also necessitate a change by performing a rapid and accurate focused review of systems to address the presenting urgent, potentially life-threatening client complaint.

The CNL will implement the nursing process to organize all nursing actions and interventions. This approach offers a systematic, problem-solving method for providing client care in all healthcare settings. The provision of client care will also be guided by the utilization of evidence-based practice concepts and practices. These concepts will promote quality client outcomes through *patient-focused interventions* of the CNL.

Holistic Assessment

The advanced physical assessment is based on a holistic approach and a systematic method of problem solving and care planning identified as the nursing process. This method is goal directed and ensures that the client receives consistent, continuous, evidence-based quality care. It also provides the foundation for professional nursing accountability while taking into account the input of the client's support persons and the entire healthcare team.

This process is put into practice to identify a client's health status and the actual or potential healthcare problems or needs of the client. It is used to diagnose and treat the human response to actual or potential health or illness problems (American Nurse Association [ANA], 1980).

The plan of care is developed for interdisciplinary and collaborative implementation with all members of the healthcare team.

A plan is developed to meet and deliver care based on identified areas utilizing the following components:

- Assessment
- Analysis/diagnosing
- Planning
- Implementation
- Evaluation (Smith et al., 2013)

Client assessment is the first step in this process. This involves the establishment of a client database, skilled observation, and documentation of the findings. This is an essential step because subsequent components depend on the precision and consistency of the initial assessment process. The plan must also include the client's health values and beliefs, individual priorities, available resources, the urgency of the current health problem, and the proposed medical and nursing treatment plan.

Assessment is followed by the formulation of applicable diagnoses. This step involves critical thinking to develop all applicable diagnoses to guide ongoing client care.

The planning process involves priority setting and establishment of client goals and outcomes based on the client response. These include both short- and long-term goals that are written on the basis of the client and the healthcare team member's plans. This is based on the healthcare needs and is specific to each client.

The implementation or intervention stage provides for execution of the plan based on scientific principles to reach specific client goals. This is established from the clinical assessment of the client, data interpretation, client needs, goals, and outcomes.

The evaluation process assesses the client outcomes and goal attainment from the implementation phase. This is the final phase of holistic care and includes any changes to the plan based on the nursing evaluation. The client's treatment plan will be continuously reevaluated to determine whether it should be continued, modified, or terminated based on the client reassessment and general response. The CNL can significantly impact a client's overall health through implementation and follow-through of the individualized plan of care. This plan can influence a client's current lifestyle, promote healthy behaviors, reduce risk factors, and prevent the development of future disease processes.

The CNL can serve in the roles of client educator and care coordinator to promote an ongoing lifestyle of health promotion for clients. The client's health literacy should be assessed prior to providing the patient with any health information. Low-literacy levels contribute to noncompliance, increased complications, and increased rates of acute care readmissions (Jarvis, 2016). The role of client educator is supported by professional standards and provides the client with consistency and individualized care. This plan of care should include mutually agreed upon client management of health, nutrition, exercise, medications, and lifestyle modifications to improve an individual's sense of well-being (Harris, Roussel, & Thomas, 2013).

Pathophysiology, Assessment, and Pharmacology

The concepts of pathophysiology, physical assessment, and pharmacology must be incorporated in each patient's plan of care across the life span. The completion of an advanced clinical assessment will provide support for diagnosing pathophysiological alterations. Health alterations may be treated with a variety of therapies to include pharmacotherapy as required.

Clinical Judgment and Decision-Making Skills in Client-Focused Care

The CNL's use of clinical judgment is constant and must be dynamic while remaining goal-directed and client-centered. It involves collaborative care that can be universally applied through the implementation of a methodical approach to client care. It is essential that this approach involve gathering input from all members of the healthcare team to form a cohesive conclusion about current and future plans of care.

CNLs are positioned, educated, and prepared to coordinate the complete care of clients within their microsystems. This coordinated effort includes the use of clinical judgment and decision-making skills to develop, coordinate, implement, and evaluate comprehensive client care. The mastery of advanced clinical assessment techniques will enhance the decision-making process of client care and provide the information necessary to support decisions related to future care.

The CNL may use multiple methods to document the advanced clinical assessment based on the clinical agency's preference for documentation. A common method for organizing a client's clinical record is the use of SOAP notes.

- S—subjective data—the primary information provided by the client.
- O—objective data—direct observations from sight, smell, touch, and hearing.
- A—assessment—interpretation, conclusions, potential diagnoses, actual and potential problems.
- P—plan—diagnostic tests, therapeutic modalities, consults, and rationales (Seidel, Ball, Dains, Flynn, & Solomon, 2014).

Illustrations can provide a better explanation than a narrative description in conveying a client's pain location, radiation, or the size, shape, or location of lesions (Figure 14.1). They can also be used to document additional information, including pulse amplitude and deep tendon reflexes (Seidel et al., 2014).

Emergency or life-threatening conditions require the CNL to complete a rapid primary assessment to determine and manage life-threatening conditions. This rapid assessment should be completed within seconds, and the priorities should be established on the basis of pathophysiological processes and the ABCDEs as follows (see also Box 14.10).

- Airway—assessment and cervical spine stabilization.
- Breathing—ventilation is assessed and assisted.
- Circulation—assessed and bleeding is controlled.

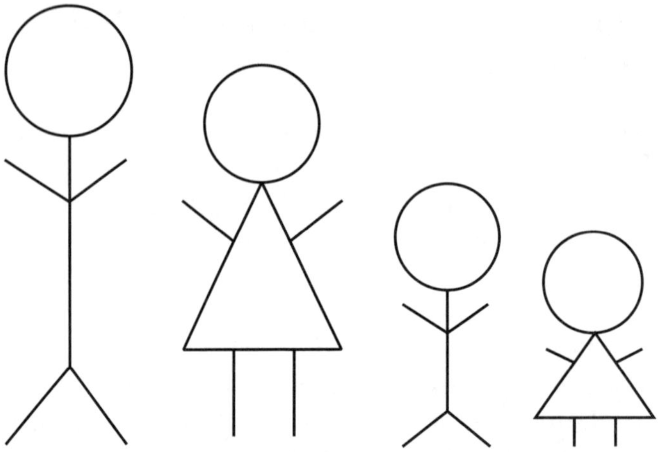

FIGURE 14.1 Put an "X" at each part of the body where you have pain.

BOX 14.10
Level of Responsiveness: AVPU

- A—Alert
- V—Verbal stimuli: responsive to
- P—Painful stimuli: responsive to
- U—Unresponsive

- Disability—assessment of neurological status.
- Exposure—complete assessment unclothed.

The secondary assessment begins when stabilization of emergency conditions is under control. The assessment will include SAMPLE:

- S—Symptoms
- A—Allergies
- M—Medications
- P—Past illnesses
- L—Last meal
- E—Events preceding the precipitating event (Seidel et al., 2014)

Evaluating the Effectiveness of Pharmacological and Complementary Therapies

The CNL will use advanced skills assessment to evaluate the effectiveness of both the pharmacological and the complementary therapies ordered

TABLE 14.1 Advanced Clinical Assessment

CATEGORY	WEIGHT
E. Advanced Clinical Assessment	**5%**
1. Designs, coordinates, and evaluates plans of care	
2. Develops a therapeutic alliance with the client as an advanced generalist	
3. Identifies client problems that require intervention, with special focus on those problems amenable to nursing intervention	
4. Performs holistic assessments across the life span and directs care based on findings	
5. Applies advanced knowledge of pathophysiology, assessment, and pharmacology	
6. Applies clinical judgment and decision-making skills in designing, coordinating, implementing, and evaluating client-focused care	
7. Evaluates effectiveness of pharmacological and complementary therapies	

Used with permission from the Commission on Nurse Certification (2011, 2014).

for his or her clients. These therapies will be monitored by use of clinical assessment techniques, diagnostics, and overall client responses to ordered therapies.

Conclusion

The role of the CNL is important for the provision of holistic care to clients. Advanced clinical assessment skills provide the CNL with valuable information to make ongoing decisions about client care. These skills correlate with the provision of quality practice and optimal client care outcomes to promote comprehensive care at all levels (Table 14.1).

Resources

American Nurse Association. (1980). *The nursing process*. New York, NY: Author.

Commission on Nurse Certification. (2011). *Clinical Nurse Leader job analysis report*. Retrieved from http://www.aacn.nche.edu/cnl/Job-Analysis-Report.pdf

Commission on Nurse Certification. (2014). *Clinical Nurse Leader (CNL®) certification exam blueprint*. Retrieved from http://www.aacn.nche.edu/leading-initiatives/cnl/cnl-certification/pdf/ExamContentOutline11.pdf

Harris, J. L., Roussel, L., & Thomas, P. (2013). *Initiating and sustaining the clinical nurse leader role* (2nd ed.). Sudbury, MA: Jones & Bartlett Learning.

Healthy People 2020 Leading Indicators. (2015). Retrieved from http://www.healthypeople.gov/2020/Leading-Health-Indicators

Jarvis, C. (2016). *Physical examination & health assessment* (7th ed.). St. Louis, MO: Elsevier.

Seidel, H., Ball, J., Dains, J., Flynn, J. A., & Solomon, B. S. (2014). *Mosby's guide to physical examination* (8th ed.). St. Louis, MO: Elsevier.

Smith, S. F., Duell, D. J., & Martin, B. C. (2013). *Clinical nursing skills: Basic to advanced skills* (8th ed.). Boston, MA: Pearson.

U.S. Preventive Services Task Force. (2014). *Guide to clinical preventive services, 2014.* Retrieved from http://www.ahrq.gov/professionals/clinicians-providers/guidelines-recommendations/guide/index.html

Wilson, S. F., & Giddens, J. F. (2013). *Health assessment for nursing practice* (5th ed.). St. Louis, MO: Elsevier.

IV

Key Certification Topics: Care Environment Management

15

Team Coordination

Bonnie Haupt

The ratio of we's to I's is the best indicator of the development of a team.
—*Lewis B. Ergen*

The *Future of Nursing: Leading Change, Advancing Health* report calls for interprofessional collaboration in healthcare: This increasing complexity in the delivery of care in a wide range of settings highlights the importance to coordinate care among the various providers; thus, developing highly efficient teams is a crucial healthcare objective (Institute of Medicine [IOM], 2010). Historically, the healthcare delivery system has functioned in a practice of hierarchical order. The physician-driven orders have long been the model for the healthcare team in decision making. Little feedback or input was sought from other team members regarding the patient's plan of care. Healthcare team members are no longer operating in silos; they are working together for better patient care outcomes. Today's healthcare system involves active participation of all interprofessional team members when coordinating and delivering care. Physicians, nurses, lab technicians, health assistants, and physical therapists are a few of the direct care professionals coming together to improve patient stays, satisfaction, and outcomes. In the healthcare setting, patients are also interfacing with indirect care professionals, who are members of the interprofessional team. Indirect team members may include dietary staff, medical clerks, pharmacists, clinical informatics, housekeepers, patient advocates, and leadership individuals, all of whom affect the patient's care.

Leading Teams

Strong leaders in nursing are needed to collaborate and build effective teams. It is essential for nursing leaders to act as full partners with direct and indirect health professionals, being accountable for establishing high-quality care outcomes while working collaboratively with members of the interprofessional healthcare team. Team-based healthcare defined by

Naylor et al. (2010) is the delivery of services to communities, families, and individuals by a minimum of two collaborative members of the healthcare team, along with caregivers and patients, to achieve identified goals through high-quality care services. Coordinating the required services streamlines the healthcare process, improves communication among providers, and improves patients' interaction with the healthcare team.

The clinical nurse leader (CNL) has emerged as a strong leader and team coordinator in the healthcare system. Introduction of the CNL role into the healthcare setting has increased nursing membership's role in collaborating for patient care outcomes. The American Association of Colleges of Nursing (AACN) white paper (2007) establishes the CNL role as designing, coordinating, and evaluating client care outcomes (p. 12). CNLs have taken a lead role in team collaboration and coordination, bringing all members of the interprofessional team together. For example, the following scenario highlights the CNL's role here.

A CNL on a 30-bed acute care unit has identified a patient who requires coordination of his care. Mr. J, a 75-year-old male patient, was admitted yesterday to the unit with weight loss and failure to thrive. The medical team believes he has been aspirating. Mr. J has a medical history of hypertension, diabetes, alcohol use, is legally blind, and smokes one pack of cigarettes per day. Mr. J's visiting nurse has logged 10 out of the last 14 days with periods of hypotensive blood pressure. Mr. J complains that he has felt dizzy at times and unsteady on his feet this past week. It is noted that he has several cigarette burns on his clothes and lower extremities. His daughter is concerned about her father's living conditions, ability to care for himself, and overall health status. Mr. J lives alone in a two-story home and has been independent and active in the community up to 3 months before this admission, when his wife of 50 years passed away. When coordinating care for Mr. J, what members of the interprofessional team should be included? The team might include a pharmacist, physician, registered nurse, care coordinator, dietician, psychiatrist, social worker, physical and occupational therapists, and let us not forget the patient and his family as active members of the healthcare team. Daily, CNLs are charged with coordinating care teams for various patients in the healthcare system. These care teams focus on patient care, patient safety, and clinical outcomes. CNLs are involved with assessing and identifying needs, formulating plans, and implementing and objectively evaluating the outcomes.

As the CNL's role expands, he or she is also focusing on facility and systems issues throughout the healthcare setting that affect patient safety, satisfaction, and outcomes. An example might include a recent reduction in nightly quiet satisfaction scores on a particular unit, as documented in hospital survey scores. The CNL must assess and identify the root cause of the decrease in scores. What factors are causes of the reduction in scores: possibly staffing, other patient noise, construction, or even equipment and unit alarms? The CNL would then build an interprofessional team to identify solutions and plan development to increase the scores. The team members again expand beyond direct care providers to indirect care team members. What members of the healthcare team would you select? The team might include nursing, housekeeping, lab personnel, engineering, patients, and even their caregivers. After assessing the data and developing, implementing, and trialing the agreed upon plan, the CNL would obtain feedback from unit members and adjust the plan as needed to meet the goals. The CNL will also monitor the unit satisfaction scores for improvements.

CNL Curriculum Framework for Client-Centered Health Care

A master's-prepared education provides the CNL with the necessary skills and leadership abilities to form and lead effective teams. AACN (2007) identifies the team coordination competencies necessary for success in the CNL curriculum framework for client-centered healthcare: delegation, supervision, interdisciplinary care, group process, handling difficult people, and conflict resolution.

Delegation

Healthcare professionals view delegation as a process of assigning a task or tasks to team members. The CNL must feel comfortable and confident in this role, whether assigning simple tasks to subordinates, or complex assignments to peers and executive leadership when working in teams. An important aspect of delegation is knowing your team members' skills, experiences, and competencies. The CNL should define interprofessional team member abilities and identify responsibilities that are appropriate to complete assigned tasks. If team members lack certain abilities, the CNL is responsible for ensuring individual team members are knowledgeable in proper processes and procedures. The CNL should model appropriate and effective delegation practices and support members of the team that struggle with a sometimes difficult, but necessary, part of teamwork.

Supervision

Supervision of team members is a vital component of the collaborative process, whether supervising the team member in a simple task or chairing a committee identifying safety issues affecting patient outcomes. The CNL, as team coordinator, is the individual who assumes accountability and responsibility for supervising and leading the team to a common goal. Acting as a coach and mentor, the CNL is responsible for not only team goals but also individual member goals. Seamless supervision leads to enhanced safety and well-being of patients and interprofessional team members in the healthcare environment.

Interdisciplinary Care

Interdisciplinary care is now referred to as interprofessional care, involving interacting, communicating, and collaborating with all members of the healthcare team. Establishing working relationships within the team is instrumental in team collaboration and coordination.

Interprofessional collaborative practice described by WHO (2010) is when diverse healthcare professionals function together to provide the utmost quality care to communities, families, and patients. Research has confirmed successes in patient satisfaction and care outcomes in teams trained in interprofessional education (Chau, Denomme, Murray, & Cott, 2009). Organizing care involves assembling personnel and other resources needed to carry out all required patient care activities, and is often managed by the exchange of information among participants responsible for different aspects of care.

Group Process and Communication

Lack of team communication can lead to medical errors. In 1999, the Institute of Medicine's (IOM, 1999) *To Err Is Human: Building a Safer Health System* reported at least 44,000 and as many as 98,000 patients died every year in U.S. hospitals because of medical errors. Recently, James (2007) identified that deaths related to medical errors exceeded 210,000 annually. Inadvertent patient harm is caused by lack of teamwork and communication failures (Leonard, Graham, & Bonacum, 2010). The CNL directs the group process and utilizes technology and evidence-based research to strengthen practice and prevent harm.

Demonstrating critical listening is instrumental in a group process. Team coordination and effective communication are essential to the delivery of optimum patient care and outcomes. Are the messages of all group members being heard? A collaborative team may be formed for any number of reasons. Once a member of the interprofessional team identifies patient safety concerns or a clinical or systems issue affecting patient care or satisfaction, a team can be formed.

The team coordinator is responsible for assessing gaps, providing solutions, and implementing process changes to improve patient care. Members of the interprofessional team come to the table for diverse reasons. Individuals may come with enthusiasm and passion for a project, with goals to promote practice changes or a personal experience compelling them to seek change. At times, it is possible that team members may be assigned by management or leadership and have no desire to participate in the project. Individual motives for participation may have an overall effect on the group. It is identified in highly effective teams that members possess five personal characteristics: creativity, curiosity, discipline, honesty, and humility (Mitchell et al., 2012). When creating an interprofessional team, it is crucial to select members who are representative of different interprofessional teams and hold high values.

A collaborative approach is a joint effort with a common goal identified to improve patient care outcomes. Tuckman and Jensen (1977) identified five stages of group development (see Box 15.1).

The first stage, known as the *forming stage*, involves the team coming together. Team members are looking to the team coordinator and CNL to set the mission and group expectations. Team members are forming relationships, identifying how they fit in, analyzing whether their goals mesh with the team goals, and exploring the team's expectations of themselves. The first stage of forming aligns with Mitchell et al.'s (2012) principle of team-based healthcare and identifying that team members share common goals that are understood, clearly articulated, and championed by team members. The team members are seeking a safe and trusting environment, where they can feel comfortable expressing their ideas and concerns. The forming stage may produce uncomfortable silence, until members establish trust. According to the U.S. Office of Personnel Management (1997), building an effective collaborative team requires establishing a common goal, trust, respect, open communication, role clarity, appreciation of diversity, and a balanced team focus.

The second stage, *storming*, is a potentially tumultuous stage, one in which conflict may occur. There may be a lack of unity, struggles over leadership, and power in the group. The team coordinator is responsible for keeping team members on track during this phase. Questions and concerns over the mission, goals, and the group's progress will come under fire. To be successful and progress to the next stage, the team members must grow together, being flexible and respectful in their views to meet the group's goals.

The third stage is called *norming*. The group is now established. The ground rules and agendas have been set and everyone is on the same page. Team members feel they are working in a safe environment, where everyone's opinions and ideas are shared openly and valued.

In the fourth stage, *performing*, tasks are being completed. Team members are working together or independently in their assigned roles while

BOX 15.1
Five Stages of Group Development

- Forming
- Storming
- Norming
- Performing
- Adjourning/mourning

still collaborating. If working independently, each member may be responsible for goals related to his or her own professional expertise (O'Daniel & Rosenstein, 2008). The group has already identified individual strengths and weaknesses of the project and is working collaboratively to manage and guide the outcomes. The team coordinator brings all expert professionals together to share their progress and successes of research in terms of meeting the team goals. Team members are focused on problem solving, seeking solutions, and finding long-term outcomes. This is the time according to Mitchell et al. (2012) where measurable processes and outcomes are implemented. The data gathered during this time will guide members in identifying opportunities and strengths of the plan. All members of the team are exhibiting responsibility and accountability for the project or team objectives during this stage.

The final stage is identified as adjourning or *mourning*. Team members have achieved the group's mission or goals that were set forth. This stage involves termination of the group. Some team members may feel a sense of loss after working so closely for many hours on a project. It is important for the group to have a final meeting that includes time for goodbyes and includes recognition to all team members for their hard work.

The IOM (2003) reports the need to "Cooperate, collaborate, communicate, and integrate care in teams to ensure that care is continuous and reliable." The CNL is continuously assessing how teams are operating in the dynamic care environment. Are team members participating and engaging fully with new and innovative strategies and ideas? Are roles with the team clarified? What characteristics does the team coordinator envision in the team members? Are there personality conflicts between team members, or, possibly, time management issues? Do team members communicate openly and effectively? Are team members exhibiting responsibility and accountability for the project or team objectives? What are the goals or strategic initiatives the team is challenged with reaching? What barriers exist in terms of accomplishing the team's goals? Are completion time frames being met?

Handling Difficult People and Conflict

Conflict occurs in teams and between individuals when there is a disagreement over views or goals. If a conflict occurs, immediate and swift resolution and actions are needed to diffuse the situation. Handling difficult situations requires enhanced communication skills. As a team coordinator, the CNL must demonstrate effective leadership qualities, including proficient communication skills. Communication is the number one means in which healthcare professionals, patients, and caregivers interact. The CNL is aware of the verbal, nonverbal, and written messages that are being portrayed to the team members. Difficult situations may arise at any time or place in the healthcare environment. Interprofessional team members are confronted not only with difficult patients, caregivers, and families; they require the skill to communicate effectively with other members of the healthcare team. Highly effective communication skills will promote a transparent and positive work environment that will build trust and a culture of retention for the interprofessional team (Box 15.2).

Conflict or other problems can arise in a group when some essential component is missing. Team leaders may want to perform a gap analysis to gain better understanding into the team's functioning. A *gap analysis* evaluates the strengths and weaknesses of the team in relation to the required outcomes. Evaluation of the disciplines represented, the skill sets possessed by team members, the goal of the team, and expected outcomes can all be explored. This analysis is sometimes supported by individuals outside of the team who may be more objective. One example might be that a project requires significant support of the information technology staff who have not been included as members of the team. Hospitals seeking recognition from the American Nurses Credentialing Centers often hire consultants to assist the nursing team to conduct a gap analysis as they begin a massive organizational initiative focused on teamwork. Despite the versatility of

BOX 15.2
Resources for Interprofessional Team Collaboration

http://www.aacn.nche.edu/education-resources/ipecreport.pdf
http://www.IHI.org
http://collaborate.uw.edu
http://www.saferpatients.com
http://teamstepps.ahrq.gov
http://www.ahrq.gov

nurses, they cannot do it all. Having the right team members involved with the needed skill set is essential to success.

Interprofessional Team Collaboration

The foundation of the CNL was based on a concept of interdisciplinary or interprofessional collaboration. The AACN white paper clearly delineates the CNL as a key figure in the support of safe and patient-centered care from all professional groups. This concept has gained tremendous attention in healthcare recently, from training professionals in an interprofessional format to training practicing care providers in the importance of team collaboration to provide a safe environment. This recent awareness in identifying the critical role of interprofessional teams has led to the emerging resources now available. From leading government healthcare agencies to private consulting firms, this topic has clearly gained national attention. Innovative strategies such as simulation are being utilized in supporting safe communication of team members and are playing a pivotal role in the future of how students and practicing professionals develop the skill necessary for high-functioning teams. Resources highlighting interprofessional education and team coordination may be useful to CNL students, practicing CNLs, and all professionals interacting with and leading teams.

Professional healthcare organizations are also supporting interprofessional collaboration by establishing competencies for interprofessional collaboration as part of formal education. This report is inspired by a vision of interprofessional collaborative practice as key to the safe, high-quality, accessible, and patient-centered care desired by all (AACN, 2011). Imagine a healthcare team that has strong understanding and respect for team collaboration upon entering their chosen field! Achieving that vision for the future requires the continuous development of interprofessional competencies by health profession students as part of the learning process, so that they enter the workforce ready to practice effective teamwork and team-based care (AACN, 2011). This restructuring of professional education can only enhance the patient-centered care teams in which the CNL functions.

Conclusion

The AACN white paper (2007) states,

> The CNL is responsible for the clinical management of comprehensive client care, for individuals and clinical populations, along the continuum of care and in multiple settings, including virtual settings. The CNL is responsible for planning a client's contact with the healthcare system. The CNL also is responsible for the coordination and planning of team activities and functions. In order to impact care,

the CNL has the knowledge and authority to delegate tasks to other healthcare personnel, as well as supervise and evaluate these personnel and the outcomes of care. Along with the authority, autonomy and initiative to design and implement care, the CNL is accountable for improving individual care outcomes and care processes in a quality, cost-effective manner.

In 2010, the World Health Organization (WHO) published a framework for action on interprofessional education and collaborative practice. CNLs are coordinators of care and processes within the healthcare team, focusing on patient safety, outcomes, and satisfaction. CNLs practice interprofessional teamwork as defined by leading teams through coordination, collaboration, and cooperation and understanding relationships between the interprofessional teams in healthcare (IPE, 2011). Research shows that teams working collaboratively improve patient care outcomes. CNLs are at the forefront of implementing change in the healthcare setting, coordinating teams, promoting evidence-based practice, and establishing quality standards to promote the overall health, safety, and satisfaction for our patients, families, caregivers, and staff. The CNL® certification exam covers many aspects of team coordination that are critical to supporting positive change (Table 15.1). Collaboration should occur within and across settings, following patients throughout the healthcare system.

TABLE 15.1 Team Coordination

CATEGORY	WEIGHT
A. Team Coordination	**6%**
1. Supervises, educates, delegates, and performs nursing procedures in the context of safety	
2. Demonstrates critical listening, verbal, nonverbal, and written communication skills	
3. Demonstrates skills necessary to interact and collaborate with other members of the interdisciplinary healthcare team	
4. Incorporates principles of lateral integration	
5. Establishes and maintains working relationships within an interdisciplinary team	
6. Facilitates group processes to achieve care objectives	
7. Utilizes conflict resolution skills	
8. Promotes a positive work environment and a culture of retention	
9. Designs, coordinates, and evaluates plans of care incorporating client, family, and team member input	
10. Leads gap analysis to create a cohesive healthcare team	

Used with permission from the Commission on Nurse Certification (2011, 2014).

Resources

American Association of Colleges of Nursing. (2007). *White paper. Education and role of the clinical nurse leader*. Retrieved from http://www.aacn.nche.edu/publications/white-papers/cnl

American Association of Colleges of Nursing. (2011). *Core competencies for interprofessional collaborative practice*. Retrieved from http://www.aacn.nche.edu/education-resources/ipecreport.pdf

Chau, J., Denomme, J., Murray, J., & Cott, C. (2009). Inter-professional education in the acute-care setting: The clinical instructor's point of view. *Physiotherapy Canada*, *63*(1), 65–75. DOI: 10.3138/ptc.2009–41

Commission on Nurse Certification. (2011). *Clinical Nurse Leader job analysis report*. Retrieved from http://www.aacn.nche.edu/cnl/Job-Analysis-Report.pdf

Commission on Nurse Certification. (2014). *Clinical Nurse Leader (CNL®) certification exam blueprint*. Retrieved from http://www.aacn.nche.edu/leading-initiatives/cnl/cnl-certification/pdf/ExamContentOutline11.pdf

Institute of Medicine. (2003). *Health professions education: A bridge to quality*. Washington, DC: National Academy Press. Retrieved from http://www.nap.edu/openbook.php?record_id=10681&page=45

Institute of Medicine. (2010). *The future of nursing: Leading change, advancing health*. Washington, DC: National Academies Press. Retrieved from http://www.rwjf.org/files/research/Future%20of%20Nursing_Leading%20Change%20Advancing%20Health.pdf

Institute of Medicine. (1999). *To err is human: Building a safer health system*. Washington, DC: National Academy Press. Retrieved from http://www.iom.edu/Reports/1999/To-err-is-Human-Building-A-Safer-Health-System.aspx

Interprofessional Education Collaborative Expert Panel. (2011). Core competencies for interprofessional collaborative practice: Report of an expert panel. *National Network of Libraries of Medicine*. Washington, DC. Retrieved from https://www.aamc.org/download/186750/data/core_competencies.pdf

James, J. T. (2007). *A sea of broken hearts*. Bloomington, IN: AuthorHouse.

Leonard, M., Graham, S., & Bonacum, D. (2010). The human factor: The critical importance of effective teamwork and communication in providing safe care. *Quality Safety Health care*. doi:10.1136/qshc.2004.010033.

Mitchell, P., Wynia, M., Golden, R., McNellis, B., Okun, S., Webb, C. E., & Von Kohorn, I. (2012). Core principles and values of effective team-based health care. *Institute of Medicine of the National Academies*. Retrieved from https://www.nationalahec.org/pdfs/VSRT-Team-Based-Care-Principles-values.pdf

Naylor, M. D., Coburn, K. D., Kurtzman, E. T., Prvu Bettger, J., Buck, H. G., Van Cleave, J., & Cott, C. A. (2010). *Inter-professional team-based primary care for chronically ill adults: State of the science*. Paper presented at ABIM Foundation meeting to Advance Team-Based Care for the Chronically Ill in Ambulatory Settings, Philadelphia, PA, March 24–25.

O'Daniel, M., & Rosenstein, A. H. (2008). *Patient safety and quality: An evidence-based handbook for nurses* (Chapter 33). Rockville, MD: Agency for Healthcare Research and Quality (US).

Tuckman, B., & Jensen, M. (1977). Stages of small group development. *Group and Organizational Studies*, *2*, 419–427.

U.S. Office of Personnel Management. (1997). Building a collaborative team environment. *Work Performance Newsletter*. Retrieved from www.opm.gov/perform/articles/072.asp

World Health Organization. (2010). *Framework for action on interprofessional education and collaborative practice*. Geneva, Switzerland: World Health Organization. Retrieved from http://www.who.int/hrh/resources/framework_action/en

16

Healthcare Finance and Economics

E. Carol Polifroni and Denise M. Bourassa

As the role of the clinical nurse leader (CNL) develops, the individual must be aware of the environment in which he or she works, the economic climate of the environment, the specific fiscal details related to the nurses (and ancillary personnel), the supplies used for care delivery, and the reimbursement expected for this care delivered. This economic lens is a challenge for most nurses, as they typically view the care they give as being separate from finance.

The average age of the nurse is well over 45 years, and many practicing nurses began work at a time when costs were not discussed (or even known). The philosophy that guided patient care delivery was "whatever the patient needs." Individuals remained in acute care facilities for weeks on end, neither short-term rehabilitation nor subacute facilities existed, and how much something cost was not a known variable. The world of retrospective payment existed for the institution and the nurse practiced within that environment.

In today's healthcare, all that has changed. With the Affordable Care Act, economics are at the forefront. It is impossible to watch the evening news without reference to the gross domestic product, the ever-escalating costs of healthcare, and the increasing percentage of every American dollar spent on healthcare. Depending on the reference used, current healthcare costs range from 15% to 19% of the annual gross domestic product in the United States. This means that for every dollar spent, 15 to 19 cents of that dollar goes toward healthcare costs in this country. Are the outcomes expected with such an expenditure delivered? The obvious answer is no, not when we live in an industrialized nation. The Centers for Disease Control and Prevention (CDC) estimates that approximately 50,000 people are newly infected with AIDS a year (CDC, 2015a). In 2005, the United States ranked 30th in infant mortality, behind most European countries—Canada, Australia, New Zealand, Hong Kong, Singapore, Japan, and Israel

(MacDorman & Mathews, 2009). And lastly, in 2009, the top four leading causes of death were heart disease, malignant neoplasms, chronic lower respiratory disease, and cerebrovascular diseases. These indicators are a reflection of lifestyle as much as they are of economics, and we continue to push death away as far as it will go (CDC, 2015b).

Thus, the context for our discussion and review is that, in the United States, we spend up to 18 or more cents of every dollar on healthcare. This is in comparison with per capita spending in other countries as noted in Figure 16.1.

In a recent study (Kwok et al., 2011), it was noted that nearly a third of elderly Americans had a surgical intervention during the last year of life, and most of these procedures occurred in the month before death. The culture of the United States is such that we aim to push death away and to avoid it at all possible costs. Regardless of your beliefs on death with dignity and a rational and dignified end to life, or the need to avoid death no matter what, the costs of such a belief need to be known and addressed (Kelly, 2011).

Is it right and is it just for finite dollars to be spent at the end of life, or is it more right and more just to spend those dollars at an earlier time in the healthcare cycle or on something altogether different? This chapter does not aim to answer these questions, but makes readers aware of the question and the components within the question, so that they understand economics and finance as they relate to healthcare.

In addition to the aforementioned statistics, total health spending has, according to recent figures, increased to 17.1% of the gross domestic product (World Bank, 2016). As a response to this, the CNL is called to make adjustments in practice that answer to reimbursement changes, staffing shortages, the increasing rate of uninsured Americans, and mandates that

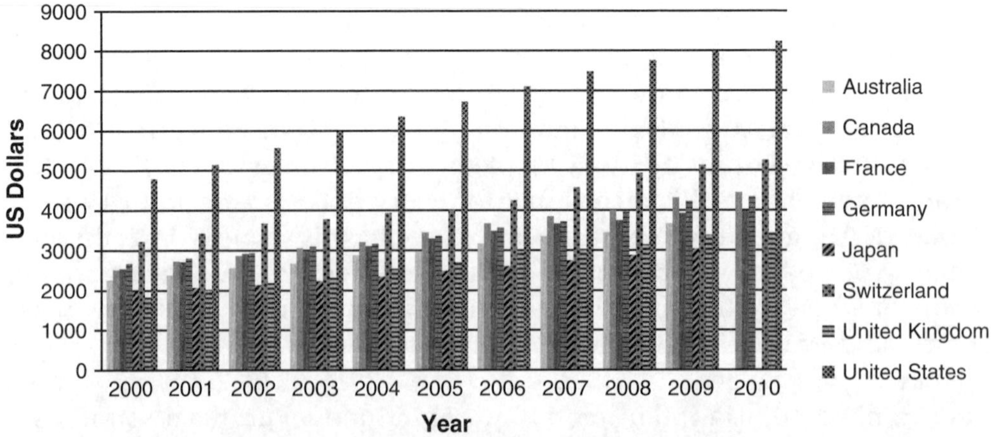

Source: OECD Health Data 2012.

FIGURE 16.1 Total expenditure on health per capita.

link quality and outcomes to reimbursement. Areas of direct potential impact that the CNL, at the frontline of healthcare delivery, can influence include cost/financial outcomes, specifically in the areas of length of stay, readmission rates, patient flow, and quality/internal process outcomes (Ott et al., 2009). As patients more often are becoming consumers and the healthcare industry is expected to perform in a fiscally prudent manner, it is important that the registered nurse of the future understand how finance and economics impact the care he or she gives at the bedside.

Cost Reduction and Standardization

Cost reduction for care delivery is a focus of a 2011 issue of *Hospitals & Health Network*'s financial fitness series. Joan Moss, Senior Vice President at SG2, a healthcare intelligence and information services firm, advises that cost reduction be addressed in four phases:

> The first is reducing variation by standardizing protocols. ... Second is removing unnecessary care, including provider errors, preventable readmissions, avoidable conditions and unnecessary diagnostic tests. Third is cost restructuring to use the lowest cost setting and provider possible for each service. ... The fourth is adopting a system of care strategy ... such as medical homes and disease management. (Larkin, 2011, p. 30)

There is a component of the CNL's role in each of the four areas. Cost reduction is not the sole focus of the CNL, but as the CNL is the system's bridge between administration and the point of care, every strategy suggested has a component for the CNL role.

It is essential to note that the CNL must work toward standardizing protocols within his or her span of control. Within the hospital setting, the CNL needs to bring the need for standardized protocols to the attention of management and to facilitate committee activity from planning through the evaluation of the protocols. In an outpatient setting, protocols will drive services provided and costs. The CNL must educate the staff about the value of protocols and what protocols bring to them, as well as what protocols add to the patient care. Reduction of provider errors is a key component of the CNL's role, as he or she creates systems of care delivery that address ease of access, accuracy of use, and appropriate charging of cost to the right individual or center. The attention to preventable readmissions and unnecessary diagnostic tests is a key reason why the CNL is prepared with coursework and practice in assessment, pathophysiology, and pharmacology. They all relate to the cost of care provided in a very direct manner. Assigning the appropriate provider to care for a patient, in an inpatient or outpatient setting, also has a correlation to costs. Thus, the CNL must be keenly aware of which level of personnel/provider can do the job and be aware of the skill level of each individual within a role category. The last element that Moss addresses is disease management and the concept of the "medical home," a term for primary contact among multiple providers. Again, these are key roles of the CNL as they directly relate to cost and financial management within whatever type of setting the CNL is employed. Before we proceed further into this review, it is time to define terms that are imperative for the CNL to know (see Box 16.1).

Finances Within a Microsystem

The relevance of the terms found in Box 16.1 should be evident in their definition. Volume is the key factor in any discussion about inpatient or outpatient healthcare finance. Volume—the number of services provided,

BOX 16.1
Definition of Terms

Acuity: Level of intensity of care required by patients.

Case mix: The mix (variety) of patients for whom care is delivered organized by specified characteristics (e.g., gender, DRG, payer).

Cost center: A microsystem responsible for providing services and monitoring the costs associated with such service provision.

Diagnosis-related group (DRG): Group used by Medicare and other payers to determine reimbursement to organizations and providers.

Direct costs: Costs that are directly related to the provision of a service; the cost can be specifically identified for an individual patient or activity.

Expenses: Dollars owed as a result of both services delivered and organizational costs incurred in the delivery.

First-party payers: Individuals responsible for payment for services rendered.

Gross domestic product: Market value of all goods and services produced (created) within a country in a specific period (https://en.wikipedia.org/wiki/Gross_domestic_product).

ICD-9-CM: *International Classification of Diseases, Ninth Revision, Clinical Manifestations*; used for documentation of diagnoses and procedures; in turn, used to assign a DRG and create patient charges.

Indirect costs: Those costs of doing business that are not directly related to a specific individual, such as heat, electricity, overhead, water, and some administrative personnel.

Length of stay: Time spent (number of days) in an organization receiving healthcare services.

(*continued*)

BOX 16.1 (*continued*)

Medicaid: A program sponsored by states and federal government for low income and/or disabled individuals; services and payment are provided.

Medical home: A concept initially designed in 1969 and now used to coordinate medical care among multiple providers.

Medicare: A governmental program related to Social Security for the elderly.

Outcome: The end product of an action.

Private insurance: Third-party payers in the private marketplace not funded by government sources.

Reimbursement: Dollars received by an organization or provider for services rendered.

Revenue: Money received through the delivery of services.

Retrospective/prospective payment: Prior to 1994, retrospective payment was a system used to reimburse hospitals for services delivered on the basis of cost without any foreknowledge; since 1994, prospective payment is a system wherein reimbursement to hospitals or other organizational entities is based on a DRG or ambulatory patient classification (APC).

Second-party payers: The agency providing the services also pays for the service.

Third-party payers: Governmental or private insurance entities who pay for all or some of the services provided.

Volume: The number of beds occupied, procedures done, cases received, visits made, or other description of amount of services provided.

patients seen, or cases addressed—dictates the dollars available for care delivery. From these available dollars, revenue and all expenses incurred by the institution to deliver the care for a patient must be found. The revenue and expenses are typically assigned to an individual cost center for ease of monitoring and reporting. A cost center is a microsystem within the larger whole such as a unit (7 W), a service (outpatient cardiac rehab), or an entity. There are both direct and indirect costs associated with care. As noted, direct expenses are those directly related to care, such as the nurse caring for the patient, the supplies used for the needed dressing, food provided, and linen provided throughout the day. Indirect costs are still charged to the patient and they are those things that indirectly service the client, such as heat, water, physical space, aesthetics of the environment, and institution-wide electricity and equipment. Therefore, it is self-evident that the CNL must know the expected reimbursement, the planned length of stay on which the reimbursement is dependent, and the costs associated with the care provided.

In a direct relationship, the CNL is responsible and accountable for outcomes within the microsystem of care. Outcomes relate to conditions, incidence, and dollars as an end of the care delivered. The focus of this chapter is to achieve the desired clinical condition as an outcome within a defined dollar amount. The dollar amount is determined by the admitting diagnosis (DRG for patients for whom Medicare is the primary payer) and the length of stay associated with that DRG. Whether the length of stay for patient Y is less than the range provided, more than the range provided, or within the range provided, the reimbursement to the facility is the same. In other words, there is an incentive to the agency (not necessarily to the patient or the provider) for the individual to be discharged earlier than the defined range, or certainly within the defined range for which reimbursement will be provided. When the patient is discharged after the defined range without an approved comorbidity, no additional payments are made to the agency nor can the individual be charged a separate bill.

Thus, the key variables for the CNL are two: length of stay and utilization of services and supplies within that length of stay. These are two variables that the CNL must understand and influence. Variation may exist in how length of stay is managed and services allocated, but the purpose here is to know that this management is essential for cost-effective care delivery.

Within the supply component, it is imperative that the CNL know the costs of all supplies, those that are deemed direct, meaning they are then appropriately charged to the patient for whom the supplies are used, and the access to the supplies. The CNL needs to ensure that all users know how the charging system—barcode or otherwise—works, when charges are appropriate, and the relationship between the charge assigned to the correct payer and the financial solvency of the organization in which the care is provided. CNLs can also influence the correct use of these charging systems by being sure that they are user friendly to those responsible for charging the patient. The CNL cannot be responsible for every charge, as it is often incurred by the specific caregiver, but the CNL can design, or redesign, the system for ease of use, so that charges are appropriately made and not circumvented. Additionally, the CNL is responsible for educating the staff on system use, monitoring its utilization, and making changes as needed.

The indirect costs, while needing modest management, are typically outside the realm of responsibility for the CNL. Indirect costs are usually allocated to a cost center's operating budget on the basis of percentage, occupancy, or a simple mathematical formula created and monitored by the finance department of the agency. The CNL, however, is accountable for just utilization of the indirect costs.

Reimbursement

Within the reimbursement component from which revenue is derived, the CNL needs to be aware of the payer mix of the patients. Payer mix, as noted earlier, is the specific combination of payment mechanisms for all patients; when combined together, they are known as the case mix. The CNL needs to be aware of who the payer is; in most instances, it will be a third-party payer of either the government (Medicare, Medicaid, VA benefit) or private insurance such as Anthem Blue Cross Blue Shield. As with indirect costs, the CNL will not be responsible for monitoring the payment, but is accountable for the knowledge of which payer is involved, so that costs are appropriately allocated, length of stay is closely monitored within the expected range, and services are delivered consistent with payer expectations and requirements. In the instance that the patient's bill is going to be paid by himself or herself (first-party payer) or the organization (second-party payer), the CNL's accountabilities remain the same; namely, knowing and implementing measures to monitor costs and utilization of services. When charitable care is provided by the agency delivering the care, this is known as second-party payer. Even though the agency is paying the bill for the care, the CNL must ensure that the care meets the required standards and can be defended fiscally.

In an outpatient setting, ICD-9 codes are used to track expenses and services provided. The CNL in these settings is responsible for educating the staff about the appropriate codes, monitoring the system for recording the codes, and auditing the code utilization as needed. These activities require diligence and a developed system to ensure that items are not missed and teaching moments are seized.

Patient acuity is the transition between revenue/expenses and the discussion of staff to provide care to the patients. Acuity determines the amount of care required. There are varied patient classification systems with which the CNL needs to be familiar. The key to all systems is validity and reliability. An external system may be adopted in its entirety and the data benchmarked with institutions of like size and patient population. If it is an internal system, the limitation is that it cannot be benchmarked against like institutions. However, with a specialized patient population, an internal system may work best. A standardized product that has been tailored/individualized to an agency may be an option as well. All systems, regardless of origin, must be reliable and valid, and the role of the CNL is to contribute to this process. If not reliable, valid, and utilized for staffing purposes, the nurses, in particular, will not see the system as useful and may sabotage its reliability through inflated assessments. Therefore, the system needs to be reassessed for reliability and validity on a regular basis. Everyone must be confident that the numbers determined by the system reflect the needs of the patients for whom the care is being delivered. When the system is reliable and individuals

BOX 16.2
Staffing Terms

FTE: Full-time equivalent based on a 40-hour work week for 2,080 hours per year; expressed as a 1.0 or a fraction thereof; a 0.5 FTE is one-half of 2,080 hours or coverage for 20 hours per week; an FTE is not an individual but a position with hours associated with it.

HCPPD: Hours of care per patient day; a numerical expression of the amount of care a type of patient receives in a 24-hour period.

Productivity: The work product of a unit or individual based on the amount of work required and the hours available to deliver that care.

Staffing matrix: The number of staff assigned to work on a given shift on a given day.

Staffing mix: The mixture of licensed and unlicensed staff as well as the type of license; a staffing mix may be 70% licensed and 30% unlicensed, with 80% of the licensed staff being RNs and the remaining 20% possessing an LPN license.

have confidence in it, the acuity system can be used to allocate staff with confidence. However, numbers are only numbers and must be used only as a guide, and the role of the CNL is to use the numbers with reasoned judgment, knowing the context of the specific situation at hand.

The role of the CNL is to educate the staff on the system and its uses as well as how to implement the system. Within this discussion, the reliability and validity of the system must be addressed. When an effective patient classification for acuity determination is implemented, the staff and patients benefit alike. Another list of words is shared, as these definitions guide the next area of discussion (Box 16.2).

Staffing and Scheduling

The outcome of this effective system is the design of a staffing matrix. The matrix is determined by the number of hours of care per patient day delivered by the system, not by each individual nurse. Most inpatient settings operate on a 24-hour basis. Inherent in this perspective is care delivered over a 24-hour period. Thus, if a patient classification system determines a patient's acuity is a category "four," this, by a previous determination, translates to requiring 6 hours of care per day. If they are at a "three," the care hours required are 4, a classification of a "two" may be 3 hours of care, and a category "one" is 2 hours of inpatient care over a 24-hour period, after which this patient is ready for transfer to another facility or to home (see Box 16.3).

BOX 16.3
Example of Staffing Determinants Based on a Classification System

Using this approach, let us say we have 24 patients; 6 in each category.

Using a simple multiplication process, we determine:

- The six category-4 patients require 36 hours of patient care (6 × 6).
- The six category-3 patients require 24 hours (6 × 4) of care.
- The six category-2 patients require 18 hours (6 × 3) of care.
- The six category-1 patients require 12 hours (6 × 2) of care.

The total hours of care required for all 24 patients is 84 hours of care in a 24-hour period.

The management of the unit has previously determined that there is a 70/30 mix of licensed to unlicensed staff. This means that 70% of the hours of nursing care required for all 24 patients must be delivered by a nurse with a license, and 30% can be delivered by a patient care assistant, a nurse's aide, or someone holding another title without a license. To further break this down, 70% of 84 is 58.8 hours.

If each nurse works 7 hours after breaks are deducted, the CNL divides 7 into 60 and knows that 8.4 licensed nurses are needed to provide the nursing care, along with an additional 3.6 nursing assistants to provide the remaining 25.2 hours of care.

For this example, the CNL knows that 12 people must be assigned to work over the 24-hour period, and the staffing mix must be a minimum of 8.4 nurses and 3.6 nursing assistants.

It is important to explain and appreciate that the hours of care required are on a per-patient basis and represent an average (Finkler, Kovner, & Jones, 2007). The categories of the classification system, as reliable and valid as they may be, are not able to capture every patient need. Thus, in a category 4 or any category, the individual patient may require a few less minutes or a few more minutes. This is one of the driving reasons that nursing care is not reimbursed on a per-nurse basis or per-treatment basis as is medical care for physician providers. Nursing care requires a holistic assessment and determination of need. The fact that an individual has a fractured hip repaired with a hemiarthroplasty means that a certain number of hours of care are required. However, if the patient has a cardiac condition as a comorbidity, additional hours may be required if the patient experiences a dramatic decrease in blood pressure. There is no known system that can capture this nuance. However, it is understood that the number of nurses and aides available on a given shift determines the maximum hours of care that can be delivered. As the CNL understands this patient/staffing matrix as a frontline contributor, he or she can and should act as an advocate for patients and staff when ratios are inadequately represented, as they can be in the real world.

A productivity ratio may be calculated to determine the effectiveness of care delivery in terms of staffing. This number is calculated as hours of care needed divided by hours of care available. Thus, if 84 hours are needed and 84 hours of care are available, the productivity is 100%. There is an inherent fallacy in productivity numbers when a clock is utilized in patient care delivery, as it is with CNLs. However, it is important to understand how hours are calculated so that the CNL can understand the ratio when presented with these data.

Conclusion

The CNL has a very powerful role to fill when it comes to economics and healthcare finance. While not the manager, the CNL must understand finance to make the most appropriate decisions in regard to services provided, by whom, and for what length of time. The CNL is on the frontline at the point of care delivery and must recognize his or her role in educating staff about resource utilization, making recommendations to management and other providers about disease management and use of standardized protocols, ensuring the systems are in place to reduce system error, assisting environments to reduce human error, assigning the appropriate provider to care delivery, and ensuring that all charges incurred are assessed and tracked to the appropriate cost center. Each of these is an essential function within the CNL role and all are directly related to finance and economics. No one factor is more important than any other. When achieved in combination, financial solvency is not assured, but it is certainly on the path to achievement. The Commission on Nurse Certification includes many topics of economics and finance in the certification blueprint for CNLs (Table 16.1).

TABLE 16.1 Healthcare Finance and Economics

CATEGORY	WEIGHT
B. Healthcare Finance and Economics	**5%**
1. Identifies clinical and cost outcomes that improve safety, effectiveness, timeliness, efficiency, quality, and client-centered care	
2. Serves as a steward of environmental, human, and material resources while coordinating client care	
3. Anticipates risk and designs plans of care to improve outcomes	

(continued)

TABLE 16.1 Healthcare Finance and Economics *(continued)*

CATEGORY	WEIGHT
B. Healthcare Finance and Economics	**5%**
4. Develops and leverages human, environmental, and material resources	
5. Demonstrates use of healthcare technologies to maximize healthcare outcomes	
6. Understands the fiscal context in which practice occurs	
7. Evaluates the use of products in the delivery of health care	
8. Assumes accountability for the cost-effective and efficient use of human, environmental, and material resources within microsystems	
9. Identifies and evaluates high-cost and high-volume activities	
10. Applies basic business and economic principles and practices	
11. Applies ethical principles regarding the delivery of healthcare in relation to healthcare financing and economics, including those that may create conflicts of interest	
12. Identifies the impact of healthcare financial policies and economics on the delivery of healthcare and client outcomes	
13. Interprets healthcare research, particularly cost and client outcomes, to policy makers, healthcare providers, and consumers	
14. Interprets the impact of both public and private reimbursement policies and mechanisms on client care decisions	
15. Evaluates the effect of healthcare financing on care access and patient outcomes	

Used with permission from the Commission on Nurse Certification (2011, 2014).

Resources

Centers for Disease Control and Prevention. (2015a). *Statistics overview*. Retrieved from http://www.cdc.gov/hiv/statistics/overview/index.html

Centers for Disease Control and Prevention. (2015b). *National vital statistics reports*. Retrieved from http://www.cdc.gov/nchs/products/nvsr.htm

Cleverly, W., Song, P., & Cleverly, J. (2011). *Essentials of health care finance* (7th ed.). Sudbury, MA: Jones & Bartlett Learning.

Commission on Nurse Certification. (2011). *Clinical Nurse Leader job analysis report*. Retrieved from http://www.aacn.nche.edu/cnl/Job-Analysis-Report.pdf

Commission on Nurse Certification. (2014). *Clinical Nurse Leader (CNL®) certification exam blueprint*. Retrieved from http://www.aacn.nche.edu/leading-initiatives/cnl/cnl-certification/pdf/ExamContentOutline11.pdf

Finkler, S., Kovner, C., & Jones, C. (2007). *Financial management for nurse managers and executives* (3rd ed.). St. Louis, MO: Saunders.

Harris, J., & Roussel, L. (2010). *Initiating and sustaining the clinical nurse leader role.* Sudbury: MA, Jones & Bartlett Learning.

Kelly, A. (2011). Treatment intensity at end of life—time to act on the evidence. *The Lancet, 378*(9800), 1364–1365. doi:10.1016/S0140-6736(11)61420-7.

Kocharek, M., Xu, J., Murphy, S., Minino, A., & Kung, H. (2014). *Deaths: Preliminary data for 2009.* Retrieved from http://www.cdc.gov/nchs/deaths.htm

Kwok, A., Semel, S., Lipsitz, S., Bader, A., Barnato, A., Gawande, A., & Jha, A. (2011). The intensity and variation of surgical care at the end of life: A retrospective cohort study. *The Lancet, 378*(9800), 1408–1413. doi: 10.1016/S0140-6736(11)61268-3.

Larkin, H. (2011, October). Smart money management. *Hospitals & Health Network.* Retrieved from http://www.hhnmag.com/articles/4508-smart-money-management

MacDorman, M. F., & Mathews, T. J. (2009, November). Behind international rankings of infant mortality: How the United States compares with Europe. *NCHS Data Brief,* No. 23.

OECD Health Data 2012: Health expenditure and financing. OECD Health Statistics (database). Retrieved from https://data.oecd.org/healthres/health-spending.htm

Ott, K., Haddock, S., Fox, S., Shinn, J., Walters, S., Haridin, J., . . ., Harris, J. (2009). The clinical nurse leader: Impact on practice outcomes in the Veterans Health Administration. *Nursing Economics, 27*(6), 363–370.

World Bank. (2016). *Health expenditure, total (% of GDP).* Retrieved from http://data.worldbank.org/indicator/SH.XPD.TOTL.ZS

17

Healthcare Systems/Organizations

Dawn Marie Nair and Stephanie Collins

The clinical nurse leader (CNL) practice model and role were developed and implemented in collaboration with leaders in nursing education and practice to address the current and future needs of the healthcare system and, most importantly, to provide quality patient care outcomes. This chapter will review the current state of healthcare systems, organizations, unit-level healthcare delivery, and microsystems, as well as CNL competencies in these areas.

Current State of Healthcare Systems/Organizations

It is no secret that our current healthcare system is in chaos. Many people are involved with patient care but working in silos, all working hard but not efficiently and not always safely. According to Lee and Mongan (2009), who elaborate on chaos in healthcare in their book *Chaos and Organization in Health Care*, the answer is organization. Yes, simply put, but not easily solved. We know additional spending in healthcare is not the answer, so where should we begin? Understanding where the center or nucleus of the healthcare environment is located may be the best place to begin organizing care. In every instance, the core of care is with a single patient, group of patients, or population of patients. It is here that change in the way we provide care will have the greatest impact in organizing the chaos.

A CNL is directly involved and responsible for many aspects of care in the healthcare environment. Being in a position to make necessary changes to improve care can be an enormous challenge. To fully assess the system or environment, a CNL must have a clear understanding of the structure, function, and goals that are in place, from the top of the organization to the bedside. The basic healthcare system can be broken down to gain perspective. First, the structure of our healthcare system is composed of three essential elements: the frontline clinical microsystems, mesosystems, and the all-encompassing macrosystems. According to Nelson et al. (2008), there are three fundamental assumptions in relation to these elements:

- Bigger systems (macrosystems) are made of smaller systems.
- These smaller systems (microsystems) produce quality, safety, and cost outcomes at the frontline of care.
- Ultimately, the outcomes of a macrosystem can be no better than the outcomes of the microsystems of which it is composed.

Leading Microsystems—A Role for the CNL

The term *microsystem* is used to describe the small, functional, frontline units that provide the most healthcare to most people—and is essential to designing the most efficient, population-based services (Godfrey, Nelson, Wasson, Mohr, & Batalden, 2003). Clinical microsystems have become the focus for improvement of healthcare within our rapidly changing healthcare system/organizations. This approach can offer senior leaders a strategy and execution framework for competing in an increasingly competitive, data transparent, and value-seeking medical marketplace.

Why is the CNL a needed role in the healthcare system? First, it is a known fact that providing continuity of care to a complex and aging population is a challenge with no available silver-bullet solution. The high cost of healthcare in this country can be contributed to fragmented care, medical errors associated with poor communication, confusion due to health professionals working in silos, frustration, poor outcomes, and increased waste. As a result, insurance companies are changing reimbursement policies for complications they deem to have resulted from poor or fragmented care. The CNL is therefore an intervention in changing the current model of healthcare that is driving up costs and waste by targeting patient care on the frontlines. The CNL will improve the current model through better control of resources, provide patient-focused care, and improve the outcomes with measurable goals. It is in achieving these goals that the CNL establishes the specific patient-focused solutions to the healthcare needs of patients, decreases medical errors and length of stay, and increases patient satisfaction. The CNL relies on research as evidence for the patient-focused healthcare solutions that are implemented.

Leadership Style

A microsystem has lots of moving parts and needs motivated leaders. This is where the CNL is needed in order to promote patient safety, retain nursing staff, and maintain quality improvement. Leadership development today includes information on both transformational and transactional leadership. A *transformational leader* must have charisma, the ability to inspire and intellectually stimulate its followers, and be able to take individual consideration of each member of the team (Bass, 1990). A transformational leader is able to spark the interests of an organization's employees while keeping a larger purpose in mind. Employees often want to identify with a transformational leader because they know they will be able to accomplish great things under the leader's guidance. There is a sense of trust in their relationship. What was once considered a problem at work changes into a challenge to be solved. When you have this type of effective leadership, organizations tend to do better financially (Bass, 1990).

A *transactional leader* is task-oriented and only intervenes when standards are not being met. The focus is given to only those who are performing well; those who are doing poorly get punished. The employees who follow the rules get financial awards and job advancement. This environment does not give much room for creativity or problem solving (Bass, 1990). When employees advance into leadership roles, they tend to replicate their leader's guidance. Followers who were inspired by their managers tend to be great motivators in leadership positions. Followers who are shaped by reward and punishment tend to continue this type of conditioning when they become managers (Watts & Corrie, 2013).

Being an exceptional clinical nurse does not necessarily mean one will be an outstanding leader. Nurses tend to take on managerial roles without adequate education or support. In today's healthcare environment, managers are required to improve standards of care and patient satisfaction scores while maintaining costs. A transformational leader is committed to a larger vision and has attachment to the organization. Employees feel a greater sense of affiliation and loyalty to the job with a transformational leader. This type of environment is conducive to problem solving and research. Employees are part of decision making and feel as though their contributions are valued. Open door policy allows for mentorship between the transformational leader and each individual employee. An optimistic leader has a positive impact on the team's morale (Curtis & O'Connell, 2011).

Understanding Complexity Theory

As far back as the 1960s, the view of healthcare systems was compared to being a machine, or, to be successful, a well-oiled machine. It followed traditional systems theory (Senge, 1990) that has roots in explaining the behavior of "dead" systems. This explains the closed system where individual organizations were not as dependent on the community. Today, healthcare organizations consist of multiple organizations dependent on each other within the system to survive. Open-ended systems have therefore taken over in healthcare with the newer metaphor of healthcare organizations being a living organism, not a machine. Such a metaphor is conveyed by the science of complex adaptive systems, which reformulates systems theory in a way that produces a "model" of the organization more closely related to reality.

Today's healthcare is an ever-changing entity. *Complexity leadership* is not just a new way to lead, but also a new way of thinking that is radically different from the linear, top-down approach many have experienced in healthcare (Crowell, 2011, p. 2). Complexity leadership is based on complexity science, the study of complex adaptive systems. It considers the pattern of relationships in the system, how they are sustained, how they self-regulate and self-organize, and how outcomes emerge (Crowell, 2011, p. 3). In this model, all things are connected and the systems thrive on this relationship (see Table 17.1).

When complexity theory is applied to today's nursing leadership, a model emerges and it draws structure from three key concepts. The complexity leadership model (Crowell, 2011, p. 4) emphasizes:

- Knowledge of complexity science and its application to the organization
- Leadership style that is transformational, self-reflective, collaborative, and relationship based
- Personal being and awareness that utilizes self-care practices to sustain the personal strength and courage needed to lead in a complex environment

These key concepts prepare a healthcare leader to expect the unexpected and model a professional life of continued improvement. When one understands the enormity of the components making up the organization, in addition to the ever-changing external factors, one can learn to survive and thrive in the constant chaos. A leader who understands and appreciates the benefits of complex organization will also appreciate the benefits of this environment. Complex adaptive systems have the following key features (Crowell, 2011, p. 34):

- Diverse independent agents interact and adapt to change locally.
- New behavior, ideas, patterns, and structure emerge from relationships.
- Results are often nonlinear, unpredictable, and surprising.
- Self-organization occurs with distributed leadership and simple rules.

TABLE 17.1 Complexity Science Versus Established Science

COMPLEXITY SCIENCE	ESTABLISHED SCIENCE
Holism	Reductionism
Indeterminism	Determinism
Relationships among entities	Discrete entities
Nonlinear relationships	Linear relationships
Critical mass thresholds	Marginal increases
Quantum physics	Newtonian physics
Influence through iterative nonlinear feedback	Influence as direct result of force from one object to another
Expect novel and probabilistic world	Expect predictable world
Understanding; sensitivity analysis	Prediction
Focus on variation	Focus on averages
Local control	Global control
Behavior emerges from bottom up	Behavior specified from top down
Metaphor of morphogenesis	Metaphor of assembly

Source: Dent (1999).

Traditional Systems Thinking

For a CNL to understand how to emerge with complex adaption principles, it is first important to understand the results of traditional systems thinking. Traditional systems thinking has created a vicious cycle of (a) designing a system and (b) when the system does not act as predicted, redesigning the system. The assumption according to Begun, Zimmerman, and Dooley (2003) is that leaders can control the evolution of complex systems by intentions and clear thinking. Complexity science leads one to ask different questions. For example, when an intended intervention does not play out as predicted, how do things continue to function? The common result is that "things get done anyway." How do patients continue to get care, and clinicians provide care, despite the machinations of formal organizations? Complexity science focuses on how this "anyway" behavior unfolds through everyday interactions and in spite of the fact that leaders continue to focus on the "systems" that attempt to secure predicted changes. The challenge for the CNL is to stick with the lateral integration approach to overseeing patient care. The CNL can intervene, facilitate, or coordinate care for individual patients, groups of patients, and populations of patients in the community using complexity theory to identify areas in need of improvement.

It is through this research that service sector leaders were identified as the source of power and scope in the frontline interface that connected the organization's core competency with the needs of an individual customer. The CNL's critical role is to lead the frontline staff in line with the organization's core competencies. How does this happen? The CNL can be guided by recent research by Donaldson and Mohr (2000a, 2000b), who identified eight dimensions that were associated with high quality in high-performing clinical microsystems:

- Constancy of purpose (goal is the same for all)
- Investment in improvement (dollars invested when needed)
- Alignment of role and training for efficiency and staff satisfaction (staff and other stakeholders give buy-in)
- Interdependence of care team to meet patient needs
- Inclusion of all members involved in the process of meeting the goal
- Integration of information and technology into workflow (utilizing benchmarks through statistics and data collection)
- Ongoing measurement of outcomes (real-time data to compare pre- and postinterventions)
- Supportiveness of the larger organization

Additionally, Nelson et al. (2008) surveyed 20 high-performing clinical microsystems (small groups of people who work together regularly to provide care to a discrete population of patients) and found that the microsystems shared a set of primary success characteristics that interacted with one another to produce a synergistic outcome:

- Leadership of microsystem
- Macrosystem support of microsystem
- Patient focus
- Staff focus
- Interdependence of care team
- Information and information technology
- Process improvement
- Performance result

Unit-Level Healthcare Delivery/Microsystems of Care

Clinical microsystems can be reduced into smaller, more manageable pieces or units that can allow for rapid diffusion of change across the nursing division. In a unit where care is generally focused on a set of patients, a CNL can integrate emerging nursing science into practice and lead efforts to enhance patient care. The American Association of Colleges of Nursing (AACN) white paper (2007) describes the competency that a CNL will execute through the following actions:

- Accountable for healthcare outcomes within a unit and in line with the meso- and macrosystems goals.
- Assimilates and applies research-based information to design, implement, and evaluate the client plans of care.
- Synthesizes data, information, and knowledge to evaluate and achieve optimal client and care environment outcomes through measures of unit outcomes.
- Uses appropriate teaching/learning principles and strategies as well as current information, materials, and technologies to facilitate the learning of clients, groups, and other healthcare professionals.

TABLE 17.2 Successful Characteristics of High-Performing Clinical Microsystems

CHARACTERISTIC	DEFINITION
Leadership	The role of leaders is to balance setting, reach collective goals, and empower individual autonomy and accountability through building knowledge, pursuing respectful action, reviewing, and reflecting.
Organizational support	The larger organization looks for ways to support the work of the microsystem and coordinates the hand-offs between microsystems.
Staff focus	There is selective hiring of the right kind of people. The orientation process is designed to fully integrate new staff into culture and work roles. Expectations of staff are high regarding performance, continuing education, professional growth, and networking.
Education and training	All clinical microsystems have responsibility for the ongoing education and training of staff and for aligning daily work roles with training competencies. Academic clinical microsystems have the additional responsibility of training students.
Interdependence	The interaction of staff is characterized by trust, collaboration, willingness to help each other, appreciation of complementary roles, respect, and recognition that all contribute individually to a shared purpose.
Patient focus	The primary concern is to meet all patient needs—caring, listening, educating and responding to special requests, innovating to meet patient needs, and offering smooth service flow.
Community and market focus	The microsystem is a resource for the community; the community is a resource for the microsystem; the microsystem establishes excellent and innovative relationships with the community.

(*continued*)

TABLE 17.2 Successful Characteristics of High-Performing Clinical Microsystems *(continued)*

CHARACTERISTIC	DEFINITION
Performance results	Performance focuses on evaluating patient outcomes, reducing avoidable costs, streamlining delivery, using data feedback, promoting positive competition, and conducting frank discussions about performance.
Process improvement	An atmosphere for learning and redesign is supported by the continuous monitoring of care, use of benchmarking, frequent tests of change, and a staff that has been empowered to innovate.
Information and information technology	Information is *the* connector—staff to patients, staff to staff, needs with actions to meet needs. Technology facilitates effective communication and multiple formal and informal channels are used to keep everyone informed all the time, listen to everyone's ideas, and ensure that everyone is connected on important topics.

Source: Nelson et al. (2007).

The CNL is positioned to mentor, coach, and lead multidisciplinary teams to evolve and sustain a culture of safety, utilizing evidence-based practices and quality improvement (Table 17.2). Nelson, Batalden, and Godfrey (2007) provide a series of questions and exercises for the CNL to incorporate in leading interdisciplinary teams through a microsystem assessment. It is necessary to establish the condition of the microsystem (health), make obvious the areas requiring attention (diagnosis), and provide the solutions (treatment) to be evaluated by the team. Here are sample questions for the CNL to answer in order to evaluate the microsystem and to develop goals in line with the macrosystem:

- What is the aim or purpose of the microsystem?
- Who is the small population of people who benefit from this aim?
- Whom do you work with daily (administratively, technically, and/or professionally)?
- What information and information technology is part of the daily work?
- How do you measure outcomes for the population?

Assessing the Microsystem

In order to assess in a systematic and thorough manner, a framework or tool is frequently employed, which makes the process more defined rather than asking a group of random questions. One specific framework that offers a deliberate structure for CNLs to assess microsystems for quality improvement is the 5P (purpose, patients, professionals, processes, and patterns) framework. Each P has a definition associated with it, and these categories set a framework for the development of themes and aims (Nelson et al., 2007). When the 5Ps are reviewed and the team has chosen the area for improvement, it is essential to identify team roles, responsibilities, and ground rules. These then become the agreed-on guiding principles, rules, and accountabilities for each member of the team. When decided, a written agreement defining what the team goal is going to accomplish and how success will be measured is recorded in a team charter (Harris & Roussel, 2013). Templates and formats can be found on the Internet if none are available in the organization. Here are some general criteria found in a charter: project title, description of the project, scope of the project, specific problem to be addressed, criteria for success, time commitment, team member roles, process to be performed, decision-making process, conflict management process, communication plans, and expectations of team members (review of minutes, checking e-mail/voicemail, response and turnaround times, preparation prior to meetings, and completing assignments).

In addition to identifying a project, there are several indirect key pieces to be considered for the project to be successful: starting with unit descriptors, skills, composition, and competence of the team members; presence of formal and informal leaders; interdisciplinary team relationships and communication; accountability and control over practice; support for education; experience with the quality improvement processes and resources; and readiness for change. The latter is one of the most important factors to consider when evaluating a microsystem and the readiness for implementing changes within the microsystem. Every microsystem is part of the larger organization that needs to be taken into consideration as a CNL prepares for a microsystem assessment.

The intent of a SWOT analysis is to determine the readiness of implementing a teamwork initiative within your facility.

Through brainstorming, answer the questions within each category and record your responses on the tool provided.

S—What **strengths** in your present operation can you draw on to facilitate a transition to a teamwork system?

W—What **weaknesses** in your present operation may hinder this transition?

O—What future **opportunities** exist for your department or unit under a teamwork system?

T—Organize a list of potential **threats** to implementing a teamwork system within your nursing home.

Source: http://www.ahrq.gov/professionals/education/curriculum-tools/teamstepps/longtermcare/sitetools/swotanalysis.html

INTERNAL	**STRENGTHS** *Examples:* *Special expertise, reputation, cost advantages, technology advantages, etc.*	**WEAKNESSES** *Examples:* *Limited service lines, marketing deficiencies, management or staff problems, etc.*
EXTERNAL	**OPPORTUNITIES** *Examples:* *New technology, lack of dominant competition, new markets or services, etc.*	**THREATS** *Examples:* *New or increased competition, insurance plan changes, adverse govt. policies, economic slowdown, etc.*

FIGURE 17.1 SWOT analysis.

CNL Assessing a Project Using SWOT

In order to identify aspects that may positively or negatively affect a project, the CNL will want to complete a strengths, weaknesses, opportunities, and threats (SWOT) assessment. This assessment is vital for the successful planning and implementation of a change in process or structure in a microsystem. A full SWOT assessment of the entire organization or healthcare system assists the team in developing strategies to deal with known forces, both internal and external, and to anticipate others. SWOT stands for strengths, weaknesses, opportunities, and threats, and a gap analysis of the three levels of the system: micro, meso, and macro. A SWOT analysis can take different forms, but it generally involves an objective view of internal processes and personnel (Figure 17.1).

A Model for Improvement

Microsystems are in need of continuous quality improvement. As new technology and knowledge enter into healthcare microsystems, the CNL will be a key leader in the achievement of quality indicators or measures. After microsystems are assessed and several areas or themes emerge that require change to meet quality and safety indicators, the CNL should utilize a model of improvement to establish a uniform method throughout the organization so that all CNLs in an organization have the ability to adapt to changes that apply universally. In this highly critical role, it is essential to understand how using an established model of improvement can make a difficult task a smooth process. Nelson et al. (2007) present a model for improvement referred to as the Deming cycle (Deming, 1986), which integrates the scientific process referred to as the *plan-do-study-act* (PDSA) method. This method is used repetitively to test changes in a disciplined and rapid fashion. This model was further adapted to include three key questions for leading change (Langley, Nolan, Norman, Provost, & Nolan, 1996; see Figure 17.2).

1. **What are we trying to accomplish?**

   AIM: A specific, measurable, time-sensitive statement of expected results of an improvement process. A strong, clear aim gives necessary direction to improvement efforts. The four-step process can be repeated each time an adjustment is made to evaluate the change by studying the results. Refer to this website for details regarding the PDSA method of improvement: www.hci.com.au/hcisite3/toolkit/pdcacycl.htm

   Plan—a specific planning phase

   Do—a time to try the change and observe what happens

   Study—an analysis of the results of the trial

   Act—devising next steps on the basis of analysis

2. **How will we know if the change is an improvement?**

   Measures are indicators of change. To answer this key question, several measures are usually required. These measures can also be used to monitor a system's performance over time. In PDSA cycles, measurement used immediately after an idea or change has been tested helps determine its effect.

3. **What change can be made that will result in an improvement?**

   Ideas for change or change concepts to be tested in a PDSA cycle can be derived from:

   - Evidence or results of research/science
   - Critical thinking or observation of the current system
   - Creative thinking

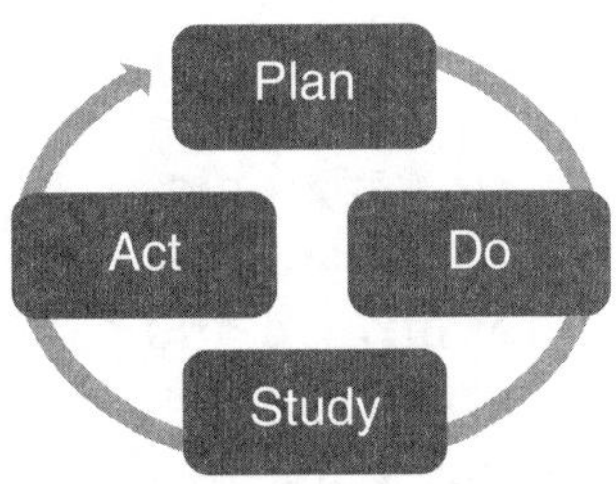

FIGURE 17.2 Continuous improvement model.

- Theories, questions, hunches
- Extrapolations from other situations

After successful PDSA cycle experimentation, a change is reached that meets the aim or goal and leads to standardization of the change throughout the microsystem. When the aim has been reached in the sample or pilot group, the adoption of this standard method is usually required throughout the microsystem. This is called the standardize-do-study-act (SDSA) cycle. The purpose of the SDSA approach is to hold the gains that were made using the PDSA cycles and to standardize the process into daily work. Often, a new or better piece of equipment or technology can come along and cause the process to shift back to the PDSA cycle again. The PDSA and the SDSA are continuous processes. Once the PDSA cycle is complete, be prepared to move back to the SDSA to refine and standardize the process. In each stage, answer questions and follow the path.

Managing Change Theory

As a CNL gathers and organizes data, the one important consideration regarding whether a change will be successful or not is to assess the readiness for change within the microsystem. To assist a CNL in organizing data in a useful way to analyze readiness and plan effectively for changes, data collection points should be based on Kotter's change theory (1996).

Kotter's theory incorporates the following eight steps:

1. Establishing a sense of urgency
2. Creating the guiding coalition
3. Developing a vision and strategy
4. Communicating the change vision
5. Empowering broad-based action
6. Generating short-term wins
7. Consolidating gains and producing more change
8. Anchoring new approaches in the culture

Kotter's theory postulates that change does not occur without adequate time placed on establishing a sense of urgency, creating the guiding coalition, developing a vision, and communicating the vision (Kotter, 1996). These first four steps in the change process are necessary to assist employees in recognizing the need for change and to embrace the process to follow. To allow time for the CNL to enact the four steps and for the employees to embrace the change, outcome data for the 3 months' postimplementation should be included in the preimplementation analysis. These baseline metrics are an important part of the evaluaton of the change. In today's data-driven healthcare environment, measures of outcomes are a crtitical component of a change process.

The Future of Microsystems With CNL Leadership

According to Lee and Mongan (2009) the sickest 5% of patients account for about 50% of healthcare dollars, with the vast majority of these patients having more than one medical issue. Cost does affect care and the ability to provide care. Microsystems are at the root of care and have therefore become the target for improving the care provided in a cost-effective way. Microsystems are currently disorganized, with providers working in silos. A potential solution is for more organized providers working together in teams. CNLs can collaborate with a shared vision to create best practice with high-quality outcomes for patients. Within each microsystem, strong leadership will be provided by a CNL, who is the steward of the ship overseeing the many improvements needed in healthcare organizations. The CNL® certification exam includes content related to general themes of healthcare systems that CNLs should be familiar with (Table 17.3).

TABLE 17.3 Healthcare Systems

CATEGORY	WEIGHT
C. Healthcare Systems	**5%**
1. Acquires knowledge to work in groups, manage change, and provide systems-level dissemination of knowledge	
2. Applies evidence that challenges current policies and procedures in a practice environment	
3. Implements strategies that lessen healthcare disparities	
4. Advocates for the improvement in the healthcare system, policies, and nursing profession	
5. Applies systems thinking (i.e., theories, models) to address problems and develop solutions	
6. Collaborates with other healthcare professionals to manage the transition of clients across the healthcare continuum, ensuring patient safety and cost-effectiveness of care	
7. Utilizes quality improvement methods in evaluating individual and aggregate client care	
8. Understands how healthcare delivery systems are organized and financed and the effect on client care	
9. Identifies the economic, legal, and political factors that influence healthcare delivery	

Used with permission from the Commission on Nurse Certification (2011, 2014).

Conclusion

A CNL is a leader in every healthcare delivery setting. It is expected that the CNL will have an understanding of the economies of care, a basic understanding of business principles, and an understanding of how to work within and effect change in systems. The CNL assumes accountability for healthcare outcomes for a specific group of clients within a unit or setting through the assimilation and application of research-based information to design, implement, and evaluate client plans of care. PDSA and SWOT are useful tools for a CNL to incorporate an organized plan of care and successful implementation of new or evidence-based interventions. Effective CNLs have the unique potential to create a new environment within the frontlines of patient care, including cost-effective, evidence-based, high-quality care within each individual microsystem.

Resources

American Association of Colleges of Nursing. (2007). *White paper on the education and role of the clinical nurse leader*. Washington, DC. Retrieved from http://www.aacn.nche.edu/cnl-certification

Bass, B. M. (1990). From transactional to transformational leadership: Learning to share the vision. *Organizational Dynamics*, *18*(3), 19–31.

Begun, J., Zimmerman, B., & Dooley, K. (2003). Health care organizations as complex adaptive systems. In S. M. Mick & M. Wyttenbach (Eds.), *Advances in health care organization theory* (pp. 253–288). San Francisco, CA: Jossey-Bass.

Commission on Nurse Certification. (2011). *Clinical Nurse Leader job analysis report*. Retrieved from http://www.aacn.nche.edu/cnl/Job-Analysis-Report.pdf

Commission on Nurse Certification. (2014). *Clinical Nurse Leader (CNL®) certification exam blueprint*. Retrieved from http://www.aacn.nche.edu/leading-initiatives/cnl/cnl-certification/pdf/ExamContentOutline11.pdf

Crowell, D. (2011). *Complexity leadership*. Philadelphia, PA: F. A. Davis.

Curtis, E., & O'Connell, R. (2011). Essential leadership skills for motivating and developing staff. *Nursing Management (Harrow)*, *18*(5), 32–35.

Deming, W. (1986). *Out of the crisis*. Cambridge, MA: MIT Center for Advanced Engineering Study.

Dent, E. B. (1999). Complexity science: A worldview shift. *Emergence*, *1*(4), 5–19.

Donaldson, M., & Mohr, J. (2000a). *Exploring innovation and quality improvement in health care microsystems: A cross-case analysis*. Technical Report for the Institute of Medicine Committee on Quality of Healthcare in America. Washington, DC: Institute of Medicine.

Donaldson, M., & Mohr, J. (2000b). *Improvement and innovation in healthcare microsystems. A technical report for the Institute of Medicine Committee on the quality of health care in America*. Princeton, NJ: Robert Wood Johnson Foundation.

Godfrey, M., Nelson, E., Wasson, J., Mohr, J., & Batalden, P. (2003). Microsystems in healthcare: Part 3. Planning patient-centered services. *The Joint Commission Journal on Quality and Patient Safety*, *29*(4), 159–170.

Harris, J., & Roussel, L. (2013). *Initiating and sustaining the clinical nurse leader role*. Sudbury, MA: Jones & Bartlett.

Kotter, J. P. (1996). *Leading change*. Boston, MA: Harvard Business School Press.

Kouzes, J., & Posner, B. (2002). *The leadership challenge* (3rd ed.). San Francisco, CA: Jossey-Bass.

Langley, G., Nolan, K., Norman, C., Provost, L., & Nolan, T. (1996). *The improvement guide: A practical approach to enhancing organizational performance*. San Francisco, CA: Jossey-Bass.

Lee, T., & Mongan, J. (2009). *Chaos and organization in health care*. Cambridge, MA/London, England: The MIT Press.

Nelson, E., Batalden, P., & Godfrey, M. (2007). *Quality by design: A clinical microsystems approach*. San Francisco, CA: Jossey-Bass.

Nelson, E., Godfrey, M., Batalden, P., Berry, S., Bothe, A., McKinley, K., …, Nolan, T. W. (2008). Clinical microsystems, part 1: The building blocks of health systems. *The Joint Commission Journal on Quality and Patient Safety*, *7*(34), 367–378.

Senge, P. (1990). *The fifth discipline: The art and practice of the learning organization*. New York, NY: Doubleday.

Watts, M., & Corrie, S. (2013). Growing the "I" and the "We" in transformational leadership: The LEAD, LEARN & GROW Model. *Coaching Psychologist*, *9*(2), 86–99.

18

Healthcare Policy

Catherine Winkler

Policy refers to standing decisions that serve as guidelines for action. *Health policy* generally denotes policy that impacts the health of the individual, families, or communities through production, provision, and financing of healthcare services. In contrast, public health policy, although it intersects health policy, can be thought of as more comprehensive, with an impact on the general population by influencing actions, behaviors, and resources through legislative, executive, and judicial branches of the government (Porche, 2012). Healthcare policy over the past 50 years focused on the medical care model and biomedical research that "medicalized" health status problems. Through this lens, policy makers assumed that the primary solution to public health problems involved medical care, which focused on financial and geographic access to personal health services for vulnerable populations (Lantz, Lichtenstein, & Pollack, 2007). Today, the emphasis in healthcare policy is on public health and population health. Policy work that targeted only medical care and access missed important opportunities to address the larger issues of poverty, nutrition, education, housing, and security. Public health policy, which is focused on social and economic causes of health vulnerability and disparities, is a better way to influence the health of the nation rather than to wait until patients fall into the "safety net" of medical care. Clinical nurse leaders (CNLs) have the opportunity to dramatically impact the changing landscape of the nation's healthcare system by merging their clinical expertise with advocacy through participation in policy.

A framework, Healthy People 2020, which identifies nationwide health improvement priorities and sets directions for health policy has expanded to population health with the goals of increasing the quality and years of a healthy life, eliminating health disparities, and creating social and physical environments that promote good health (U.S. Department of Health and Human Services, n.d.).

CNLs who use theory and research in coordinating care in an interdisciplinary healthcare team have the skill set to advise and develop policy that will be needed as the healthcare system evolves. A united voice and more strategic alliances, along with leadership and added education in policy, will be needed for CNLs to increase their influence in organizations, communities, and in national and international healthcare.

Healthcare Policy Intentions

Policy is developed with specific intentions to regulate behaviors and actions and/or allocate resources. A policy with regulatory intent proposes to prescribe and control the behavior of a particular population. A policy that is allocation focused aims to provide resources such as income, services, or goods to ensure implementation of a policy. The Patient Protection and Affordable Care Act (PPACA or ACA) P.L. 111-148 is an example of both, with the intent to improve access, decrease waste and costs, and support quality through process changes and improved outcomes. The principal stakeholders that affect policy decisions are consumers (patients and their families), providers (hospitals, physicians, nurses, pharmacists, etc.), payers (employers, insurance companies), and regulatory bodies (Department of Public Health, Centers for Medicare and Medicaid Services [CMS], etc.). Policy making is a complex, layered, and dynamic process that is influenced by the values of these stakeholders. The phases of the public policy making process include:

- Issue identification and agenda setting
- Policy formulation
- Policy adoption
- Policy implementation
- Policy evaluation
- Policy revision or amendment

Medicare is an example of a federal program that was introduced as policy through the Social Security Act of 1965 that has been evaluated and amended numerous times since its inception 50 years ago (Social Security Administration, 2014).

Policy and politics are interdependent, and this relationship is central to understanding their importance in healthcare delivery systems as well as their relevance to the nursing profession. Politics is a neutral term, although it raises negative connotations such as corruption, unethical compromises, and payoffs. Politics is actually the process of influencing the allocation of scarce resources; therefore, it is important in the process of policy development and implementation. Values are at the foundation of policy and politics. Consequently, CNLs need to be clear about the values that they hold and how they shape the policies and political strategies in which they will engage when working to improve conditions. Nursing has been voted as the most trusted profession in America for the 15th year since it was added to the Gallup poll in 1999 (Riffkin, 2015). All nurses inclusive of CNLs are in an excellent position to assume a leadership role in advancing the healthcare agenda because they are patient advocates, and the public has a high level of trust in the profession.

Policy is more important than politics, but politics were involved in healthcare reform. The present-day issue in the government is how to manage and finance the PPACA (P.L. 111-148) and the Healthcare and Education Reconciliation Act (P.L. 111-152) signed into law in 2010. This law, referenced as the Affordable Care Act (ACA), made changes in federal programs and tax policies in healthcare that included modifications affecting insurance coverage, affordability and accessibility of insurance, financing medical care, and operation of the Medicare and Medicaid programs. The ACA had and continues to have influence on the individual states in the regulation of the insurance industry, the healthcare exchanges, and the Medicaid program. The combined legislation extends coverage to an estimated 30 million uninsured Americans. This overhaul of healthcare delivery, which started in 2010, will roll out over approximately 10 years and extend access to healthcare for most, though not all, Americans.

The Congressional Budget Office (CBO) had analyzed the effects of the act under current law and the effects of proposals to change the law back in 2008–2009. The U.S. government estimated a cost of $938 billion over the next decade while reducing the federal deficit by $143 billion (CBO, 2011). However, today the CBO and the Joint Committee on Taxation (JCT) indicate that they are unable to provide a retrospective analysis and cost estimate of the ACA because they cannot separately identify costs using the agencies' normal estimating procedures. Nonetheless, one would imagine that their initial projections have likely increased in costs. On an interesting note, the CBO is able to estimate the effects of repealing the ACA, indicating that it would increase federal budget deficits by $137 billion over the 2016 to 2025 period (CBO, 2014). The repeal of the ACA has been discussed in Congress numerous times due to the expense of the program, the concern that the federal government is overstepping into state jurisdiction as it relates to Medicaid monies, and the concerns of some that the quality of healthcare will suffer. Further, the CBO goes on to qualify this estimate by stating that there is uncertainty surrounding their estimate and that, in actuality, the effects of repealing the ACA could differ substantially and move in either direction, with a reduction in deficits just as likely to occur as an increase (CBO, 2014). Both doubters and supporters of the law will continue to have concerns as the ACA regulations and appropriations are implemented and applied over the next 5 years.

Becoming skilled at influencing the legislative processes as well as the regulatory processes is important. Legislation is a law proposed by a legislative body, whereas a regulation is a specific requirement or rule within legislation. Legislation tends to be broad while the regulations reflect the details that are needed to give the law traction and allow it to be carried out. The ACA is an example of a law in effect through the legislation, but relies on regulations that guide its implementation at the state and federal levels.

The process of policy development, analysis, and implementation occurs in the context of political diplomacy and negotiation. Once the problem is identified, an agenda set, and a proposal drafted, it will be introduced into the process through the executive branch, members of the legislative branch, and/or by citizens, organizations, or special interest groups that petition the government and elected officials. Once the bill becomes a law, it moves from policy formation to implementation with a proliferation of regulations followed by operationalization. During policy development, careful analysis is compulsory to promote policy success. Nurses are in the unique position of being particularly effective in policy making because it is a natural extension of their role as an advocate and an educator in their practice. Health service's research unites with policy analysis; again, nurses inclusive of CNLs are well positioned to systematically analyze the issues and develop strategies for advancing their agenda. As Leavitt, Chaffee, and Vance (2012) state, nurses bring value to the discussions of any health policy issue because they understand how such policies affect the delivery of care and patient outcomes and can anticipate unintended consequences. Any political analysis analogous to a clinical assessment involves problem identification, a plan for possible solutions, an understanding of the history and previous attempts to correct the problem, and knowledge of the stakeholders, values, and, finally, the resources required to secure the best outcome (Table 18.1).

Healthcare Delivery System

The U.S. healthcare system is complex, involving patients, providers, and payers. It is also a mix of private and public initiatives with institutions that employ millions of workers in multiple settings to deliver healthcare services to a diverse population. The latest estimation of healthcare spending since 2013 ranges from 17.4% to 19.6% of the gross domestic product (GDP) in 2014 (CMS, 2015). According to the U.S. Census Bureau, the percentage of people with health insurance for all or part of 2013 was 86.6%, with 13.4% (or 42 million) without insurance (Smith & Medalia, 2014). Health insurance is provided through the private insurance industry (estimated at 64.2%) and by the government, with approximately 34.3% of healthcare financed by Medicare, Medicaid, TRICARE, the Children's Health Insurance Program, and the Veterans Health Administration (Smith & Medalia, 2014). The principal type of health insurance in 2013 was employment-based health insurance, which covered 53.9% of the population (Smith & Medalia, 2014). Most of the healthcare dollars spent go to hospitals (38%) and physicians (23.8%), with the balance of spending to pharmaceutical companies (11%), extended care facilities (6%), and the rest on other clinical services and administrative overhead (CDC, 2014).

The healthcare delivery system is disjointed with incentives misaligned, competing priorities, and many Americans uninsured or underinsured. An example of a misaligned incentive is in the hospital setting, where reimbursement is based on capitated payments made by Medicare called *DRGs* (diagnosis-related groups) and case rates preestablished by insurance companies. The practice of sending patients home quickly to maximize reimbursement through a shortened length of stay has an unintended consequence. Discharged patients who are still acutely ill or not fully recovered require a readmission to the hospital. In the past, the hospital had received

TABLE 18.1 Political Analysis and Clinical Assessment Parallels

STEPS	POLITICAL ANALYSIS	CLINICAL ASSESSMENT
Problem identification	Heart failure program needed	Diagnosis of heart failure
Possible solutions	Assemble team	Symptom management
	Contact experts	Education
	Develop program	Goal setting
History	Poor transition in care	Problem with fluid overload
	Patients readmitted often	Confused about medicines
	Long length of stay	
	Frequent readmission	
Stakeholders	Patient	Patient
	Family	Family
	Healthcare professionals	Healthcare professionals
Values	Cost-effective	Enhanced quality of life
	Decrease readmission rates	Independence
	Increase access	Cost-effective care
Resources needed	Time	Affordable medicines
	Money	Clear direction for symptom management
	Staff	
	Literature	Transportation
	Chronic bundle checklist	Diet assistance
Outcomes	Decrease readmissions to 10%	Improved quality of life

an additional fee for the new inpatient stay. Now, there is a disincentive or financial penalty that hospitals will incur if patients are readmitted within 30 days of discharge. This new policy will be a challenge because, although hospitals will be able to manage those patients who may have been sent home too soon, it will be quite another thing to prevent a readmission for patients who need hospitalization for another medical reason, as well as those who have broader social issues such as poverty (cannot afford medications), transportation limits (cannot make follow-up appointments), and lack the knowledge to self-manage (complexity of illness or medical regimen). Beginning in 2012, CMS carefully examined the readmissions of those patients who were diagnosed with heart failure, acute myocardial infarction, and pneumonia within 30 days of discharge. Interdisciplinary teams together with CNLs came together to carefully plan each discharge. Patients may need to stay longer in the hospital setting to begin with, require follow-up assessment and education in their home or rehabilitation facility immediately, and have continuous communication with all healthcare professionals to avoid a readmission. Medical homes, outpatient clinics, and the addition of telemedicine in remote areas have also been added to better meet the demand of patients who require ongoing care after discharge. However, even with intensive observation and care tracked and moving with the patient to the outpatient setting, some will be readmitted because of the often unavoidable disease trajectory.

The healthcare system has to deliver care on many fronts and often fails to manage the challenging needs of emergency care, urgent care, preventive care, chronic care, acute care, extended care, and home care. Each care setting, although related to each other in an episode of care, is separated financially, through payments made to each individual organization, and clinically, through breaks in communication during a transition of care period. There are plans under way to move from this payment structure (fee-for-service) to value-based purchasing and bundling of care (more discussion later in this chapter). Symptom management difficulties, complications, and readmissions follow when there is a break in the continuum of care. These two factors contribute to less efficient, more expensive care being rendered to our patients in the best-case scenario and potential harm in the worst-case scenario. CNLs need to actively engage in systems of care improvements and follow the idea that "form follows function." The form that the healthcare system takes will be the healthiest if it follows the functions or set of actions that factor in when we actively try to make a patient well. CNLs can be the catalyst of change by connecting care for the patient being discharged via comprehensive W10 forms, follow-up phone calls, and very clear medication reconciliation lists.

The traditional medical model involved complex hospital systems that focused on "sick care" with a plethora of technologies. The healthcare system of the future needs to address the continuum of care that ranges from prevention services to hospice care over multiple settings, with more targeted use of technology. Accordingly, reimbursement is moving in this direction with new incentives that promote *accountable care organizations* (ACOs) in which physicians and hospitals work together to improve outcomes and share in cost savings; as another example, medical homes tightly coordinate a patient's care within the system. Communication will be critical, whether it is between caregivers when transitioning patients across levels of care or through electronic medical records that are seamless and timely. Organizational and systems theories relate effectiveness of a system with the ability to adapt to internal and external factors to remain relevant and to survive (Chuang & Inder, 2009) as well as one that seeks to establish operational control of the patient (Brown, 2015). Operational control involves "system safety" where there is an infrastructure comprised of six safety attributes:

1. Establishment of responsibility for the system, process, or procedure
2. Authority to make changes
3. Procedures that outline instructions for routine and the nonroutine
4. Controls or checks that are real-time for the system, process, or procedure
5. Process measurements (quality assurance)
6. The interfaces or coordination of systems, processes, and procedures (Brown, 2015).

Brown's (2015) description of the system safety in aviation applies well to healthcare where there is a need to design system safety into operations with focus not only on outcomes but the process of care. The typical hierarchy in healthcare today begins with the patients and community at the base, the hospital-level healthcare system layered next, followed by standard-setting, accreditation, quality measurement, and reporting systems, with government and regulation at the top (Chuang & Inder). In 1996, Venegoni realized that change was coming in the delivery of services and identified five significant factors that would transform the healthcare system. Many of the proposed changes have occurred. The first, the site of delivery, has changed from, predominately, the hospital to other settings, including the home environment, outpatient clinics, and rehabilitation centers. The second involves diverse types of people who receive care with needs that vary in kind and intensity of care: from being well but needing a physical exam, to acutely ill requiring extensive diagnostic and therapeutic interventions. The other factor related to the second is the shift from illness to wellness care aimed at averting costs that can occur because of lack of early identification and intervention in a disease process.

Quality and customer satisfaction are also significant elements in today's healthcare climate. *Value-based purchasing*, the method of payment by CMS for in-hospital stays, which began in 2012, pays on the basis of hospital scores in patient experience or the Hospital Consumer Assessment of Healthcare Providers and Systems (HCAHPS); the processes of care (clinical guidelines, order sets, etc.) and outcomes, such as core measures; and morbidity and mortality rates. Process involves modern technology, which is ever present through the introduction of electronic medical records and the ability to send and store diagnostic testing data, as well as the overall structure for healthcare delivery (Table 18.2). Changes will continue to occur as the system expands to involve other entities contingent on the model of care that is adopted by a community, state, or government.

With the prospects of a capitated method of payment for an episode of care, the reimbursement period might be grouped. It could include a visit to a clinic, a brief hospital stay if the patient's condition worsens, and a follow-up home visit by a visiting nurse. All of this care would need to be coupled with planned communication between all caregivers; again, application of system safety would provide the infrastructure for care.

To achieve the aim of evaluating the healthcare system, there needs to be a better integration of patient safety and quality into the system, which has established links between the layers with good control and communication (Brown, 2015; Chuang & Inder, 2009). It is commonplace today to evaluate healthcare systems on the basis of how well they provide safe and effective care at a cost that is reasonable and evenly disseminated in access, quality, and cost (Russell, 2011). However, such measures remain elusive because of fragmented care that lacks synergy between the principals (patients, healthcare professionals, and payers), the organizations (hospitals, extended care facilities, physician offices, etc.), and the payers (Medicare, Medicaid, private insurance, etc.). Of course, there are many entities that evaluate healthcare systems at a global level, such as the World Health Organization (WHO); on a private level, such as The Joint Commission; and on a state level, such as the Department of Public Health. Other professional organizations, such as the American College of Surgeons, will evaluate care for trauma designation, or the American Nurses Credentialing Center will evaluate hospitals for Magnet status. Nevertheless, refining the delivery of care requires daily process improvements in practice to facilitate systemic progress in any healthcare organization. CNLs stand at the crossing where the patient enters the system needing direct care and within the system itself, which is a matter of public interest.

Economic, legal, and political factors that affect healthcare are the reasons that brought the American government and its citizens to the table to negotiate for a better future. We needed to decide whether healthcare was a human right, much in the same way that we, as a country, decided that education was a right many years ago. Americans have decided that is a "right" with the passage of the ACA and collectively, as a nation we

TABLE 18.2 Five Factors of Change Underway in Healthcare Delivery

FACTOR	CURRENT	CHANGE
Site of care	Hospital	Extended care facility Home Rehabilitation center Rural Medical home
Type of patient	Homogenous and ill	Heterogeneous and either well or ill
Healthcare model/focus	Sickness model of care Acute care	Wellness model of care Acute and chronic
Quality	Uncoupled with reimbursement	Linked to reimbursement—value-based purchasing
Technology processes	High-tech interventions	High- and low-tech interventions Electronic medical records E-mail between healthcare professional and patient

are working to decide how to regulate and finance healthcare to then implement the changes that are needed to deliver quality, cost-effective, integrated care.

Healthcare Economics

Over the next 5 to 10 years, there will be a significant shift in health plan enrollment. Fewer people will be covered by profitable private plans or employer-based plans (decreasing to 8 million), while more will join government-sponsored programs (25 million) by 2018 (CBO, 2014). Expanded coverage for the uninsured who will need to obtain insurance through state exchanges may not be enough to offset the growing number of Medicare and Medicaid beneficiaries. For many years, the hospital industry had subsidized losses incurred by Medicare and Medicaid by demanding higher premiums from commercial payers. It is estimated that the aggregate payment-to-cost ratio from Medicare was 87.9%; from Medicaid, 89.8%; and from commercial payers, 143.6% (American Hospital Association [AHA], 2015). It is estimated that this will require most healthcare systems to reduce their current operating budgets by 10% to 15%, due to the underpayments by both Medicare and Medicaid, as these patients make up more than half of the patients in the system. Uncompensated care occurs in circumstances when Medicare pays only 90 cents on a dollar and Medicaid only 89 cents on a dollar, along with services provided to those who are either underinsured or uninsured where hospitals provide care and no payment is received (AHA, 2014). States once supported hospitals when they bridged the finance gap by delivering uncompensated care to communities through tax breaks. This, too, is no longer the case when states are taxing hospitals without considering uncompensated care. Further, the anticipated rise in the number of people with health insurance coverage were expected to increase the demand for care at hospitals, as well as patient revenue from insured patients, and reduce the amount of uncompensated care that hospitals provide. Based on these assumptions, the ACA reduced Medicaid Disproportionate Share Hospital (DSH) payments to hospitals that serve a large number of Medicaid and uninsured patients to help cover the costs of uncompensated care.

This is problematic because this phenomenon only happened in states that expanded Medicaid (some states opted out due to state budget financial concerns); although there may be more patients, the reimbursement is low and often does not cover the cost of care. Medicare in 2015 also is set to decrease payments for bad debt expenses from a rate of 65% to only 25%. Since cost shiftingcost shifting does not occur as it once did, more patients need to be prepared to pay a percentage of their healthcare costs. Already, it is anticipated that high-income Medicare beneficiaries will need to pay more beginning in 2018. Taken together, this may result in further bad debt and lowered utilization of health services. Recently, many health insurance companies raised their rates; sometimes the percentage of increase was double-digit. This change caused a number of states to enact legislation to block or reduce premium increases. In addition, the federal government, through Health and Human Services (HHS), spent $150 million to regulate the insurance industry to prevent excessive rate increases. As of 2015, a few insurance companies are in the process of merging for the purposes of efficiency and to promote innovation. However, there is a concern that this will result in a monopoly with higher premiums occurring as the result and providers losing their ability to negotiate fair contracts if it results in only one local insurance carrier, which could very well be the case.

The cost of physician integration into an *accountable care organization* (ACO) may decrease the cost of care through increased efficiencies and cost sharing between the principles; however, the initial expense associated with contract negotiations, acquisition of office equipment and space, and work redesign as it relates to the staff may increase expenses due to the change in structure. Nonetheless, hospitals are acquiring physician practices to secure patient volumes. The ACA states that the ACO will only be rewarded for improving quality and increasing cost savings. This will undoubtedly be done through reducing specialty consultations, high-tech procedures, and hospital admissions as well as through health promotion and disease prevention interventions. The difficult problem with this model is that there is no evidence or previous experience with it to know if shared savings from working together will be enough to balance the loss in volume and revenue or the political capital invested in the effort.

CNLs and administrators will be critically important influences in the system for setting the course and holding all staff accountable for performance-based budgets based on best practice. Services that do not generate a profit or reduce expenses will be under consideration for discontinuation, and workforce reductions can only be avoided through work redesign efforts to eliminate waste and inconsistencies in care. In addition, a programmatic approach to chronic illnesses such as heart failure and diabetes must be taken to address the complications and comorbidities associated with these illnesses. The complexity of these chronic conditions with the education requirements to keep these patients well is in line with the CNL's role to promote health and reduce risk.

Since there are limited resources in healthcare, it is necessary to continually evaluate the intervention options. By applying six techniques to clinical decisions, it is possible to decide on the best approach in terms of priority level to treatment, intervention, and outcome (Box 18.1). When looking at the cost of illness, investigators compare one or more illnesses to determine the primacy of the condition. The investigators compare the expenditures using cost identification and minimizing techniques and, once determined, select a condition where reducing expense might be possible through the intervention type. Cost-consequence and cost-effectiveness analysis, as well as cost–benefit analysis, help to measure the pros and cons of competing interventions. As an example, pilot projects are now underway through the ACA to determine the best model for healthcare service delivery models. Rural healthcare clinics and medical homes are other currently funded projects seeking to determine their effectiveness in delivering care to segments of the population. Grant funding is available to investigate the application of navigator services to coordinate care and demonstration programs for chronically ill Medicare beneficiaries, using home-based teams as well.

In addition to a macroeconomic perspective of healthcare, CNLs are charged with integrating this knowledge into unit-level and patient-level budgeting. All too often in hospitals and healthcare organizations, budgeting, cost accounting, strategic planning, and financial and clinical analytics are disconnected, making budgeting and staffing to meet patient needs all but impossible. The case mix, census, and length of stay are a few of the variables that need to be considered when staffing a unit 24 hours a day, 7 days a week. Staffing a unit is dependent on the level of practitioner that is assigned as well as support staff, transporters, aides, and technicians. The acuity and the activity of the unit are variables that should be considered, too. A unit with very acute patients or one that has a large

BOX 18.1
Techniques for Healthcare Economic Decision Making

Cost of illness—total expenses related to care
Cost identification—summary of each expense
Cost minimization—analysis of costs and possible reductions
Cost–consequence analysis—expense associated with illness beyond care
Cost-effectiveness analysis—comparing two types of possible intervention
Cost–benefit analysis—comparing intervention versus not using it

number of admissions and discharges and short-stay observation patients will need the staff to flex to meet one-to-one direct care and/or the many admission orders and discharge instructions on any given shift. Databanks to help with calculating staffing ratios are available through the National Database for Nursing Quality Indicators® (NDNQI), with oversight by the American Nurses Association (ANA; Montalvo, 2007).

Healthcare Policy and Professional Ethics

To frame a discussion of healthcare, policy involves consideration of professional ethics. Ethics broadly has to do with right and wrong and adherence to principles. Politics, which influences the allocation of scarce resources, balances power, human rights, integrity, and equality; it is also involved when there is an occasion involving justice in the distribution of social goods, fairness and equity in relationships, and access to education, healthcare, and assistance. Professional ethics has to do with how personal norms apply or conflict with the promises and duties of one's profession (Curtain, 2012). As Curtain outlines, professional ethics is composed of its purpose or responsibility to meet society's needs, the conduct expected of the professional, and the skills and expected outcomes in professional practice. Society demands that professionals such as nurses uphold an elevated moral standard, because their clinical decisions can and do have a significant impact on the lives of others. Curtain lists the following areas where ethics come into play: human rights and the degree to which the patient exercises them; when technical options are available and choice is possible; the extent of research and learning on people; resource allocation in situations of scarcity; in futile care and patient's autonomy; in self-interest when exposed to hazards, biologic or otherwise; and with law and regulations. When considering the areas where ethics factor into clinical care, it is important to note that this too translates into policy in the exploration of public initiatives that target broad public health concerns, such as better environmental conditions, nutrition, education, and economic viability.

The most common principles encountered in ethics are beneficence (weighing benefit versus risk of an action), nonmaleficence (doing no harm), justice, and autonomy. *Values clarification* is a process used to promote clarity regarding personal and professional values that will intersect thoughts and actions in relation to policy and politics (Porche, 2012). Additionally, in 2015 the American Nurses Association (ANA) published an updated Code of Ethics which serves as a guide to nurses carrying out their responsibilities while providing quality care and meeting their ethical obligations (ANA, 2015). CNLs who are familiar with clarification of values and the ethical decision-making process will recognize that the same practice is required in the political process to avoid a conflict of interest, to problem solve, and to promote public trust.

Quality and Safety in Healthcare

Quality of care is the extent to which healthcare services for individuals and the population increase the likelihood of preferred outcomes that are consistent with current knowledge (Russell, 2012). There are two landmark documents that address quality and safety. In the first, dimensions of the healthcare system are outlined in the report *Crossing the Quality Chasm: A New Health System for the 21st Century* by the Institute of Medicine (IOM, 2001). The dimensions listed are safety, effectiveness, timeliness, efficiency, equity, and patient-centeredness. The second, *Bridge to Quality* (IOM, 2003), a follow-up to the initial recommendation for change, provides direction related to oversight, training, research, public reporting, and leadership. In the United States, we continue to spend more health dollars than any other nation, yet spending amounts and quality seem ever farther apart. When the United States is compared with other industrialized nations on equity, efficiency, and healthy life years, our scores are surprisingly poor. In fact, according to Davis and colleagues (2014) despite having the most costly healthcare system, the United States ranked last overall among 11 industrialized countries on measures of health system quality, efficiency, access to care, equity, and healthy lives. The report indicates that the United States stands out for having the highest costs and lowest performance, which seems to relate mostly to lack of adequate access to primary care, inequities, and inefficiencies (Davis et al., 2014). To enhance care there are certain attributes that are conducive to positive changes. Organizations need to build human resources through investment and training, they must deliver services, and they must finance all these activities. These organizations act as the overall stewards of the resources and powers entrusted to them. These attributes are important for policy makers as they make choices to improve health system performance. By translating research into practice, developing patient-specific evidence for effectiveness of care, and promoting needed policy change, CNLs will contribute to public health improvements.

In 2005, the Patient Safety and Quality Improvement Act was enacted to increase protection for those who reported errors. The intention of this act was to encourage reporting of medical errors to enable healthcare professionals to become more aware of problems, trend issues, and work to make system and process changes quickly to avoid error recurrence. Although there has been a shift from fear to accountability, healthcare professionals still struggle with reporting medical errors because of liability concerns or loss of work and the associated shame. *Patient safety* is the freedom from harm while receiving healthcare. Preventing avoidable harm is really the first level of quality. Institutions that demonstrate a culture of safety often have daily unit-based safety committees or huddles that serve as a forum for communication to avoid errors and secure safety. Hudson, Sexton, Thomas, and Berenholtz (2009) outline three distinct dimensions of safety that overlap to generate a safety profile for a unit. These dimensions are safety climate (compliance with rules and no-fault error reporting), teamwork climate (collaboration and communication), and positive perceptions of management (working conditions, opinions of management; Hudson et al., 2009). The safety culture with reliability and team training efforts, as well as staffing and scheduling, are part of the day-to-day work for many CNLs.

The federal government continues to put a high priority on quality through funding and has enacted legislation with the Recovery and Reinvestment Act, which allocates $1.1 billion for comparative effectiveness research. This type of research evaluates the impact of intervention options available for treating specific conditions in a particular group of patients. This research is in response to the ongoing variability that we continue to see in clinical practice as well as the concern over healthcare costs. Some see this type of research as timely, given the current depressed economic climate, whereas others worry that this will lead to fixed coverage benefits and rationing of care. As referenced earlier in this chapter, the establishment of patient operational control through a system safety approach facilitates proactively identifying, assessing, and eliminating or controlling safety-related hazards (Brown, 2015). Healthcare systems must be designed to depend on the system of care, which is established proactively rather than relying retrospectively on individuals. The "processes of care" are as important as outcomes.

Typically report cards or scorecards measure outcomes, while hospital performance and quality measures for specific indicators relate to processes. There is a current problem with the lack of standardization and regulation when it comes to quality and performance reports. The public uses them to make healthcare decisions. Still, public disclosure is generally viewed as positive because of transparency and purported accountability associated with this action. Associated ethical implications, due to lack of standardization, have led to an absence of control for data integrity, quality, or timeliness, or for the motivation and bias of quality and performance reports that are purchased by the hospital for hospital consumption (Suchy, 2010). Richard, Rawel, and Martin (2005) propose a framework for report card development and dissemination that incorporates the principles of legitimacy, unbiased data, enhanced transparency, consumer education, equitable information that is offered free of charge, and secure and private reporting of healthcare data. These activities are collaborative in nature with accountability and continuous improvement built into them. Agencies that lead the way in quality measures include the National Quality Forum, Agency for Healthcare Research and Quality, American Nurses Association, the American Medical Association, and regulatory groups such as The Joint Commission and CMS. Several other respected organizations such as the WHO, the IOM, and the Commonwealth Fund evaluate quality, access, and costs when they evaluate a healthcare system. Using external benchmarks to track and trend nurse-sensitive indicators are very important. Nurses must be at the forefront of the work to reduce adverse events and deliver patient-centered care. The NDNQI delivers evidence to support the work of the nurse by providing a national database to examine relationships between nursing care and patient outcomes.

The contribution of nurses and CNLs to the quality of care and safety of patients is significant although it is in the context of a system that is very large and where there are many moving parts that factor into the healthcare equation. Value-driven healthcare with nurse-sensitive indicators will be an area where nursing contributions can be noted and appreciated distinctly from the other dynamics. CNLs as information managers and system analysts can work at the unit level to sort out the actions that are needed to comply with HCAHPS, nurse-sensitive indicators, core measures, and other scoring procedures.

Health Services Research: Translating Research Into Practice

Healthcare research is very important to raise awareness about important healthcare issues, mobilize communities to action, and influence and inform public policy. Research can be used most effectively when it is relevant to a particular policy and local in its significance to the issue, because it helps to make the community or state official more accountable to the constituent base. Policy makers also need a reasonable solution to the problem that does not necessarily need to include the results from a robust, randomized clinical study, but they would recognize the value of surveys and pilot studies. A strong, simple message needs to be developed to communicate the problem, the effect, and the policy solution to the public and the legislators so that it can be prioritized and addressed by the right people. The relationship between the researcher and the advocate should be balanced to avoid conflict when analyzing the information and promoting a particular solution. The reason that this affiliation requires a thoughtful approach is to avoid working at cross purposes. At times the researcher will work to maintain objectivity, taking time to describe the strengths and limitations of the research, whereas the advocate might subjectively summarize the data to get to the heart of the problem as quickly as possible and to advance the issue with a solution (Goldstein, 2009). As Philpott, Mahur, and GrossKurth (2002) state, "when researchers and policy makers form strategic alliances it is possible to shift policy." It works best when the relationship is started early, the data is in a form that is easy to understand, and the environment is conducive to obtaining credible results (Philpott et al., 2002).

Research can be used as a political instrument. However, translating public health and clinical science evidence into not only practice but policy requires a strategy. As an example, Ryan, Card-Higginson, McCarthy, Justus, and Thompson (2006) were able to translate research into a policy to fight childhood obesity. This work required a four-step framework that included assessing the problem, implementing individual- and population-level interventions, and conducting surveillance to monitor progress (Ryan et al., 2006).

In a policy roundtable report published in *Health Services Research* in 2005, Mitch Greenlick, PhD, who is also a Democratic representative from Oregon, indicated that it was important to develop the answer years before the question is asked. As he points out, often the questions are the same ones asked years before that had been left unsolved even though they were important. He also indicated that there is a difference between a policy expert and an advocate because a researcher needs to be careful not to wrap science in values or in the position that one is advocating. Subsequently, it is important to know the difference between a point estimate and a confidence interval and that it is not the details of the sample size or confidence interval that are needed or even wanted, but rather a solid estimate so that focus can move off of the data and onto the solution to the problem (Foltz, 2005).

CNLs who use evidence-based research to inform their practice should use this same approach when participating in public health policy and health services research. In health services research, where the emphasis is on controlling costs, increasing efficiencies, expanding access to care, and improving quality and safety, CNLs who are familiar with qualitative and quantitative research methods and publicly available datasets (U.S. Department of Health and Human Services, Centers for Disease Control, American Hospital Association, American Nurses Association, etc.)

are very competent in conducting research and addressing healthcare problems. Box 18.2 includes a list of policy institutes, resources, and journals that are helpful for healthcare policy research.

BOX 18.2
Examples of Resource References in Health Policy for the CNL

POLICY INSTITUTES
Brookings Institute
The Commonwealth Fund
Kaiser Family Foundation
Institute for Higher Education
Robert Wood Johnson
Institute of Medicine
POLICY RESOURCES
Centers for Disease Control and Prevention: www.cdc.gov
Healthy People 2020: www.healthypeople.gov
The Joint Commission: www.jointcommisssion.org
Department of Health and Human Services: www.hhs.gov
Centers for Medicare and Medicaid Services: www.cms.gov
U.S. Congressional Budget Office: www.cbo.gov
POLICY JOURNALS
Health Affairs
Journal of Public Health
Journal of Healthcare Management

TABLE 18.3 Health Policy Certification Exam Content

CATEGORY	WEIGHT
D. Healthcare Policy	**4%**
1. Acknowledges multiple perspectives when analyzing healthcare policy	
2. Recognizes the effect of healthcare policy on health promotion, risk reduction, and disease and injury prevention in vulnerable populations	
3. Influences regulatory, legislative, and public policy in private and public arenas to promote and preserve healthy communities	
4. Understands the interactive effect of health policy and healthcare economics and national and international health and health outcomes	
5. Accesses, critiques, and analyzes information sources	
6. Incorporates standards of care and full scope of practice	
7. Articulates the interaction between regulatory controls and quality control within the healthcare delivery system	

(*continued*)

TABLE 18.3 Health Policy Certification Exam Content *(continued)*

CATEGORY	WEIGHT
D. Healthcare Policy	**4%**
8. Creates a professional ethic related to client care and health policy	
9. Understands the political and regulatory processes defining healthcare delivery and systems of care	
10. Evaluates local, state, and national socioeconomic and health policy issues and trends as they relate to the delivery of healthcare	
11. Participates in political processes and grassroots legislative efforts to influence healthcare policy on behalf of clients and the profession	
12. Understands global healthcare issues (e.g., immigration patterns, pandemics, access to care)	
13. Understands the effect of legal and regulatory processes on nursing practice	

Used with permission from the Commission on Nurse Certification (2011, 2014).

Conclusion

Rising healthcare costs and patients who present with several comorbidities will need care that the CNL is responsible for and able to deliver across the practice settings. The CNL who bridges the gap between the world of clinical care and that of health policy will be able to navigate patients and other stakeholders such as physicians, hospital administrators, and members of the team through tumultuous times. Educating themselves and their patients about important health system issues and participating in healthcare reform processes are central CNL responsibilities. The system desperately needs CNLs in all practice settings to educate and involve patients in their own care, to coordinate clinical needs, to communicate effectively with professional colleagues, and to assess and monitor changes in the healthcare delivery system. The certification exam covers a broad range of healthcare policy concepts that reflect the diverse role of CNLs in this area (Table 18.3).

Resources

American Hospital Association, (2015). *Trendwatch chartbook 2015*. Retrieved from http://www.aha.org/research/reports/tw/chartbook/2015/15chartbook.pdf on 1-191-16.

American Hospital Association. (2014). Uncompensated hospital care cost fact sheet. *Health Forum, AHA Annual Survey Data, 1980–2012*. 1–3. Retrieved from www.aha.org

American Nurses Association. (2015). *Code of ethics for nursing*. Retrieved from http://www.nursingworld.org/codeofethics

Brown, J. (2015). Adverse events do not happen by accident. *Biomedical Instrumentation & Technology, 49*(23), 216.

Center for Disease Control and Prevention. (2014). *Health, United States, 2014: With special feature on adults ages 55–64.* Retrieved from http://www.cdc.gov/nchs/data/hus/hus14.pdf#102

Centers for Medicare and Medicaid Services. (2015). *National health expenditures 2013 highlights.* Retrieved from http://www.cms.gov/Research-Statistics-Data-and-Systems/Statistics-Trends-and-Reports/NationalHealthExpendData/Downloads/highlights.pdf

Chuang, S., & Inder, K. (2009). An effectiveness analysis of healthcare systems using a systems theoretic approach. *BMC Health Services Research, 9*(195), 1–11.

Commission on Nurse Certification. (2011). *Clinical Nurse Leader job analysis report.* Retrieved from http://www.aacn.nche.edu/cnl/Job-Analysis-Report.pdf

Commission on Nurse Certification. (2014). *Clinical Nurse Leader (CNL®) certification exam blueprint.* Retrieved from http://www.aacn.nche.edu/leading-initiatives/cnl/cnl-certification/pdf/ExamContentOutline11.pdf

Congressional Budget Office. (2011). *CBO's analysis of the major health care legislation enacted in March 2010.* Retrieved from http://www.cbo.gov/sites/default/files/03-30-healthcarelegislation.pdf

Congressional Budget Office. (2014). *What is CBO's latest estimate of the budgetary effects of the ACA?* Retrieved from https://www.cbo.gov/faqs

Curtain, L. L. (2012). Health policy, politics, and professional ethics. In D. J. Mason, J. L. Leavitt, & M. W. Chaffee (Eds.), *Policy and politics: In nursing and health care* (pp. 77–87). St. Louis, MO: Elsevier.

Davis, K., Stremikis, K., Squires, D., & Schoen, C., (2014). *Mirror, mirror on the wall. How the performance of the U.S. healthcare system compares internationally.* (Update 2014, The Commonwealth Fund.) Retrieved from http://www.commonwealthfund.org/publications/fund-reports/2014/jun/mirror-mirror

Folz, C. E. (2005). Health policy roundtable. View from the state legislature: Translating research into policy. *Health Services Research, 40*(2), 337–346.

Goldstein, H. (2009). Translating research into public policy. Commentary. *Journal of Public Health Policy, 30,* S16–S20.

Hudson, D. W., Sexton, J. B., Thomas, E. J., & Berenholtz, S. M. (2009). A safety culture primer for the critical care clinician: The role of culture in patient safety and quality improvement. *Contemporary Critical Care, 7*(5), 1–13.

Institute of Medicine. (2001). *Crossing the quality chasm: A new health system for the 21st century.* (Executive Summary). Retrieved from https://iom.nationalacademies.org/~/media/Files/Report%20Files/2001/Crossing-the-Quality-Chasm/Quality%20Chasm%202001%20%20report%20brief.pdf

Institute of Medicine. (2003). *Health professions education: Bridge to quality.* Retrieved from http://www.ncbi.nlm.nih.gov/books/NBK221528/pdf/Bookshelf_NBK221528.pdf

Lantz, P. M., Lichtenstein, R. L., & Pollack, H. A. (2007). Health policy approaches to population health: The limits of medicalization. *Health Affairs, 26*(5), 1253–1257.

Leavitt, J. K., Chaffee, M. W., & Vance, C. (2012). Learning the ropes of policy, politics, and advocacy. In D. J. Mason, J. L. Leavitt, & M. W. Chaffee (Eds.), *Policy and politics: In nursing and health care* (pp. 19–28). St. Louis, MO: Elsevier.

Montalvo, I. (2007). The national database of nursing quality indicators™ (NDNQI®) *OJIN: The Online Journal of Issues in Nursing, 12*(3), Manuscript 2.

Philpott, A., Maher, D., & GrossKurth, H. (2002). Translating HIV/AIDS research findings into policy: Lessons from a case study of "the Mwanza trial." *Health Policy and Planning, 17*(20), 196–201.

Porche, D. J. (2012). *Health policy: Application for nurses and other healthcare professionals*. Sudbury, MA: Jones & Bartlett Publishers.

Richard, S. A., Rawel, S., & Martin, D. K. (2005). An ethical framework for cardiac report cards: A qualitative study. *BMC Medical Ethics*, *6*(1), 3–13.

Riffkin, R. (2015). *Americans rate nurses highest on honesty, ethical standards. Gallup Poll.* Retrieved from http://www.gallup.com/poll/180260/americans-rate-nurses-highest-honesty-ethical-standards.aspx

Russell, G. E. (2012). The United States healthcare system. In D. J. Mason, J. L. Leavitt, & M. W. Chaffee (Eds.), *Policy and politics: In nursing and health care* (pp. 122–134). St. Louis, MO: Elsevier.

Ryan, K. W., Card-Higginson, P., McCarthy, S. G., Justus, M. B., & Thompson, J. W. (2006). Arkansas fights fat: Translating research into policy to combat childhood and adolescent obesity. *Health Affairs*, *25*(4), 992–1004.

Smith, J. C., & Medalia, C. (2014). *Health insurance in the United States: 2013 current population reports*. U.S. Department of Commerce Economics and Statistics Administration. Retrieved from https://www.census.gov/content/dam/Census/library/publications/2014/demo/p60-250.pdf

Social Security Administration Office of Retirement and Disability Policy Office of Research, Evaluation, and Statistics. (2014). *Annual statistical supplement to the Social Security bulletin, 2014*. SSA Publication No. 13-11700. Released: April 2015. Retrieved from http://www.socialsecurity.gov/policy/docs/statcomps/supplement

Suchy, K. (2010). A lack of standardization: The basis for ethical issues surrounding quality and performance reports. *Journal of Healthcare Management*, *55*(4), 241–251.

U.S. Department of Health and Human Services, Office of Disease Prevention and Health Promotion. (n.d.) *Healthy People 2020 framework*. Retrieved from http://www.healthypeople.gov/

Venegoni, S. L. (1996). Changing environment of healthcare. In J. V. Hickey, R. M., Ouimette, & S. L. Venegoni (Eds.), *Advanced practice nursing: Changing roles and clinical applications* (pp. 77–90). Philadelphia, PA: Lippincott Williams & Wilkins.

World Health Organization. (2015). *Health expenditure ratios, all countries, selected years: Estimates by country*. Retrieved from http://apps.who.int/gho/data/node.main.75

19

Quality Improvement and Safety

Kathryn B. Reid and Soraya Rosenfield

The clinical nurse leader roles of *quality improvement, risk reduction*, and *patient safety* provide the basis for point-of-care clinical leadership. Advanced knowledge of quality-safety principles and methodologies is core to CNL practice. This chapter reviews the underpinnings of the role of the CNL with respect to quality improvement, risk reduction, and patient safety. Environmental factors that support quality and safety are identified, and key terms are defined. Measures of quality and safety, including nurse-sensitive, safety, and core measure indicators, are described. Processes used for quality and safety improvement are highlighted. The use of informatics and a *dashboard* in relation to quality and safety outcomes management is discussed.

Background

National mandates emphasize the need for advanced nurses who are skilled in point-of-care clinical leadership to address critical problems in patient safety and quality care delivery. These include:

- A 2013 study published in the *Journal of Public Safety* estimating the number of premature deaths associated with preventable harm to patients at more than 400,000 (James, 2013).
- *Crossing the Quality Chasm* (IOM, 2001), which calls for professionals and organizations to promote healthcare that is safe, effective, client-centered, timely, efficient, and equitable (p. 6).

- *Health Professions Education: A Bridge to Quality* (IOM, 2003), which states, "All health professionals should be educated to deliver patient-centered care as members of an interdisciplinary team, emphasizing evidence-based practice, quality improvement approaches, and informatics" (p. 3).

In response to these broad mandates for healthcare delivery reforms, the role of the CNL, an advanced master's-prepared nurse, was envisioned by key stakeholders within the nursing profession. "The nursing profession must produce quality graduates who, among other things, are prepared to implement outcomes-based practice and quality improvement strategies" (AACN, CNL White Paper, 2007, p. 1). The focus of the CNL as a frontline leader at the point of care (*microsystem*) fulfills a critical role necessary to re-engineer healthcare delivery systems to improve quality and safety in today's complex care environments. A core role competency of the CNL is that of a "systems analyst/risk anticipator" who participates in system reviews to evaluate/anticipate client risks in order to improve patient safety (AACN, 2007). The Quality Improvement Task Elements in the CNL role are delineated in Box 19.1 (Tan, 2011).

BOX 19.1
Quality Improvement Task Elements in the CNL Role

1. Evaluates the healthcare outcomes through the acquisition of data and the questioning of inconsistencies
2. Leads the redesign of client care after root cause analysis (RCA) of sentinel events
3. Gathers, analyzes, and synthesizes data related to risk reduction and patient safety
4. Analyzes systems and outcome datasets to anticipate individual client risk and improve quality care
5. Understands economies of care, cost-effectiveness, resource utilization, and effecting change in systems
6. Evaluates the environmental impact on healthcare outcomes
7. Collaborates and consults with other health professionals to design, coordinate, and evaluate client care outcomes
8. Evaluates the quality and use of products in the delivery of healthcare
9. Identifies opportunities for quality improvement and leads to improvement activities utilizing evidence-based models

Source: AACN Clinical Nurse Leader Job Analysis Report (2011, p. 38).

Environmental Factors Supporting Quality and Safety

The CNL fulfills critically important linkages between the larger organization's quality–safety initiatives and implementation of these initiatives at the point of care (unit or microsystem). Several key factors provide the basis for effective quality improvement and maintenance of safe care environments at the unit level. These include concepts related to a Healthy Work Environment (HWE), described in Box 19.2, and a culture of safety, described in Table 19.1.

The American Nurses Association's (ANA) National Center for Nursing Quality also provides resources related to quality professional practice and healthcare delivery environments. More information can be accessed at www.nursingworld.org/MainMenuCategories/ThePracticeofProfessionalNursing/PatientSafetyQuality. Additional information about the National Center for

BOX 19.2
Hallmarks of a Healthy Work Environment (HWE)

- Skilled communication
- True collaboration
- Effective decision making
- Appropriate staffing
- Meaningful recognition
- Authentic leadership

Source: AACN (2005).

TABLE 19.1 Subcultures Present in a Culture of Safety and Related CNL Role Competencies

CNL ROLE FUNCTION	CNL COMPETENCIES	SAFETY SUBCULTURE CONTRIBUTION
Advocate	Effects change through advocacy for the profession, interdisciplinary healthcare team, and the client	*Leadership*
	Communicates effectively to achieve quality client outcomes and lateral integration of care for a cohort of clients	*Just* *Leadership* *Teamwork* *Communication* *Patient centered*
Member of a profession	Actively pursues new knowledge and skills as the CNL role, needs of clients, and the healthcare system evolve	*Leadership* *Learning*

(*continued*)

TABLE 19.1 Subcultures Present in a Culture of Safety and Related CNL Role Competencies *(continued)*

CNL ROLE FUNCTION	CNL COMPETENCIES	SAFETY SUBCULTURE CONTRIBUTION
Team manager	Properly delegates and utilizes the nursing team resources (human and fiscal) and serves as a leader and partner in the interdisciplinary healthcare team	*Leadership*
	Identifies clinical and cost outcomes that improve safety, effectiveness, timeliness, efficiency, quality, and the degree to which they are client centered	*Teamwork* *Communication* *Learning* *Patient centered*
Information manager	Uses information systems and technology at the point of care to improve healthcare outcomes	*Evidence based* *Communication*
Systems analyst/ risk anticipator	Participates in systems review to critically evaluate and anticipate risks to client safety to improve quality of client care delivery	*Communication* *Learning*
Clinician	Assumes accountability for healthcare outcomes for a specific group of clients within a unit or setting, recognizing the influence of the meso- and macrosystems on the microsystem	*Patient centered*
	Assimilates and applies research-based information to design, implement, and evaluate client plans of care	*Evidence based* *Learning*
Outcomes manager	Synthesizes data, information, and knowledge to evaluate and achieve optimal client and care environment outcomes	*Evidence based*
		Learning *Patient centered*
Educator	Uses appropriate teaching/learning principles and strategies as well as current information, materials, and technologies to facilitate the learning of clients, groups, and other healthcare professionals	*Leadership* *Teamwork* *Communication*

Source: Sammer et al. (2010).

Nursing Quality is discussed later in this chapter. Through advocacy for the professional practice environment itself, the CNL advances quality-safety initiatives designed for continuous outcome improvement.

Measures of Quality and Safety

Indicators of quality and safety that fall within the scope of CNL practice and oversight include safety measures, nurse-sensitive quality and safety indicators, and disease-specific core measures. The Joint Commission provides national direction for major patient safety issues through the National Patient Safety Goals (NPSG), which are updated annually (http://www.jointcommission.org/assets/1/6/2015_HAP_NPSG_ER.pdf). The NPSG for 2015 are listed in Box 19.3. The National Quality Foundation (NQF) provides national leadership to establish national priorities and goals ensuring that healthcare delivery is safe, effective, patient centered, timely, efficient, and equitable. The NQF establishes standards for measuring and reporting as well as providing education and outreach to drive continuous quality improvement in the nation's healthcare system. More information, including the complete quality standards information, is available through the NQF website at www.qualityforum.org/Home.aspx.

BOX 19.3
National Patient Safety Goals for 2015

Improve accuracy of patient identification.

- Use at least two patient identifiers when providing care, treatment, and services.
- Eliminate transfusion errors related to patient misidentification.

Improve the effectiveness of communication among caregivers.

- Report critical results of tests and diagnostic procedures on a timely basis.

Improve the safety of using medications.

- Label all medications, medication containers, and other solutions on and off the sterile field in perioperative and other procedural settings.
- Reduce the likelihood of patient harm associated with the use of anticoagulant therapy.
- Maintain and communicate accurate patient medication information.

Reduce the risk of healthcare-associated infections.

- Comply with either the current Centers for Disease Control and Prevention (CDC) hand hygiene guidelines or the current World Health Organization (WHO) hand hygiene guidelines.
- Implement evidence-based practices to prevent healthcare-associated infections due to multidrug-resistant organisms in acute care hospitals.

(*continued*)

BOX 19.3 *(continued)*

- Implement evidence-based practices to prevent central line-associated bloodstream infections.
- Implement evidence-based practices for preventing surgical site infections.
- Implement evidence-based practices to prevent indwelling catheter-associated urinary tract infections (CAUTI).

The organization identifies safety risks inherent in its patient population.

- Identify patients at risk for suicide.

Universal Protocol for Preventing Wrong Site, Wrong Procedure, Wrong Person Surgery™.

- Conduct a preprocedure verification process.
- Mark the procedure site.
- Perform a time-out before the procedure.

Source: The Joint Commission (2015).

The Centers for Medicare & Medicaid Services (CMS) also advances national quality initiatives through various mechanisms, such as the Hospital Quality Initiative (HQA). The American Nurses Association (ANA), in conjunction with the University of Kansas, maintains the National Database for Nursing Quality Indicators® (NDNQI); these indicators are listed in Box 19.4 (Montalvo, 2007). Many of these indicators are also endorsed by the NQF (as noted in the box).

Processes Used for Quality and Safety Improvement

With the CNL focus on point-of-care leadership, the use of a microsystem framework provides a valuable organizing framework. Microsystem improvement processes center on a comprehensive microsystem assessment using the "5Ps" approach (Box 19.5), followed by careful analysis of the "metrics that matter," as previously described. Processes used for point-of-care quality and safety improvement include application of a systematic methodology. Eight common steps in quality improvement are listed in Box 19.6 (Harris & Roussel, 2010). Other commonly used quality improvement methodologies include Plan-Do-Study-Act (PDSA), Lean, and Six Sigma. Continuous quality improvement processes are enhanced by the use of a quality-safety dashboard system, which the CNL accesses to track and monitor quality-safety data on a regular basis to help inform staff and drive change.

BOX 19.4
National Database of Nursing Quality Indicators® (NDNQI)

1. Patient falls*
2. Patient falls with injury*
3. Pressure ulcers
   a. Community
   b. Hospital-acquired*
   c. Unit-acquired
4. Skill mix*
5. Nursing hours per patient day*
6. RN surveys
   a. Job satisfaction
   b. Practice environment scale*
7. RN education and certification
8. Pediatric pain assessment cycle
9. Pediatric IV infiltration rate
10. Psychiatric patient assault rate
11. Restraints prevalence*
12. Nurse turnover*
13. Hospital-acquired infection (HAI)
    a. Ventilator-associated pneumonia (VAP)*
    b. Central line-associated bloodstream infection (CLABSI)*
    c. Catheter-associated urinary tract infection (CAUTI)*

*NQF-endorsed standard.

Source: Montalvo (2007).

BOX 19.5
Microsystem Assessment: The "5Ps"

1. Purpose: What is the purpose or overall mission of the setting?
2. Patients: What are the characteristics of the patients served by the setting?

(*continued*)

BOX 19.5 (*continued*)

3. Professionals: Who are the individuals involved in delivering care in the setting?
4. Processes: What are the processes involved in delivering care?
5. Patterns: What are the patterns observed in care delivery?

The New Age of Quality Improvement and Patient Safety

In the past, there have been many internal and external factors driving organizations to pursue optimal outcomes for consumers of healthcare in many settings. Recent implementation of pay-for-performance initiatives have put new and urgent focus on quality, safety, and risk reduction, directly affecting the role of CNLs. Unlike some quality programs that identify nursing quality indicators, the implications of healthcare reform have a compelling financial impact on organizations and are truly associated with all disciplines. The implications for the CNL are many. The CNL competencies related to a culture of safety (Table 19.1) are perfectly suited to enable CNLs to lead or significantly contribute to the emerging role of interdisciplinary improvement teams.

Let us take, for example, the issue of avoidable rehospitalizations. The CMS has identified this issue as one of the first areas to implement pay-for-performance mandates for Medicare patients. The rationale for this prioritization stems from data that indicate up to 20% of Medicare patients discharged from hospitals are readmitted within 30 days, and of those readmissions, up to 76% are potentially avoidable (Hackbarth, Reischaucer, & Miller, 2007). It is worth noting that a 2013 study showed that the most recent rate of readmission has been 19.2% nationally (Gerhardt et al., 2013). Healthcare systems across the country are addressing this issue with renewed enthusiasm, knowing that this is only the beginning of a new era of quality outcomes that will impact the organization's bottom line.

A topic such as the readmission of patients requires an understanding of both the larger system and the microsystems in which patients receive care as well as the global and specific aims of the group. It also requires the ability to develop a structured process of improvement (such as PDSA) with an established timeline. Academic preparation coupled with clinical expertise enables this master's-prepared generalist to bring a multitude of skills and talents that can be utilized in the team approach to reducing readmissions. The CNL is well versed in the benefits and challenges of working with an interdisciplinary team and can utilize and develop leadership skills to then cultivate a highly functional team of professionals, in which all voices are valued, but the top priorities of the team are addressed.

One of the key elements to any quality improvement initiative is the establishment of metrics to measure the success of the initiative. Vast amounts of data are collected in today's healthcare world based on the use of electronic medical records and other informatics advances. The role of informatics is exploding in today's healthcare, and all healthcare disciplines can benefit from working closely with informatics experts to understand the complicated world of healthcare technology. In the future of pay for performance, there will be ever increasing roles for informatics and the electronic medical record in proving compliance with accepted standards of practice. Although the CNL is not required to be the expert on all data, he or she will understand the benefit of including a data and informatics expert on the team and utilizing the skill and knowledge of that individual to support the team's knowledge of the metrics involved. The CNL should continually expand on this knowledge and facilitate increasing knowledge of informatics in both nursing and nonnursing disciplines.

Once a group of professionals has been assembled and common professional aims established for the improvement initiative, the CNL must then create a way to tackle the vastness of a topic such as hospital readmissions. The area of quality improvement has many tools that the CNL can utilize in supporting the team as it examines the task at hand. For example, a flowchart could help map patient care from the primary care setting to the emergency department (or other inpatient access point) to the inpatient areas and back to the discharge destination. A Pareto chart could help identify top readmission rates and guide the group in a focus on the top readmission issues. Cause and effect diagrams may aid in the analysis of particular problems that are identified to categorize them and address such categories. *Root cause analysis* (RCA) can be used as a tool to evaluate a particular situation and determine what happened, as well as how and why it happened. All the previously mentioned strategies serve to achieve the same goal of making changes to prevent future events. Many options are available for groups and a CNL will utilize his or her knowledge to lead the group in focusing on the specific aims and making the best use of time.

There are many areas of quality, safety, and risk reduction that have comprehensive, scholarly, and interdisciplinary work available to interested organizations. Publications regarding quality improvement, evidence-based practice, and improving patient safety are abundant. The CNL should conduct or contribute to a literature search in the area of interest. Many professional organizations have been mentioned in this chapter as excellent resources for quality work. The CNL should work with other group members to identify the most useful and highly regarded materials. Even publications of initiatives that did not lead to improved metrics by a particular group can be valuable to a team.

The CNL's ability to critically review available resources is vital. On the topic of hospital readmissions, the Institute for Healthcare Improvement (IHI) has provided extensive resources in the form of a "how-to" guide for improving transitions from the hospital to the outpatient setting in order to reduce avoidable rehospitalizations (IHI, 2011). It is a comprehensive, interdisciplinary body of work that could be a critical component to a time-efficient, productive team. The example provided here, which utilizes common practices of quality improvement as listed in Box 19.6, will eventually inform a structured plan of action. For more information on the resources to prevent readmissions, visit www.IHI.org.

The example of preventing hospital readmissions illustrates the value of the CNL throughout the team improvement process. Just a few elements of that value have been described in relation to getting the improvement team started in the right direction. CNLs have had both the academic and clinical preparation to support the success of interdisciplinary groups as they move through each phase of the project and then onto the challenge of sustainability. A key element of quality and safety is the ongoing presence of the CNL in the clinical setting, supporting direct care members as they attempt to improve outcomes as well as sustaining multiple improvement initiatives. The CNL serves as the vital link between information from various sources and its utilization by frontline caregivers, a link so critical to the culture of safety.

BOX 19.6
Eight Common Steps in Quality Improvement

1. Establish a clear and defined aim or purpose
2. Review the literature
3. Examine current resources available to facilitate quality improvement
4. Map current processes
5. Analyze root cause
6. Select appropriate tools for process analysis
7. Select measures and metrics (baseline and outcome)
8. Conduct rapid cyclical review of the plan, data, interventions, and outcomes

Sources: Solecito and Johnson (2006); Harris and Roussel (2010).

Conclusion

There is a vital connection between the CNL and the new era of quality and safety. The master's-prepared clinical expert is perfectly equipped to be a driving force, facilitator, and valued team member in the work that is to be done. Even in the few years since the CNL was envisioned and became a reality, major changes to healthcare and the financial implications of quality improvement have created a new world of opportunities for CNLs to be the link between the front line of care and the chief officers of the organization. CNLs will impact quality and safety in every healthcare setting and support safe and patient-focused transitions of care. The certification exam for CNLs covers many aspects of quality improvement and the various competencies involved in improved outcomes for patients (Table 19.2).

TABLE 19.2 Quality Management

CATEGORY	WEIGHT
E. Quality Improvement	**6%**
1. Evaluates healthcare outcomes through the acquisition of data and the questioning of inconsistencies	
2. Leads the redesign of client care following RCA of sentinel events	
3. Gathers, analyzes, and synthesizes data related to risk reduction and patient safety	
4. Analyzes systems and outcome datasets to anticipate individual client risk and improve quality care	
5. Understands economies of care, cost-effectiveness, resource utilization, and effecting change in systems	
6. Evaluates the environmental impact on healthcare outcomes	
7. Collaborates and consults with other health professionals to design, coordinate, and evaluate client care outcomes	
8. Evaluates the quality and use of products in the delivery of healthcare	
9. Identifies opportunities for quality to improvement and leads improvement activities utilizing evidence-based models	

Used with permission from the Commission on Nurse Certification (2011, 2014).

Resources

American Association of Colleges of Nursing. (2005). *AACN standards for establishing and sustaining healthy work environments*. Retreived from http://www.aacn.org/wd/hwe/docs/hwestandards.pdf

American Association of Colleges of Nursing. (2007). *White paper on the education and role of the clinical nurse leader*. Retrieved from http://www.aacn.nche.edu

Commission on Nurse Certification. (2011). *Clinical Nurse Leader job analysis report*. Retrieved from http://www.aacn.nche.edu/cnl/Job-Analysis-Report.pdf

Commission on Nurse Certification. (2014). *Clinical Nurse Leader (CNL®) certification exam blueprint*. Retrieved from http://www.aacn.nche.edu/leading-initiatives/cnl/cnl-certification/pdf/ExamContentOutline11.pdf

Gerhardt, G., Yemane, A., Hickman, P., Oelschlaeger, A., Rollins, E., & Brennan, N. (2013). Data shows reduction in Medicare hospital readmission rates during 2012. *Medicare and Medicaid Research Review 3*(2), E1–E12.

Hackbarth, G., Reischaucer, R., & Miller, M. (2007). *Report to congress: Medicare payment policy*. Washington, DC: Medicare Payment Advisory Committee.

Harris, J., & Roussel, L. (2010). *Initiating and sustaining the clinical nurse leader role: A practical guide*. Sudbury, MA: Jones & Bartlett Publishers.

Institute for Healthcare Improvement. (2011). *How-to guide: Improving transitions from the hospital to the clinical office practice to reduce avoidable rehospitalizations*. Retrieved from http://www.ihi.org/resources/Pages/Tools/HowtoGuideImprovingTransitionsHospitaltoOfficePracticeReduceRehospitalizations.aspx

Institute of Medicine. (2001). *Crossing the quality chasm: A new health system for the 21st century*. Washington, DC: The National Academies Press.

Institute of Medicine. (2003). *Health professions education: A bridge to quality*. Washington, DC: The National Academies Press.

James, J. (2013). A new, evidence-based estimate of patient harms associated with hospital care. *Journal of Patient Safety*, *9*(3), 122–128.

The Joint Commission. (2015). *Hospital national patient safety goals*. Retrieved from http://www.jointcommission.org/assets/1/6/2015_hap_npsg_er.pdf

Montalvo, I. (2007). The National Database of Nursing Quality Indicators. *Online Journal of Issues in Nursing, 12*(3). Retrieved from http://www.nursingworld.org/MainMenuCategories/ANAMarketplace/ANAPeriodicals/OJIN/TableofContents/Volume122007/No3Sept07/NursingQualityIndicators.html.

National Association of Clinical Nurse Specialists. (2008a). *National Association of Clinical Nurse Specialists update on the clinical nurse leader. September 2005*. Retrieved from http://www.nacns.org

National Association of Clinical Nurse Specialists. (2008b). *National Association of Clinical Nurse Specialists position statement on the clinical nurse leader. March 2004*. Retrieved from http://www.nacns.org

Reid, K., & Dennison, P. (2011). The clinical nurse leader (CNL)®: Point-of-care safety clinician. *Online Journal of Issues in Nursing*, *16*(3), 4.

Sammer, C. E., Lykens, K., Singh, K., Mains, D. A., & Lackan, N. A. (2010). What is a patient safety culture? A review of literature. *Journal of Nursing Scholarship*, *42*(2), 156–165.

Solecito, W. A., & Johnson, J. K. (2006). *McLaughlin and Kaluzny's continuous quality improvement in health care*. Burlington, MA: Jones and Bartlett Learning.

Tan, R. (2011). *CNL job analysis report, 2011*. Schroeder Measurement Technologies, Inc. Retrieved from http://www.aacn.nche.edu/cnl/Job-Analysis-Report.pdf

20

Healthcare Informatics

Carol A. Fackler

Never before has the utilization of healthcare information technology been so important to the delivery of safe, quality care to the citizens of the United States. Since the groundbreaking report *To Err Is Human* (Institute of Medicine [IOM], 1999), highlighting 98,000 medical errors annually in the United States, stakeholders in healthcare from clinicians to policy makers have focused on designing better systems to measure the delivery of quality care and evaluate the outcomes of that care in ways that lead to improvement. The six aims of quality care proposed by the IOM in their report *Crossing the Quality Chasm: A New Health Care System for the 21st Century* (2001) provide a blueprint for improvement. These six aims are safe, timely, patient-centered, effective, efficient, and equitable. Implementation of the clinical nurse leader (CNL) role is one way to provide the clinical expertise needed to address the ability to achieve these aims. With the CNL's focus on quality, safety, monitoring, and evaluating the processes and outcomes of healthcare delivery, a nurse in this leadership role may serve as both a facilitator and a catalyst in improving quality care and ensuring client safety.

Now well into the second decade of the 21st century, the confluence of healthcare information technology utilization with the work of the CNL positions nursing as a key player in deciding how technology is developed, implemented, and evaluated. Health information technology is not new to the nursing profession; nursing has been involved with informatics in healthcare for a long time. As early as the 1970s, nurses were involved in interdisciplinary work developing technology to assist in the delivery of healthcare (Ozbolt & Saba, 2008). Nurses' involvement in defining nurses' work in ways that could be documented and evaluated with a variety of technology tools led to the creation of a nursing minimum dataset (NMDS; Ozbolt & Saba, 2008). Other explication of nursing work resulted in nursing diagnoses developed by the North American Nursing Diagnosis Association (NANDA) and the development of the Nursing Interventions Classification (NIC), the Nursing Outcomes Classification (NOC), and the National Database for Nursing Quality Indicators (NDNQI). Despite challenges in standardizing the language defining nursing work and operationalizing data elements reflecting the work for input into computer software, nurses have moved forward both nationally and internationally in developing and describing nursing nomenclature in ways that capture the important role that nurses play in promoting quality healthcare and client safety.

The federal government is currently taking a lead role in coordinating major efforts to implement the use of electronic health records (EHRs) across the healthcare delivery system. These efforts require the expertise of informaticists, engineers, computer specialists, healthcare administrators, and nursing leaders such as the CNL. Now more than ever, the CNL is in a position to influence what information technology is implemented as well as its ongoing evaluation. Most importantly, the increasing availability of, and variety of, technology that can be utilized, as well as the data collection that technology makes possible for assessing, monitoring, implementing, and evaluating the care of clients, enhances the CNL's ability to effect changes in clinical care processes to improve client outcomes. Technology such as the EHR makes data more available in real time to assist the CNL in making decisions at the point of care related to client outcomes. In addition, the CNL can serve as a role model to nurses in leveraging clinical data from the EHR to enhance clinical care and client outcomes using that data to "optimize workflow and support clinical decision making: tell the patient's story; collaborate to foster knowledge transaction; leverage analytics to extract actionable knowledge; use sharable, comparable data; [and] build evidence out of nursing practice" (Sensmeier, 2015, p. 24).

The purpose of this chapter is to examine the ways by which the CNL should approach the use of healthcare information technology; these include but are not limited to:

- Assessing and monitoring clients
- Planning and delivering care
- Evaluating outcomes of care
- Disseminating healthcare information among team members
- Safeguarding the privacy and confidentiality of client information
- Meeting the needs of geographically remote clients
- Recognizing the advantages and challenges of consumer use of health technology
- Analyzing existing systems to identify supports and gaps
- Participating in the development of new technologies

The CNL and the Role of Informatics

In order to serve clients in today's healthcare system, the use of information technology is essential. Today's CNL may work alongside many others with expertise in information systems, including *informatics nurse specialists* (INS). An INS must be able to understand and utilize the integrated knowledge of many elements including nursing science, information science, computer science, cognitive science, and others appropriate to specific issues (Nelson & Staggers, 2015). While this specialty of nurses with expertise in healthcare information technology is emerging, there are many settings where nurse informaticists are not employed. In the absence of an INS, it is up to the CNL to have knowledge of, and become involved with, available healthcare information technology. That knowledge includes an understanding of the relationship between nursing science, information science, computer science, and cognitive science. The CNL should be aware of what the American Nurses Association (ANA, n.d.), in its current official position statements, notes as nursing's responsibilities related to the use of health information technology. This includes the Ethics and Human Rights Position Statement on Privacy and Confidentiality, as well as the Nursing Practice Position Statements on the following:

- Electronic health record
- Electronic personal health record
- Inclusion of recognized terminologies within EHRs and other health information technology solutions
- Standardization and interoperability of health information technology—supporting nursing and the national quality strategy for better patient outcomes

Because the use of health information technology is becoming more prevalent, it is also important for the CNL to be knowledgeable about resources that provide ongoing updates of the state of the science in this discipline. Therefore, in addition to reading this chapter, prospective CNLs are encouraged to read the references cited here and refer to the web-based resources referenced in this chapter. These resources are a source of helpful information about the state of the current efforts in bringing this country's healthcare information technology into the 21st century.

Setting the Stage: The Current Climate in Health Information Technology

Since 2009, with the passage of the American Recovery and Reinvestment Act (ARRA; Pub.L. 111-5), there has been increasing attention to how the country's providers of healthcare use health information technology.

Under ARRA, monies available through the Health Information Technology for Economic and Clinical Health (HITECH) Act were earmarked for the development of the EHR. Regional Extension Centers across the country, coordinated by the Office of the National Coordinator for Health Information Technology (ONC; www.healthit.gov), are assisting healthcare providers in the implementation of certified EHRs.

Educational resources that are helpful to implement EHRs, in ways that meet federal certification guidelines, are available for both institutions and individual providers from a number of sources. For example, the ONC coordinates and supports a number of initiatives that support not only EHR development and implementation, but also other aspects of health IT (www.hhs.gov/healthit). These include initiatives related to *clinical decision support* (CDS), *cyber security*, *rural health IT*, and state-level health initiatives for *health information exchange* (HIE). The Healthcare Information and Management Systems Society (HIMSS), a global nonprofit organization with a majority of its 44,000 individual members working in healthcare, promotes the optimal use of information technology and management systems through its content expertise, professional development, research initiatives, and media vehicles (www.himss.org).

The importance of delivering healthcare using evidence-based practices makes other health information technology such as CDS essential as institutions and providers work to comply with governmental guidelines and professional practice standards. Current federal guidelines require that clinical information systems be interoperable; for example, clinical decision support systems (CDSS) developed today must be capable of being embedded into any EHR. The goal is to have all health information technological tools and systems be able to "talk" to each other.

HIEs are organizational or geographical entities that manage health information electronically across organizations or regions (McGonigle & Mastrian, 2012). Organizational and/or regional management of *protected health information* (PHI) makes it possible for the information to reside in one central location, available to all providers of care requesting that information at any point in time. Before a scheduled visit or at the time of an unscheduled visit, the patient gives consent for healthcare providers to access PHI or to send PHI to the exchange.

Consumers are becoming increasingly involved in the use of health information technology. To document and manage their personal health information, some consumers are now using a personal health record. This record, which can be managed on mobile devices as well as personal computers, may be maintained by an individual, or may be collaboratively maintained by an individual and his or her healthcare provider and/or healthcare organization. Use of a personal health record brings information and knowledge about an individual's health directly to the individual consumer, thereby addressing the quality aim of patient-centeredness.

One form of the personal health record now provided by healthcare organizations is the patient portal. The patient portal, a window into the healthcare record of an individual, is made possible through an encrypted link to an individual's primary care organization. Once registered for the portal, an individual client can access portions of his or her electronic health record such as laboratory results, problem lists, and immunization records. Patient portals also provide such functionality as the ability for the individual client to make appointments online, as well as to communicate with his or her healthcare provider.

For those who have challenges accessing the healthcare delivery system because of factors such as distance or means of transportation, *telehealth* is an alternative mechanism of delivering healthcare using state of the art technology. With this technology, consumers can share subjective and objective data with healthcare providers from the comfort of their homes, or at small clinics close to home communicating with larger medical centers. Telehealth technologies and the emerging use of mobile applications such as smartphones represent exciting possibilities for healthcare delivery to remote populations, addressing such issues as access to care, chronic care management, and client satisfaction.

It is incumbent upon the CNL to remain informed of the ever-changing climate in health information technology, a climate that is evolving as new technologies, new applications of current technologies, and increasing consumer use of information systems emerge.

Assessing and Monitoring Clients

The integration of clinical data into computer systems allows for the input and retrieval of large amounts of data on clients. That data, viewed in the context of the environment in which care is delivered, yields important information about processes and outcomes involving clients. Just a few years ago, much of the information collected on clients in any healthcare delivery system reflected only demographic, scheduling, and billing information. Today, health information technology includes the input, management, and retrieval of clinically important data. With the emergence of EHRs as the preferred method of individual health record documentation, it has become obvious just how much data are generated within the healthcare system. With the data already available since the widespread adoption of EHRs, clinicians and researchers have become aware of the potential for utilizing "big data" to evaluate processes of care and implement changes in care delivery.

Large healthcare systems have created data repositories, called data warehouses, from which important clinical indices can be retrieved to examine the processes and outcomes associated with care delivery. One notable example of such a system is the U.S. Department of Veterans Affairs Clinical Case Registries (CCR), a program that supports the delivery and evaluation of care for thousands of clients in this large national healthcare delivery system (Backus et al., 2009). Lessons learned from managing registries of clinical data from clients with HIV and hepatitis C virus (HCV) include the need for manual confirmation of electronic data, for updating software to reflect changes in clinical diagnostic and laboratory test coding, and for monitoring updated software for missing critical data elements (Backus et al., 2009). The experience of the Department of Veterans Affairs in maintaining their clinical registries underscores the significance of the human–computer interface in managing electronic information.

Access to clinical data stored in data warehouses also allows large healthcare systems to conduct rigorous research related to processes and outcomes; one example is the work of Intermountain Healthcare of Salt Lake City. Working with data collected from multiple facilities in its large network, this healthcare system has been able to examine processes such as the relationship between the amount of nursing care clients receive and client outcomes (Hall et al., 2009).

The meaningfulness of clinical data is recognized in the development, adoption, and implementation of the EHR. *Meaningful use* is the term used to denote the standards defining what meaningful data should be included in the EHR; however, challenges exist related to how to make clinically relevant data available for collection, management, and retrieval within the EHR. Data reflecting nursing care remains some of the most difficult data to capture. How to embed language reflective of nursing care into the EHR continues to be a challenge. What data should be collected has been informed by efforts such as the development of the Systematic Nomenclature of Medicine (SNOMED; www.ihtsdo.org), the Nursing Minimum Data Set (NMDS), the Nursing Interventions Classification (NIC; www.nursing.uiowa.edu), and the Nursing Outcomes Classification (NOC; www.nursing.uiowa.edu), as well as by organizations such as the North American Nursing Diagnosis Association (NANDA; www.nanda.org).

The CNL, in managing the care of a subpopulation of clients, should play an active role in decision making about what clinical data should be collected in and from the EHR and other technology tools, how that data should be managed, and who should have access to the data for the purpose of analyzing and improving care delivery processes and client outcomes. The CNL also needs to be vocal about the importance of standardizing nursing terminology in healthcare information technology. In the absence of such standardization, data that could be meaningfully related to nurses' contribution to quality, safe healthcare may be lost. As Ozbolt and Saba (2008) explain:

> Faced with the bewildering array of choices and the licensing fees required for the use of NANDA, NIC, NOC, and SNOMED, many health care organizations adopting nursing information systems opted to use their own or vendor-provided, non-standard terms. This approach allowed entry of data via familiar terms, but because the terms were not consistent in definition or usage, investigators could not retrieve meaningful data to analyze for quality improvement or research. (p. 202)

Therefore, nursing needs to be aware of and collaborate with the other professionals in understanding standard terminology used in varied disciplines and, where possible, agree on standardized nomenclature. The CNL should have an understanding of terminology used in standards not normally reviewed by nurses, such as ICD-10 coding, CPT coding, and the LOINC.

Planning and Delivering Care

The process of delivering safe, quality care requires ongoing collection, management, and analysis of clinically relevant data. The CNL may have data requiring analysis from a number of sources, including individual paper medical records, unit-based computerized reports, or aggregate data from a data warehouse. In addition, nationally benchmarked data analysis may be available from recognized sources such as the National Database of Nursing Quality Indicators® (NDNQI; www.nursingquality.org) and Press Ganey (www.pressganey.com).

Once data analysis is complete, the CNL can then share the results with the unit's interdisciplinary team, encourage feedback, and involve those on the team in decision making about change that positively impacts client outcomes. That change may come in the form of alterations in processes to deliver care or the development of new processes to address a clinical problem. Recognized approaches to implementing change may include quality improvement processes such as continuous quality improvement with its *plan-do-study-act* (PDSA) process. Guidelines for evidence-based practice changes as described by experts like Melnyk and Fineout-Overholt (2014) also serve nursing leaders and educators well in advocating for improving outcomes based on current evidence.

In the delivery of healthcare to clients, healthcare information technology itself offers a number of modalities with which to prevent errors in real time. *Computerized physician order entry* (CPOE) is a feature of the EHR that assures standardized, legible communication of the medical plan of care to other members of the healthcare team. CDSS may be embedded in the EHR, prompting clinicians in their assessment and ongoing monitoring of clients to address deficits in documentation; to consider potential outcomes related to their decision making (e.g., drug–drug interactions); or as reminders to order, for example, standard screening tests for clients. This CDS may be passive, consisting of pop-up reminders or alerts on the computer screen, or it may be more active. In an active system, the clinician is not only reminded of a drug–drug interaction, but also advised by the system about what to monitor and what other care to consider when two interacting drugs are being utilized simultaneously.

Evaluating and Improving Outcomes of Care

Evaluating outcomes of care requires an interdisciplinary approach. The CNL is in a key position to orchestrate the evaluation process, because he or she is in constant interaction with the healthcare team at the point of patient care. Evaluation of unexpected outcomes may use processes such as *root cause analysis* (RCA). Analyses resulting from such processes result in identification of changes needed to improve outcomes of care.

The CNL can foster both collaborative and collegial approaches to the delivery of safe, quality care to patients. Educated as a nurse, the CNL's educational background includes a holistic approach to care, reflecting knowledge from multiple disciplines including medical science, psychology, public health, nutrition, and information technology. Additional graduate preparation as a CNL affords further opportunities for exposure to principles underlying clinical microsystems, leadership, and the change process. This background provides the CNL with the knowledge and skills needed to identify problems, analyze data, communicate findings to other healthcare team members, and lead the change process. Only through an educated, systematic approach to addressing deficiencies in the delivery of client care can the healthcare team improve processes and outcomes.

Analyzing and Disseminating Healthcare Information Among Team Members

The availability of and ability to use "big data" is one of the positive outcomes of the adoption of the electronic health record. More data are being collected in the healthcare system than ever before. Big data have been described as referring to the volume, variety, and rapid accumulation of data, as well as to the analytics being used to evaluate that data for the discovery and communication of patterns within and between data (Bates, Saria, Ohno-Machado, Shah, & Escobar, 2014).

The availability and use of big data is one indication of the complexity of today's healthcare system. The Institute of Medicine (2012) describes two overarching imperatives for what it believes should be a "learning health care system" in America "to manage the health care system's ever-increasing complexity"; and "to curb ever-escalating costs" (p. 7). In their report *Best Care at Lower Cost: The Path to Continuously Learning Health Care in America*, the IOM goes on to note the opportunities, well known to the CNL, that are available to meet the imperatives noted above:

- Vast computation power that is affordable and widely available
- Connectivity that allows information to be accessed in real time virtually anywhere
- Human and organizational capabilities that improve the reliability and efficiency of care processes
- The recognition that effective care must be delivered by collaboration between teams of clinicians and patients, each playing a vital role in the care process (p. 7).

A nurse who is effective in the role of a CNL brings together the healthcare team to assess, implement, and evaluate initiatives aimed at delivery of safe, quality care to a subpopulation of clients. The CNL has an obligation and is accountable for timely dissemination of the analysis of client data to members of the healthcare team. That analysis may include frequency distribution of data, trends in the clinical data, probability statistics, and the interpretation of run and control charts. Working with information technology specialists and statisticians, the CNL may also use some of the emerging analytics being developed to interpret the meaning of big data.

In addition to the dissemination of client care data and analysis for the particular subset of clients with whom the CNL is working, this nursing leader also has an obligation to remain current with the peer-reviewed published literature on quality, safety, and healthcare outcomes. The CNL should be an active member of organizations that examine and monitor quality outcomes in healthcare and keep the healthcare team abreast of new developments, current research, and nationally recognized guidelines.

CNLs should remain informed about the work of such organizations as:

- Agency for Healthcare Research and Quality (AHRQ; www.ahrq.gov)
- National Quality Forum (NQF; www.qualityforum.org)
- Institute of Medicine (IOM; www.iom.edu)
- Quality and Safety Education for Nurses (QSEN; www.qsen.org)

Safeguarding Privacy and Confidentiality of Client Information

Both clients and healthcare providers are understandably concerned about how the privacy and confidentiality of clients' PHI will be assured as more and more technology is utilized to collect and manage data, as well as use data to evaluate healthcare processes and outcomes. Assurances from the federal government are not enough. There must be a commitment by those interacting directly with clients to safeguard client information, making it available on a need-to-know basis only. Clinical nurse leaders as well as other members of the nursing community must be aware of laws and regulations that govern how PHI is utilized and shared with others, and the gaps in protection of consumer privacy related to HIPAA (McGraw, 2009). These gaps have implications related to how much consumers do and will trust the healthcare system as it attempts to implement technology in individual and regional care settings.

The development of HIEs has elevated the level of concern of both clients and providers. HIEs allow for multiple healthcare organizations serving a client to share health information across electronic networks. This has the potential to contribute to continuity of care and client satisfaction. The exchange of information addresses the IOM aims of timeliness, effectiveness, and efficiency. The electronic transmission of client information from one organization to another is more timely than the transfer of paper records. The receiving provider has more rapid access to information with which to plan care and make decisions; this timeliness may therefore achieve greater benefit (effectiveness). Having timely access to client information also avoids unnecessary retesting, thereby enhancing efficiency. The sharing of client information, however, requires a level of electronic encryption to assure the security necessary to avoid breaches in confidentiality. It demands a level of trust in information technology experts that leads clients and clinicians to feel assured that privacy and confidentiality are being maintained.

According to one nurse scholar, nurses involved in the development, use, and evaluation of information systems in healthcare should be guided by nursing theoretical frameworks, principles, and concepts when expressing their thoughts about the ethical issues related to the privacy and confidentiality of PHI (Milton, 2009). Others will look to nurses, placing their trust in the input nurses have in this important area of concern around the use and potential abuse of information available as a result of healthcare information technology.

Meeting the Needs of Geographically Remote Clients

As the country embraces the increased use of health information technology, no longer will the issue of access be so dramatically affected by the lack of geographic proximity to large healthcare institutions. With the advent of telehealth technologies, clients can now be cared for without needing to be face-to-face with a clinician. Across the continuum of wellness to illness and recognizing especially the needs of those with chronic illnesses, remote assessment, monitoring, and decision making are now possible through the use of technology.

In rural communities, where expertise in critical care medicine and nursing may be concentrated in metropolitan areas far removed, the ability to remotely monitor critically ill clients through live streaming video has enabled clinicians to have available 24-hour consultation with critical care specialists in the care of those clients. Furthermore, where a shortage of clinicians exists in more remote areas of the country, having the ability to remotely monitor very ill clients on the "off shift" in small hospitals has been invaluable to critical care nurses at the bedside during those times. This remote monitoring is called the electronic ICU or E-ICU.

In managing subpopulations of chronically ill patients, today's technology makes it possible for at-home clients to communicate with clinicians and for clinicians to assess clients through live video viewing. If managing a large cohort of clients with chronic illness, computer systems have the ability, when programmed, to triage incoming data from clients so that clinicians have a prioritized list of clients to contact. By redefining the location of care using healthcare information technology, programs such as the Department of Veteran Affairs' Care Coordination/Home Telehealth (CCHT) program have reported that benefits of such a program include the reduction in the numbers of hospital admissions, reduction in the number of hospital bed days of care, and improvement in veterans' satisfaction with services (Darkins et al., 2008).

Advantages and Disadvantages of Consumer Use of Health Technology

Consumers today are active users of technology, both in their workplace and in their personal lives. It is not surprising that consumers are increasingly turning to the Internet for healthcare information. There are a number of applications consumers may use in accessing computers for their healthcare needs, and there are many reasons consumers choose to use web-based resources; these include information-seeking, communication and support, the maintenance of personal health records, decision support, and disease management (Zielstorff & Frink, 2012). In a review of 12 studies on healthcare consumers' experiences with healthcare information technology, Akesson, Saveman, and Nilsson (2007) found that consumers were empowered by the perceived knowledge and support they gained in using technology. The ONC agrees, making consumer access to timely summaries of healthcare visits and other healthcare information part of the "meaningful use" criteria that must be met in adopting EHR technology. However, while efforts are ongoing to make healthcare more patient-centered by the availability of patient portals for consumer access, not as many consumers are taking advantage of the increasing options for accessing and managing their healthcare information. In a study of New York State communities, consumers were much more likely to believe that personal health records may improve the quality of their care than to actually use a personal health record (Abramson, Patel, Edwards, & Kaushal, 2014). While this information is helpful, more research needs to be done in this area.

There are issues of concern regarding consumers' use of computers for health. These include, but are not limited to, the issues of variability in quality of available information, privacy, and security of data on the Internet; the digital divide; educational, ethnic, and cultural barriers; physical and cognitive disabilities; and the impact on consumers' relationships with healthcare providers (Zielstorff & Frink, 2012). The digital divide may reflect both access to and comfort with computer use. Educational and literacy barriers associated with the ability to use computers need to be areas of focus for intervention and research as we move forward as a nation toward a more fully computerized healthcare delivery system.

Analyzing Systems to Identify Supports and Gaps

As healthcare institutions examine their existing health technology products to assess whether they meet national standards, the CNL has the opportunity to provide input on how those products might best meet the need for quality improvement and control. Using the standards set by the federal government and available on the website of the ONC (www.healthit.gov), the CNL is in a position to assess whether the organization's EHR meets the standards set for a comprehensive quality-outcome-driven electronic portal. Also in need of evaluation is whether CDSS in use in the organization reflect the application of evidence-based clinical practice in the delivery of quality care. If not already embedded as part of the EHR, CDS should be interoperable with the existing EHR. For ongoing monitoring or follow up of patients with chronic disease, telemedicine in the form of remote monitoring and mobile applications for ongoing assessment should also be considered by the organization for delivering comprehensive, patient-centered care.

Improvements in quality and safety related to client outcomes can be achieved with health information technology if human–technology interfaces are effective (Effken, McGonigle, & Mastrian, 2015). Human factors that influence the performance of clinicians within the human–machine system include human capabilities and the environment (Alexander, 2012). Human capabilities include physical and sensory characteristics, including functions such as attention, perception, learning, memory, recall, reasoning, making decisions, and transmitting information (Alexander, 2012). The environment includes organizational structures and processes, tasks (cognitive and physical), and feedback mechanisms (Alexander, 2012).

The CNL plays a role as an advocate for user involvement early in the design and implementation of technology, with particular attention to human–technology interfaces. The CNL is also in a position to prevent workarounds by being involved as a coach and cheerleader for members of the multidisciplinary team. Aware of the human factors that might impede successful implementation and consistent use of technology, this involvement may include orientation to the technologies, continuing education, and other methods of achieving and maintaining "buy-in" from colleagues.

Development of New Technologies

The recent IOM report, *The Future of Nursing: Leading Change, Advancing Health* (2010), highlights the role nursing must play in the current and future healthcare delivery system. One of the IOM's key messages is that nurses "should be full partners, with physicians and other health professionals, in redesigning health care in the United States" (IOM, 2010, p. 4). Much of that change is now integrated with industry-wide efforts to incorporate information technology into all aspects of client care. In order to remain current with all the new developments in the field of electronic assessment, management, and outcome evaluation of the country's health, it is incumbent upon the CNL to be an active member in ongoing development, implementation, and evaluation of healthcare information technologies. This includes participation in research.

CNLs are encouraged to participate in the information technology-oriented organizations that currently exist to educate, support, and provide leadership opportunities for its members. These organizations include, but are not limited to, the American Nursing Informatics Association (www.ania.org) and the Health Information and Management Systems Society (www.himss.org). Participating in the TIGER Initiative (www.himss.org/professional-development/tiger-initiative) also affords a way to remain current with what nurses are doing to educate healthcare professionals about healthcare information technology. The organization Technology Informatics Guiding Education Reform (TIGER) was formed by a group of nurses who believe in the importance of nursing's role in the implementation of information technology. TIGER's mission is to help develop the nursing workforce's capabilities in the utilization of

EHRs, to engage clinicians in the development of the national healthcare information technology infrastructure, and to assist in accelerating the interdisciplinary adoption of technologies that will improve and enhance the delivery of safe, timely, efficient, and accessible healthcare (www.himss.org/professional-development/tiger-initiative).

The CNL should also embrace and be engaged in assisting nurse researchers and others involved in information technology research in addressing important issues related to the use of healthcare information technology. Bakken, Stone, and Larson (2012), evaluating what needs to be done related to research in this area, propose a research agenda for nurses:

> A nursing informatics agenda for 2008 to 2018 must expand users of interest to include interdisciplinary researchers; build upon the knowledge gained in nursing concept representation to address genomic and environmental data; guide the reengineering of nursing practice; harness new technologies to empower patients and their caregivers for collaborative knowledge development; develop user-configurable software approaches that support complex data visualization, analysis and predictive modeling; facilitate the development of middle-range nursing informatics theories; and encourage innovative evaluation methodologies that attend to human–computer interface factors and organizational context. (p. 286)

Conclusion

There has never been a better time for the CNL to be engaged in the development, implementation, and evaluation of healthcare information technology. Experts at multiple levels of intersecting sciences are moving at an exhilarating pace to bring our healthcare delivery system into the 21st century with regard to the use of information technology. As knowledgeable, skillful, and trusted members of the healthcare team, CNLs have the opportunity to drive important change, keeping in mind the issues of access, support, education, and confidentiality. Since the middle of the last century, nurses have worked to highlight the importance of capturing the delivery of nursing care as healthcare information technologies have been designed. This nursing care data, carefully collected and analyzed, holds the key to improving the quality and safety of the care we deliver. There is no better leader to continue this important work than the CNL. The certification exam blueprint lists a number of concepts related to informatics in relation to the CNL role (Table 20.1). There is also a wide range of resources and organizations available to support knowledge in this complex area (see Box 20.1).

TABLE 20.1 Healthcare Informatics

CATEGORY	WEIGHT
F. Healthcare Informatics	**4%**
1. Analyzes systems to identify strengths, gaps, and opportunities	
2. Applies data from systems in planning and delivering care	
3. Evaluates clinical information systems using select criteria	
4. Incorporates ethical principles in the use of information systems	
5. Evaluates impact of new technologies on clients, families, and systems	
6. Assesses and evaluates the use of technology in the delivery of client care	
7. Validates accuracy of consumer-provided information on health issues from the Internet and other sources	
8. Synthesizes healthcare information for client-specific problems	
9. Refers clients to culturally relevant health information	
10. Demonstrates proficiency in the use of innovations such as the electronic record for documenting and analyzing clinical data	
11. Individualizes interventions using technologies	
12. Identifies and promotes an environment that safeguards the privacy and confidentiality of patients and families	
13. Leads the quality improvement team and engages in designing and implementing a process for improving client safety	
14. Utilizes information and communication technologies to document, access, and monitor client care; advance client education; and enhance the accessibility of care	
15. Aligns interdisciplinary team documentation to improve accessibility of data	

Used with permission from the Commission on Nurse Certification (2011, 2014).

BOX 20.1
CNL Resources Related to Informatics

- American Nursing Informatics Association (www.ania.org)
- Health Information and Management Systems Society (www.himss.org)
- TIGER Initiative (www.himss.org/professional-development/tiger-initiative)
- Office of the National Coordinator for Health Information Technology (ONC; www.healthit.gov)

(continued)

BOX 20.1 *(continued)*

- Systematic Nomenclature of Medicine (SNOMED; www.ihtsdo.org)
- Nursing Interventions Classification (NIC; www.nursing.uiowa.edu)
- Nursing Outcomes Classification (NOC; www.nursing.uiowa.edu)
- North American Nursing Diagnosis Association (NANDA; www.nanda.org)

Resources

Abramson, E. L., Patel, V., Edwards, A., & Kaushal, R. (2014). Consumer perspectives on personal health records: A 4-community study. *The American Journal of Managed Care, 20*(4), 287.

Akkesson, K. M., Saveman, B.-I., & Nilsson, G. (2007). Health care consumers' experiences of information communication technology—A summary of literature. *International Journal of Medical Informatics, 76*, 633–645. doi:10.1016/j.ijmedinf.2006.07.001.

Alexander, G. L. (2012). Human factors. In V. K. Saba & K. A. McCormick (Eds.), *Essentials of nursing informatics* (5th ed., pp. 119–132). New York, NY: McGraw-Hill.

American Nurses Association. (n.d.). *Official ANA position statements.* Retrieved from http://www.nursingworld.org/positionstatements

Backus, L. I., Gavrilov, S., Loomis, T. P., Halloran, J. P., Phillips, B. R., Belperio, P. S., & Mole, L. A. (2009). Clinical case registries: Simultaneous local and national disease registries for population quality management. *Journal of the American Medical Informatics Association, 16*, 775–783. doi:10.1197/jamia.M3203.

Bakken, S., Stone, P. W., & Larson, E. L. (2012). A nursing informatics research agenda for 2008–2018: Contextual influences and key components. *Nursing Outlook, 60*(5), 280–290. doi:10.1016/j.outlook.2012.06.001.

Bates, D. W., Saria, S., Ohno-Machado, L., Shah, A., & Escobar, G. (2014). Big data in healthcare: Using analytics to identify and manage high-risk and high-cost patients. *Health Affairs, 33*(7), 1123–1131. doi:10.1377/hlthaff.2014.0041.

Commission on Nurse Certification. (2011). *Clinical Nurse Leader job analysis report.* Retrieved from http://www.aacn.nche.edu/cnl/Job-Analysis-Report.pdf

Commission on Nurse Certification. (2014). *Clinical Nurse Leader (CNL®) certification exam blueprint.* Retrieved from http://www.aacn.nche.edu/leading-initiatives/cnl/cnl-certification/pdf/ExamContentOutline11.pdf

Darkins, A., Ryan, P., Kobb, R., Foster, L., Edmonson, E., Wakefield, B., & Lancaster, A. (2008). Care Coordination/Home Telehealth: The systematic implementation of health informatics, home telehealth, and disease management to support the care of veteran patients with chronic conditions. *Telemedicine and e-Health, 14*(10), 1118–1126. doi:10.1089/tmj.2008.0021.

Effken, J. A., McGonigle, D., & Mastrian, K. (2015). The human–technology interface. In D. McGonigle & K. G. Mastrian (Eds.). *Nursing informatics and the foundation of knowledge* (3rd ed., pp. 201–216). Burlington, MA: Jones & Bartlett Learning.

Hall, E. S., Poynton, M. R., Narus, S. P., Jones, S. S., Evans, R. S., Varner, M. W., & Thornton, S. N. (2009). Patient-level analysis of outcomes using structured labor and delivery data. *Journal of Biomedical Informatics, 42*, 702–709. doi:10.1016./j.jbi.2009.01.008

Institute of Medicine. (1999). *To err is human: Building a safer health system.* Washington, DC: National Academies Press.

Institute of Medicine. (2001). *Crossing the quality chasm: A new health system for the 21st century*. Washington, DC: National Academies Press.

Institute of Medicine. (2010). *The future of nursing: Leading change, advancing health*. Washington, DC: National Academies Press.

Institute of Medicine. (2012). *Best care at lower cost: The path to continuously learning health care in America*. Washington, DC: National Academies Press.

Mastrian, K. G., & McGonigle, D. (2012). Nursing science and the foundation of knowledge. In D. McGonigle & K. G. Mastrian (Eds.), *Nursing informatics and the foundation of knowledge* (2nd ed., p. 5). Burlington, MA: Jones & Bartlett Learning.

McGonigle, D., & Mastrian, K. G. (2012). *Nursing informatics and the foundation of knowledge* (2nd ed.) Burlington, MA: Jones & Bartlett Learning.

McGraw, D. (2009). Privacy and health information technology. *Journal of Law, Medicine & Ethics Supplement, 2*(37), 121–149. doi:10.1111/j.1748-720x2009.00424.x

Melnyk, B., & Fineout-Overholt, E. (2014). *Evidence-based practice in nursing & healthcare: A guide to best practice* (3rd ed.). Philadelphia, PA: Wolters Kluwer/Lippincott Williams & Wilkins.

Milton, C. L. (2009). Information sharing: Transparency, nursing ethics, and practice implications with electronic health records. *Nursing Science Quarterly, 22*(3), 214–219. doi:10.1177/0894318409337026

Nelson, R., & Staggers, N. (2015). Overview of nursing informatics. In D. McGonigle & K. G. Mastrian (Eds.), *Nursing informatics and the foundation of knowledge* (3rd ed., pp. 95–108). Burlington, MA: Jones & Bartlett Learning.

Ozbolt, J. G., & Saba, V. K. (2008). A brief history of nursing informatics in the United States of America. *Nursing Outlook, 56*, 199–205.

Sensmeier, J. (2015). Big data and the future of nursing knowledge. *Nursing Management, 46*(4), 22–27. doi:10.1097/01.NUMA.0000462365.53035.7d

Zielstorff, R. D., & Frink, B. B. (2012). Consumer and patient use of computers for health. In V. K. Saba & K. A. McCormick (Eds.), *Essentials of nursing informatics* (5th ed.). New York, NY: McGraw-Hill.

21

Ethics

Sally O'Toole Gerard

Contemporary nurses have a unique set of ethical and moral issues, a result of rapidly changing healthcare policies, technology explosions, and increases in longevity. Nursing stems from the work of Florence Nightingale (1820–1910) who focused on responsible obedience to physicians. The American Nurses Association (ANA) first published a code of ethics for nurses in the 1950s, a model that addressed collaborative relationships with members of the health professions and other citizens in order to meet the needs of the public. Accountability and professional responsibilities have received more emphasis in the most recently revised document. The *Code of Ethics for Nurses With Interpretive Statements* (ANA, 2001) has nine provisions regarding the professional practice of nursing and serves the following purpose: It is a succinct statement of the ethical obligations and duties of every individual who enters the nursing profession, it is the profession's nonnegotiable ethical standard, and it is an expression of nursing's own understanding and commitment to society (Guido, 2010).

The clinical nurse leader (CNL) has a unique opportunity to model ethical professionalism, support the ethical challenges of direct care nurses, raise ethical concerns in the care of patients, and influence ethical practices on an organizational level. The CNL, as a highly educated, expert clinician intimately involved with patient care, has been named as a guardian of the nursing profession (American Association of Colleges of Nursing [AACN], 2007). This guardianship considers the intentions of Florence Nightingale, the ANA, and others who consider nursing to be a profession with profound respect for patients and their complex needs. The CNL has a specific charge to identify actual and potential ethical issues arising from practice and to help address such issues (AACN, 2007). For this reason, the CNL must have knowledge of ethical issues, decision making, organizational perspectives of ethical considerations, legal guidelines, advocacy, and conflict resolution.

A good place to begin is with a review of terms related to this content:

- **Ethics**—involves the principles or assumptions underpinning the way individuals or groups should conduct themselves and is concerned with motives and attitudes and the relationship of these attitudes to the individual.
- **Values**—personal beliefs about the truths and worth of thoughts, objects, or behavior.
- **Autonomy**—personal freedom and self-determination.
- **Beneficence**—supporting actions that promote good.
- **Nonmaleficence**—the concept that one should not do harm.
- **Justice**—the concept that all people should be treated fairly.
- **Respect for others**—acknowledgment of the rights of individuals to make decisions and live or die on the basis of those decisions.
- **Codes of ethics**—formal statements that serve to articulate the values and beliefs of a given discipline, serving as a standard for professional actions and reflecting the ethical principles shared by its members.

Personal and Organizational Decision Making

There is no better way to consider ethical issues than in practice.

> *SCENARIO:* Sue is a senior charge nurse assigned to a surgical unit. She is waiting to care for Mr. L, who is about to come back from the postanesthesia care unit after vascular bypass surgery. Claire is a newer nurse on the unit, who observes as charge nurse Sue prepares a morphine injection, stating it is for Mr. L when he arrives. Ten minutes later the newer nurse observes Sue return to the medication room to discard an empty syringe, stating that she discarded the medication in the room when Mr. L. refused it. Claire is asked to "witness" the waste although she did not actually see Sue discard the narcotic. Claire had been put in this situation with Sue once before and asked that Sue please show her the actual wasting of the drug. Sue's response this time is, "Oh yeah, I forgot you're not used to how things are done on this unit." Claire is left feeling very uncomfortable and legally responsible for a narcotic she did not see properly discarded.

Many ethical concerns are raised in the day-to-day practice of nursing. Some involve patients, families, colleagues, and organizations. The desire to maintain an ethical perspective in all areas of practice includes the examination of our duties, obligations, or responsibilities to other health-care professionals and staff. But how do we make decisions about ethical concerns? In daily life an individual draws on knowledge, life experience, values, and a variety of circumstances to arrive at a decision. When it comes to complex ethical decisions, many decision-making frameworks have been described. When making ethical decisions, nurses need to combine all the elements using an orderly, systematic, and objective method (Guido, 2010). One such model that describes this process is the MORAL model, most recently applied to nursing by Halloran (1982).

- M—Massage the dilemma. Identify and define issues in the dilemma. Consider the opinions of other players as well as their value system.
- O—Outline the options. Examine all options fully, including less realistic and conflicting ones. Make a list of pros and cons.
- R—Resolve the dilemma. Review the issues and options, applying basic ethical principles to each option. Decide the best option based on the views of those concerned in the dilemma.
- A—Act by applying the chosen option. This step is usually the most difficult because it requires actual implementation versus dialogue and discussion.
- L—Look back and evaluate the entire process, including the implementation. No process is complete without a thorough evaluation.

A process allows time for a deeper understanding of the issue, related issues, and considerations of others who may be involved in the situation. Some issues are easier to reach than others, and it is important to allow sufficient time for a supportable option to be reached (Guido, 2010).

Healthcare, by virtue of the complexity of caring for human life, may benefit from a model of decision making adapted to the environment. Thompson and Thompson (1981) describe a *bioethical decision* model of using a 10-step process:

Step 1: Review the situation to determine health problems, decision needed, ethical components, and key individuals
Step 2: Gather additional information to clarify the situation
Step 3: Identify the ethical issues in the situation
Step 4: Define personal and professional moral positions
Step 5: Identify moral positions of key individuals involved
Step 6: Identify value conflicts, if any
Step 7: Determine who should make the decision
Step 8: Identify range of actions with anticipated outcomes
Step 9: Decide on a course of action and carry it out
Step 10: Evaluate/review results of decision/action

There are an infinite number of ethical dilemmas that can occur in healthcare, some mildly complex and some profoundly complex. Nurses need to realize the need for process to allow for inquiry, reasoning, and thoughtful consideration of the multiple aspects involved in a particular situation. The CNL can support nurses of varied levels of experience to recognize their important role in assuring ethical care in all healthcare settings. A CNL can also support nurses who face moral distress, confusion, and professional fear when dealing with issues that present themselves daily in our healthcare system.

Ethics Committees

Healthcare organizations put many systems into place to maintain proper care that adheres to governing laws, standards of best practice, regulations of the health department, and a plethora of human resource policies to ensure just treatment of patients and employees. The legal system is founded on rules and regulations, whereas ethics are subject to philosophical, moral, and individual interpretations (Guido, 2010). Ethics committees are common in healthcare organizations as a mechanism to address and process the inevitable issues that arise. Ethics committees can provide structure and guidelines for potential problems, serve as an open forum for discussion, and function as a true patient advocate (Guido, 2010). Despite the existence of ethics committees in many organizations, staff nurses may not have access to these meetings or even know they exist. In many settings, any member of the healthcare team can request an ethics review of a case. This is a valuable resource to nurses that many may be unaware of. The CNL, as an advanced generalist who is very involved with supporting direct care nurses, can make this resource available to nurses.

Advocacy and the CNL

The AACN specifically describes the CNL as an advocate. The CNL advocates to ensure that clients, families, and communities are well informed and included in planning of care (AACN, 2007). The CNL also ensures that the voice of the vulnerable, frail, inexperienced, and incapacitated is represented throughout the life span. Although all persons have the ability to advocate for a cause or another individual, the nurse is uniquely suited to guard the standards of the profession to ensure ethical care. The CNL plays a natural role of advocate in the spectrum of healthcare and especially for direct care nurses supported by the CNL. Perhaps never before has this CNL support of direct care nurses been so necessary as now, in an age of rapid change.

> *SCENARIO:* Missy is an RN who has been working on a surgical unit for 2 years. She is caring for Mrs. Brown, who has just returned from surgery to remove an abdominal mass. Mrs. Brown's family has been

> waiting in the room for her to return and is very happy to have the surgery over and to sit with Mrs. Brown in the room as she sleeps. After about 1 hour, the family shares with the nurses that they had expected the surgeon to have been in to tell them the outcome of the surgery. After the second inquiry from the family, the nurse phones the surgeon and inquires about his plans to see the family. The surgeon states that he spoke to Mrs. Brown (the patient) in the recovery holding area and he did not plan to visit the family as he had left the hospital and was off duty. The nurse shares that she is quite confident the family was expecting to speak with him, but the physician is terse and ends the conversation. Missy speaks to a sleepy Mrs. Brown, who states she does not remember whether the physician spoke to her or not. The family is very upset and not consoled by the news that the surgical resident would be seeing Mrs. Brown that evening on rounds. Missy does her best to support the family but feels a significant deal of distress in the poor communication that this family has received. Missy contemplates providing the family with the physician's personal phone number, to which the charge nurse has access.

Why is advocacy so important? What more could Missy do for the Brown family and for her own sense of wrongdoing? Without advocacy and effective protection of rights, there are no rights. The nurse carries the role of securing the patient's interests by every means at her disposal. The nurse understands that the advocacy role promotes, protects, and makes every effort to promote healing. This healing extends to families. Situations in which nurses are advocates in subtle and deliberate ways for patients and families happen daily. It is the cumulative effect of these many battles that can diminish a nurse's personal and professional satisfaction. The CNL can help to protect the direct care nurse by supporting the moral stress encountered. *Moral stress* most often occurs when faced with a situation in which two ethical principles compete (Guido, 2010). The CNL can be supportive by assisting the nurse to approach ethical decisions and situations in a thoughtful and knowledgeable manner. Utilizing one of the models previously mentioned could support a best outcome to the situation.

In addition to supporting the use of a decision-making model, the CNL can also model the guidelines for acting as a patient advocate or provide them directly to nurses at appropriate times. Guido (2010) shares five guidelines for acting as a patient advocate:

1. Nurses should be aware of hospital policies and protocols, as well as acceptable standards of care. They should question physician orders when they are contrary to accepted standards of care or when they believe the order could harm the patient. They should not be intimidated into following orders, but use professional and independent

judgments. If physicians persist or refuse to change orders, they should consult a nursing supervisor.

2. In emergency situations in which the nurse believes that following the physician's order could result in harm to the patient, the nurse should refuse to follow the order, ensure patient safety and appropriate care, and notify the nursing supervisor and administrators.
3. If the patient is prescribed care that could cause direct harm, the nurse should voice his or her concern to the physician and nursing supervisor.
4. In transitioning from one area of care to another, the patient/family should be fully informed, prepared, and educated regarding the situation. Patient teaching and discharge teaching are often a primary responsibility of nurses and they should prepare patients with sufficient teaching regarding symptoms and complications and provide adequate resources/instruction. If the nurse feels the patient is not being safely transitioned from the area of care, she should notify the physician and supervisor.
5. The patient is the nurse's primary concern, and nurses have an affirmative duty to serve as patient advocates.

SCENARIO—FOLLOW UP: The CNL on Missy's floor overhears her vent her frustration over what she feels is poor treatment of this patient/family and also that she is spending so much time and energy trying to console this family's anxiety. Missy states, "I don't care if they fire me; I'm going to give them the surgeon's cell phone number." The CNL speaks to Missy to review the details of the situation. The CNL supports Missy's moral stress and offers the following input: "Why don't we call the nursing supervisor and explain the situation, and provide her with the surgeon's cell phone number so that she can call him and request a call to the family as soon as possible. In the meantime, let's call the surgical resident and request that she come see the family at the beginning of her evening rounds to review how the surgery went and the next steps."

End-of-Life Care Decisions

Nurses are so often a critical factor in the ethical treatment of people at the end of their life. End-of-life care is a general term that refers to the medical and mental care given in the advanced or terminal stages of illness. Choices regarding invasive treatments, resuscitation, hydration, nutrition, and so on, are often left to emotionally charged relatives if specific planning has not been put into place. Conversations about end-of-life choice are often some of the most difficult for families and caregivers. Mentoring of a CNL can support care that is patient centered, holistic, and humane.

Advance directives are a valuable tool in the planning of end-of-life care. Advance directives are a way for patients to communicate their wishes to family, friends, and healthcare professionals, but they are often misunderstood. Some patients may be fearful of creating a living will, thinking it will give permission to potentially "pull the plug" at a premature time in the illness. Landmark cases of end-of-life controversies can make national headlines and often provide a forum for discussion in many circles, among both professional and private citizens. Often confusion and uncertainty surface in these complex situations. Nonetheless, professionals understand the importance of considering patient preferences in clinical decision making and often must advocate with patients, families, and professional colleagues.

Advance directives are legal documents, such as a living will, durable power of attorney, and healthcare proxy. These documents allow people to convey their decisions about end-of-life care. Advance directives are a way for patients to communicate their wishes to family, friends, and healthcare professionals. The use of these documents can help avoid confusion, turmoil, and guilt and promote a person's choices for care. They are often developed with an attorney and can be modified as a patient's situation changes. Unfortunately, these critical documents often do not exist or are misunderstood by patients and families.

The federal Patient Self-Determination Act of 1991 supported the patient's right to determine the medical care he or she receives. The law requires hospitals to provide information about advance directives to adult patients on admission for any condition (Tilden et al., 2011). Although this law supported the integration of advance directives into hospital care, these documents continue to be underutilized, misunderstood, and possibly feared by some. The American Academy of Nursing issued a policy calling for advance care planning as an urgent public health concern. With the aging American population and misunderstandings about advance care planning in the healthcare reform debates, this organization has made a strong call for attention to this issue (Tilden et al., 2011). The organization has put forth recommendations as a part of this statement to support advance care planning, which is holistic and patient centered. The following four recommendations of Tilden and colleagues (2011) are:

1. The time invested in advance care planning by qualified health professionals for patients with life-limiting illness should be reimbursed by all payers.
2. Health information technology offers promise for documenting advance directives care planning and making such information more readily available with and between patients' care settings. As electronic medical records (EMRs) are developed, the approach to documenting advance care planning, advance care, and advance directives must be built into

electronic systems so that this information is prominent and readily available for use in care decisions.

3. The 1991 Patient Self-Determination Act should be updated and expanded beyond the clerical function of providing forms to patients on hospital admission. Expanded requirements upon hospital admission should facilitate the components of advance care planning to include initiating conversations, providing information and assistance to patients, and facilitating patients' determination of their preferences.
4. Health professions education and training are critical to the knowledge, skills, and attitudes that future clinicians bring to the clinical care of patients with life-limiting conditions. Health professionals' education programs must include content on advance care planning.

So why is this area of care so fraught with conflict and turmoil and why must the CNL be knowledgeable about the major concepts involved? This area of healthcare offers some of the most challenging clinical situations and also some of the most rewarding opportunities. Hopefully, every experienced nurse can recall one example of supporting a patient in a peaceful, holistic death where the patient's wishes were known, respected, and communicated to family members. This can be one of the most satisfying and profound experiences, and for newer nurses, it can be a surprise that, although entering a profession to support healing, a peaceful death can be a proud component of a nursing career. Unfortunately, these situations are sometimes less common and the end-of-life path can be filled with conflict and confusion.

Addressing the issue of end-of life choices requires a person to consider his or her own mortality. The spectrum of how individuals respond to this is as varied as human beings. Some people want to assure from a young age and with no immediate health concerns that legal documents are in order. Some people at advanced ages and with serious medical conditions refuse to address these issues. The timing of developing these documents is also complex. Those who are healthy do not feel the need or urgency to develop them. Those who are older or sick may be upset or emotional to consider this topic for fear it will make some impact on their current health situation. Ideally, advance care planning among clinicians, patients, and patients' families has occurred over time; patients have expressed and clarified their preferences verbally and in writing (Tilden et al., 2011). A lack of this preparation often causes great conflict, anxiety, and turmoil for families when an individual can no longer express them. Siblings, especially, can have significant guilt and conflict when they are trying to come to a consensus on emotionally charged issues.

Living wills, in particular, are valuable documents but are misunderstood and woefully underutilized. A majority of adults do not have living wills, and if they have one in which a surrogate has been designated, often the surrogate is not aware of having been designated as a decision maker (Mahon, 2010). Although it seems logical to discuss one's wishes, the emotional, spiritual, religious, and psychological responses to this topic are powerful. Many patients have not acclimated to being asked questions about advance directives on admission to hospitals, and despite the illness at hand, it is often not seriously contemplated.

Misinformation about advance directives is an excellent opportunity for CNLs to support patients, families, and direct care nurses. A knowledge of hospital policies, state laws, and resources is key for CNLs and nursing staff. As previously stated, based on legal changes in 1991 and the Patient Self-Determination Act, adults entering the hospital must be asked for such documents and have information about these documents available for healthcare personnel. Without attention to detail and tracking by organizations, these documents, if not available on admission, may not be followed up on. Many systems may also need to have patients bring the document with each admission to the organization to guard against changes that may have been made to these documents. Patients would often not understand the logic or importance of providing these documents with each admission. Some patients are naïve with regard to the complexity of modern healthcare and may feel: "My doctor knows I don't want any of those machines to keep me alive." They do not realize that full resuscitation will routinely take place on any individual who does not have specific orders to the contrary.

A key misunderstanding around living wills is when they become effective. Patients may not understand that these documents do not come into play until they have become unable to make a decision for themselves and are deemed to be in a terminal condition. This judgment of terminal illness can be subjective and controversial among families and caregivers. Many nurses have worked with professionals treating terminal patients, but the provider communications to families are focused on continued medical treatment, interventions, and seemingly unnecessary suffering. This is often an ethical dilemma for staff nurses and requires a level of advocacy that can be supported by the CNL.

SCENARIO: A patient with advanced Alzheimer's disease is brought to the emergency department from a nursing home with fever and dyspnea. A chest x-ray confirms severe pneumonia, which will require antibiotics, oxygen therapy, and possibly mechanical ventilation. The patient has an advance directive that indicates that she does not want intubation if she is in a terminal condition. The nurses share with the physician the existence of the living will and the patient's wishes. The physician responds that pneumonia is not a terminal condition and therefore the advance directive does not come into effect. The nurse is surprised and distressed at this response as she cares for the demented and agitated patient. The patient is already being physically restrained to protect the intravenous line, and the nurse is morally distressed at the thought of intubating this patient with limited cognitive function.

Patients and families face difficult decisions across the course of a lifetime, and especially in a time of illness. Many factors affect these decisions such as understanding of the disease, experiences, hopes, and goals; the desire to please healthcare providers; family support; beliefs about quality of life; religious or spiritual beliefs; practicalities of daily living; and more (Mahon, 2010). The following four dimensions of decision making have been proposed: medical indications, patient preferences, quality of life, and contextual features (Jonsen, Siegler, & Winslade, 2006). At times, caregivers impart their own values and beliefs into patient/family discussions. This is usually quite unintentional. One approach to this level of communication seeks to keep the information from caregivers factual and objective. This decision making describes the healthcare team as bringing the raw data of the situation and the patient/family adding the meaning and values around the choices and consequences of the decision (Jonsen et al., 2006).

Palliative Care

Palliative care is an interdisciplinary approach to care in which nursing is the core discipline. Palliative care is a field of nursing that is unique in its approach, focus, and goals of patient interaction. This approach to care concerns patients whose diseases are not responsive to curative treatment, where control of pain, symptoms, psychological distress, and spiritual distress is paramount (Kuebler, Berry, & Heidrich, 2002). This model is the ultimate in patient-centered care and places additional emphasis on family support. The palliative care nurse frequently cares for patients experiencing major stressors: physical, psychological, and spiritual. Many of these patients recognize themselves as dying, and it is the role of a palliative care nurse to maximize all resources to support this process.

CNLs can assist patients and staff nurses by having a solid knowledge of what is palliative care, what the resources are in the care setting, and when to encourage conversations around this program of care. Because hospice may equate to death for some patients and families, these are often difficult conversations for healthcare members to initiate. The National Hospice and Palliative Care Organization (1999) describes hospice in the following way:

> Hospice provides support and care for persons in the last phases of incurable illness so that they may live as fully and comfortably as possible. Hospice affirms life and neither hastens nor postpones death. Hospice exists in the hope and belief that through appropriate care

> and the promotion of a caring community sensitive to their needs, that individuals and their families may be free to attain a degree of satisfaction in preparation for death. Hospice programs provide state-of-the-art palliative care and supportive services to individuals at the end of their lives, their family members, and significant others, 24 hours a day, 7 days a week, in both the home and facility-based care settings.

Many organizations also have palliative care advanced practice registered nurses (APRNs) who specialize in supporting the appropriate and holistic care at the end of life. CNLs with access to this type of professional are wise to collaborate as often as possible. CNLs can model therapeutic communication with patients and families around this topic as well as advocacy for patients in leading the interdisciplinary team to focus on patient choice and preference.

Pain assessment and management can be a significant consideration in all patient care but especially in end-of-life care. CNLs can support nursing in a variety of ways, such as proper assessment of pain, knowledge of pharmaceutical and nonpharmaceutical interventions, and knowledge of organizational resources and advocacy. There are a variety of barriers to optimal pain management that the CNL can support. These involve professional barriers, healthcare barriers, and patient/family and societal barriers. Support for nurses who are strong advocates of proper pain management is growing. Increasingly, feedback from patients regarding pain relief and assessment by healthcare organizations is gaining significance as a quality indicator of care. Organizational outcomes regarding quality indicators are becoming more transparent and accessible to the public via the Internet. Additionally, these quality outcomes are being evaluated in relation to reimbursement in a new era of "pay for performance." This new approach to pain relief as a quality indicator of care should support those who advocate for comfortable and humane care, especially at the end of life.

Active knowledge of professional organizations that support the ethical healthcare of all persons is another resource for CNLs and staff nurses. In 2010, the ANA published a position statement to support nurses, as a profession, who are involved in end-of-life care. The document was created to articulate the roles and responsibilities of registered nurses in providing expert end-of-life care and guidance to patients and families concerning treatment preferences and end-of-life decision making (American Nurses Association [ANA], 2010). This valuable document addresses practice issues, healthcare reform issues, and hospice and palliative care together with nurses' guidance and support of patients and families. Also included is specific mention of the advancing technology of healthcare and appropriate use of resources. The organization calls for reshaping and redirecting away from the overuse of technology-driven, acute, hospital-based services to a model of balance between high-tech treatment, community resources, and preventative services (ANA, 2010).

Clearly, the support of professional organizations and nurse experts will be critical in the decades ahead, as the number of aging Americans grows along with technology focused on prolonging life. Who will help patients and families navigate the healthcare system, make informed choices, and address emotionally painful issues of illness? Nurses have and will continue to be an integral part of the team trusted with this responsibility. And how will the role of the CNL help to support, nurture, and model the professional finesse required to connect with patients at this difficult time? The emotional and spiritual toll of caring for patients, advocating for basic rights, and, at times, battling against colleagues can incapacitate our direct care nurses and drive them from the profession. The CNL has the opportunity to partner with these nurses, assure proper resources are considered, and support the development of moral courage.

The Ethical Considerations of Patient Safety

One of the most significant improvements in healthcare has been the prioritization of patient safety. It was this emphasis on patient safety, highlighted by publications of the Institute of Medicine and The Joint Commission, that spurred a national conversation and the advent of the CNL role. The complexity and fragmentation of the healthcare system have set the stage for patients to experience injury and possible death as a result of medical errors. The CNL is in a unique position to advocate for a safe environment that is supported by all members of the healthcare team.

Assessments of microsystems and macrosystems show that variation in best practice procedures can cause errors. Recent attention to measures that standardize care such as best practice order sets, procedural time-outs, and checklists has been implemented. Checklists, in particular, have received particular attention for success in reducing errors and infection rates and improving patient outcomes (Gawande, 2009). Although issues of patient safety and quality improvement are detailed in other chapters of this book, there is an ethical responsibility of all nurses, especially the CNL, to be instrumental in implementing these important initiatives and sustaining them over time.

Ethical considerations of healthcare can be illustrated in any setting. Nurses as a whole have a responsibility that includes protecting patients from falls, from injuring themselves, from abuse, from medication-related unsafe conditions, or from unsafe treatment by members of health-related disciplines (Guido, 2010). National initiatives to motivate organizations to address these patient safety issues have spurred an onslaught of improvement initiatives. The CNL can be a model of ethical decision making and advocacy and can support the development of moral courage. By maintaining a patient/family focus, he or she can often direct the interdisciplinary team in a way that is congruent with the care we would all desire for our own family. Nationally, organizations are supporting a culture of safety and empowerment that encourages all members to speak up and have a voice when patient safety is being compromised. This change in culture will not come without conflict, the need for open communication, and leaders who set the tone for the patient as the highest priority. Opportunities for CNLs in this culture will be numerous, although not clear cut and not without controversy.

> *SCENARIO:* One of the least experienced nurses in a busy surgical ICU has expressed distress to the unit's CNL regarding the behavior of some of the surgical residents. A checklist has been put into place for the insertion of central line catheters, and yet when the nurse attempts to incorporate the checklist into the care of the patient as she assists with the procedure, she is ignored. The following week in report the CNL learns that this nurse's patient will be having a central line catheter placed by the surgical service. The CNL discusses the issue with the young nurse, and they prepare the checklist for the procedure. Later that morning, the residents arrive to begin the procedure. The CNL accompanies the staff nurse into the room to prepare the patient and the necessary supplies. The CNL announces to the group assembled that all the supplies for the procedure are available, including the checklist for this procedure. The surgical resident makes a disparaging remark. After an attempt to remind the resident of best practice and hospital policies, he continues to refuse. The CNL discreetly shares that she and the staff nurse will not assist in this procedure and will be immediately contacting the hospital administrators. The shocked and angry surgical resident agrees to utilize the procedural checklist for the procedure.
>
> Following this exchange, the CNL and staff nurse debrief about the situation. They discuss the often difficult situations in which nurses must advocate for patients and the courage to find that voice. The CNL assures the newer nurse that almost all members of the healthcare team are very committed to a safe culture and would support the actions taken. The CNL also requests a meeting with the manager of the unit, medical director of the ICU, and the chief of surgery to discuss the bigger issue of patient safety, compliance with best practice initiatives, and the role of the staff nurse as a patient advocate despite objections of others.

The CNL can be a role model in advocating for the patient and the development of moral courage. Nurses often struggle with their role in taking a stand against improper care and disregard for policies put in place to protect patients, staff, and the organization. The moral stress can result in moral distress when nurses are put in a painful state of imbalance when they are unable to implement a decision because of real or perceived institutional constraints (Guido, 2010). This moral distress can be generated by a wide variety of clinical and professional situations and can exact a toll on the individual. Is it acceptable for me to question more experienced health professionals? Is it acceptable for me to refuse to assist with this procedure that is not following the standards and policies of the organization? What will the repercussions be if I refuse? Will this person dislike me? Will my peers mock me? Finding the moral courage to stand up to professional issues is a development in the professional life of a nurse. A CNL can model, facilitate, and support the healthy decision making, coping skills, and often difficult communications that may be necessary to keep patients safe.

Ethical Considerations of Health Information

Advances in technology have made dramatic changes to the accumulation of health information and issues of access. Never before has so much information been available, and the future will continue to expand in this area in ways we can probably not imagine. Health information professionals, as a community, have an established code of ethics or code of conduct and cannot function in today's environment without a clear understanding of ethical principles (Harmon, 2006). Many of the values of this industry's code of ethics can easily be shared with nursing and should be embraced. Those values include providing service, protecting medical/social information, promoting confidentiality, securing health information, promoting quality, reporting data with accuracy, and promoting interdisciplinary collaboration (Harmon, 2006).

The protection of patient information has long been a responsibility of nurses as well as all members of the team. Prior to the advent of the EMR, this issue may have been more clearly delineated. In today's world of electronic data, a patient's health information could be viewed by countless individuals at a variety of locations in one day. The development of these EMRs by information specialists has a clear connection to ethical principles of privacy and confidentiality. Likewise, nurses must approach the protection of a patient's privacy with a strong ethical regard and respect. As more and more data are collected on individuals over time, access to this information will take on greater significance and the protection of this information will become more challenging.

> *SCENARIO:* Lisa, a nurse on the telemetry unit, has a chronically ill father. Lisa's peers are all quite familiar with her father's long medical history and his general status, as they have provided emotional support for their friend over the past few years. This past week Lisa's father was admitted to the medical unit for treatment of a urinary tract infection. After morning report, the staff asks Lisa about her father's status. Lisa gives her colleagues an update, including a summary of his lab results from that morning. It is clear to the CNL that Lisa is accessing the EMR to follow her father's care. Is this a problem? What should the CNL do?

Many protections can be put into place to help safeguard the EMR, and these safeguards will be of even greater significance as the technology continues to advance. Some of these securities include restricted access to health records based on security clearance and scope of practice, monitoring of EMR access by organizations to identify misuse and violations, high-level passwords changed on a regular basis, termination of access to EMRs when employment is terminated, and confidentiality statements signed by employees. Future security will most likely continue to be more sophisticated and focused on bioidentification, utilizing fingerprints or retinal images.

One of the most significant issues in healthcare information was the introduction of the Health Insurance Portability and Accountability Act (HIPAA) in 1996. This law provides for the portability of healthcare coverage; antifraud and anti-abuse programs; streamlining of the transfer of patient information between insurers and providers; incentives toward the acquisition of health insurance; and establishment of the federal government as a national healthcare regulator (Guido, 2010). All nurses working at this time saw significant changes in the practice environment in order to comply with this new law. Patient names could no longer be posted on the units for room assignments, clipboards used in everyday assignments needed to be altered, information sent to other agencies required cover sheets, and other provisions were enacted to protect patient information. Shredding of health information became the norm, as any information with patient information would no longer be placed in the traditional garbage. Organizations as a whole scrambled to reorganize systems to maintain patient confidentiality. Policies and procedures were created and implemented to integrate these new regulations into the practice environment from acute care to rehabilitation, home care, and long-term care. Nurses and CNLs, especially, must be aware of the policies and procedures around health information, privacy issues, access issues, and all facets of protecting healthcare information. How does a CNL advise a nurse when a patient requests to see his or her medical record? What are the resources within the organization for questions related to privacy? Is there a privacy officer? Some issues of privacy are straightforward and some pose ethical concerns.

The age of information presents some unique challenges with the increasing use of e-mail, the Internet, and social media networks. This area can pose potential ethical and liability issues for organizations and nurses (Guido, 2010). With the advent of social networks, the Internet, and the majority of individuals having cellular telephones with picture-taking capabilities, the issues of privacy and patient information have taken on an added dimension. Most organizations have needed to introduce new policies regarding any reference to patients, patients' families, or patient information in these venues. One organization instituted a new social media policy after a patient's family complained that they recognized that nurses from the hospital were referring to their family member on a social media site, even though the patient's name was not used. Derogatory information about the patient and family were shared between nurses on the site, which was a clear violation of ethical care. Nurses and other healthcare workers may not recognize that ethical lines are being crossed, especially in a generation raised on sharing information on social media sites.

Without a code of ethics, issues of privacy, patient information, and patient rights can be obscure. A code of professional ethics supports beneficence, nonmaleficence, and justice. A common respect for others should be the guide for all healthcare workers, but often that value of respect can be lost when workers become desensitized by their surroundings and the daily interactions of a healthcare environment. The CNL can help nurses develop a voice of advocacy for the proper treatment of patients and clearly can be a guardian of information, especially in a world of access to a plethora of information venues.

Resources for Ethical Concerns

Most organizations have a plethora of policies, procedures, and provisions of practice. Despite a system put in place to provide order, there will always be complex ethical situations that require support and reflection. Most healthcare organizations have established ethics committees to advise healthcare professionals when difficult decision points are reached. The ethics committee is usually an interdisciplinary team composed of physicians, nurses, ethicists, social workers, chaplains, dieticians, and others with experience with ethical deliberation in healthcare (Harmon, 2006). These groups are meant to be unbiased professionals who facilitate communication in emotionally charged issues (Harmon, 2006). Often, these groups will meet after a situation has occurred, as an opportunity to reflect and deliberate possible opportunities to provide the best possible care.

Many direct care nurses may not know that an ethics committee exists in their institution or that they can request an ethics consult by the team.

A CNL is an excellent medium of making nurses aware of resources such as an ethics committee. Oftentimes, nurses will have lingering conflict and possible moral distress over a patient's or family's situation. An ethics committee can provide that support needed for frontline nurses to see the many complex dimensions of some patient situations. There may also be open ethics discussions or seminars at an organization, and the CNL can raise the awareness of staff nurses to the importance of understanding these resources and having a voice in the interdisciplinary team, in which nursing is a key member.

Other resources for ethical dilemmas and concerns can be supervisors, administrators, and advanced practice nurses. Many facilities have nurses who specialize in palliative care and pain management. These nurses can be a valuable resource of knowledge of clinical issues when facing issues of patient advocacy and ethical dilemmas. Some areas of healthcare are more prone to dilemmas and conflict, and it is critical for nurses to be aware of any support available for their professional development, rather than wrestle with moral conflict. These resources can often provide support for a direct care nurse who may make decisions solely on the basis of the needs of the patient but may not be popular with members of the healthcare team.

Ethics and the Affordable Care Act

Some would say that a driving force of the Affordable Care Act (ACA) was based on ethics. The ACA represents a new social contract of healthcare through access, market choice, and individual responsibility. The new emphasis to allow Americans to reach their full potential for health with a great emphasis on preventative services represents a more just and ethical system (Koh & Sebelius, 2010). There have been long-standing concerns with a payment system in which providers profit from disease treatment rather than illness prevention. The shifting system of pay for performance may be more preferable for society but is causing turbulence in many healthcare systems in an effort to evolve into a more just system.

In every organization, the ACA and other significant changes to healthcare will impact the CNL's practice. New ethical concerns may emerge. Moral distress is likely to be shifted rather than eliminated. As in all major areas of healthcare, the CNL must be educated, informed, and prepared for the impact to his or her particular setting. CNLs should be a strong voice in the design of new systems of care in which the patient is the central focus. Collaboration with other disciples is a hallmark of the CNL and will be a critical skill as changes continue. As patient responsibility and shared decision making are emphasized, CNLs will be key advocates for individuals (Oshima Lee & Emmanuel, 2013). With millions more Americans having access to healthcare, CNLs need to be vigilant to identify areas in which their own role may change to best support positive patient outcomes.

Conclusion

The care of complex human beings will never be without areas of ethical concern and conflict. As technology advances along with easy access to information through the EMR, Internet, and other avenues, nurses will have a critical role in protection and advocacy of patient care. End-of-life issues are common for nurses to encounter across the continuum of healthcare and will always have gray areas of providing care versus prolonging suffering. Despite a growing population of older adults, advance directives are often underutilized and misunderstood. A lack of clear planning and sharing of wishes in the event of a terminal illness can send families into a crisis. Regardless of what circumstances come together to cause this crisis, the nurse is often integrally involved. The CNL provides leadership, guidance, role modeling, and support for frontline nurses in this venture. Awareness of hospital policies, resources, and strategies that can optimize patient outcomes is essential. The Commission on Nurse Certification includes many ethical areas in the certification blueprint for CNLs (Table 21.1).

TABLE 21.1 Ethics

CATEGORY	WEIGHT
G. Ethics	**7%**
1. Evaluates ethical decision making from both a personal and an organizational perspective and develops an understanding of how these two perspectives may create conflicts of interest	
2. Applies an ethical decision-making framework to clinical situations that incorporates moral concepts, professional ethics, and law and respects diverse values and beliefs	
3. Applies legal and ethical guidelines to advocate for client well-being and preferences	
4. Enables clients and families to make quality-of-life and end-of-life decisions and achieve a peaceful death	
5. Identifies and analyzes common ethical dilemmas and the ways in which these dilemmas impact client care	
6. Identifies areas in which a personal conflict of interest may arise and proposes resolutions or actions to resolve the conflict	

Used with permission from the Commission on Nurse Certification (2011, 2014).

Resources

American Association of Colleges of Nursing. (2007). *White paper on the education and role of the clinical nurse leader*. Washington, DC. Available at http://www.aacn.nche.edu/Publications/WhitePapers/ClinicalNurseLeader07.pdf

American Nurses Association. (2001). *Code of ethics for nurses with interpretive statements*. Retrieved from http://nursingworld.org/MainMenuCategories/EthicsStandards/CodeofEthicsforNurses/Foundational-and-Supplemental-Documents

American Nurses Association. (2010). *Registered nurses' roles and responsibilities in providing expert care and counseling at the end of life*. Retrieved from http://nursingworld.org/MainMenuCategories/EthicsStandards/Ethics-Position-Statements/etpain14426.pdf

Commission on Nurse Certification. (2011). *Clinical Nurse Leader job analysis report*. Retrieved from http://www.aacn.nche.edu/cnl/Job-Analysis-Report.pdf

Commission on Nurse Certification. (2014). *Clinical Nurse Leader (CNL®) certification exam blueprint*. Retrieved from http://www.aacn.nche.edu/leading-initiatives/cnl/cnl-certification/pdf/ExamContentOutline11.pdf

Gawande, A. (2009). *The checklist manifesto: How to get things right*. New York, NY: Henry Holt.

Guido, G. (2010). *Legal and ethical issues in nursing* (5th ed.). Upper Saddle River, NJ: Pearson Prentice Hall

Halloran, M. (1982). Rational ethical judgments utilizing a decision-making tool. *Heart and Lung, 11*(6), 566–570.

Harmon, L. (2006). *Ethical challenges in the management of health information* (2nd ed.). Sudsbury, MA: Jones & Bartlett.

Jonsen, A., Siegler, M., & Winslade, W. (2006). *Clinical ethics: A practical guide to ethical decisions in clinical medicine* (6th ed.). New York, NY: McGraw-Hill.

Koh, H., & Sebelius, K. (2010). Promoting prevention through the Affordable Care Act. *The New England Journal of Medicine, 363*, 1296–1299.

Kuebler, K., Berry, P., & Heidrich, D. (2002). *End of life care. Clinical practice guidelines*. Philadelphia, PA: Springer.

Mahon, M. (2010). Clinical decision making in palliative care and end of life care. *Nursing Clinics of North America, 45*, 345–362.

National Hospice and Palliative Care Organization. (1999). *Standards of accreditation committee, hospice standards of practice*. Author: Arlington, VA.

Oshima Lee, E., & Emmanuel, E. (2013). Shared decision making to improve care and reduce costs. *The New England Journal of Medicine, 368*, 6–8.

Thompson, J., & Thompson, H. (1981). *Ethics in nursing*. New York, NY: Macmillan.

Tilden, V., Corless, I., Dahlin, C., Ferrell, B., Gibson, R., & Lentz, J. (2011). Advance care planning as an urgent public health concern. *Nursing Outlook, 59*, 55–56.

Online Resources

American Nurses Association
http://www.ana.org
http://nursingworld.org/MainMenuCategories/EthicsStandards
http://nursingworld.org/MainMenuCategories/Policy-Advocacy/Positions-and-Resolutions
Compassion and Support at the End of Life

http://www.compassionandsupport.org
Hospice and Palliative Nurses Association
http://www.hpna.org
Pain Management Guidelines
http://www.guideline.gov/content.aspx?id=9744
Promoting Excellence: Advanced Practice Nursing: Pioneering Practices in Palliative Care
http://www.promotingexcellence.org/apn
The Center for Ethics and Advocacy in Healthcare
http://www.healthcare-ethics.org
The National Center for Ethics in Healthcare
http://www.ethics.va.gov

V

Test Questions, Answers, and Rationales

22

Multiple-Choice Questions and Case Studies

Coordinator of Item Writers

Carla Gene Rapp, PhD, RN
Adult Gerontology Nurse Practitioner and Consultant
Durham, North Carolina

Item Writers

Chris Blackhurst, MS, RN, CNL
Adjunct Faculty
The University of Portland;
Pediatric Nurse
Providence Center for Medically Fragile Children
Portland, Oregon

Laura Carmichael Blackhurst, MS, RN, CNL
Adjunct Nursing Instructor
Clark College
Vancouver, Washington;
Inpatient RN
Peace Health
Longview, Washington

Stephanie Collins, MSN, RNC-MNN, CNL
Clinical Nurse Leader
Stamford Hospital
Stamford, Connecticut

Deborah Foll, MSN, RNC-MNN, CNL
Clinical Nurse Leader
Stamford Hospital
Stamford, Connecticut

Heather Helton, MSN, RN, CMSRN, CNL
Clinical Nurse Leader
Carolinas Medical Center
Charlotte, North Carolina

Valerie Short, MSN, RN, CMSRN, CNL
Clinical Nurse Leader
Carolinas Medical Center
Charlotte, North Carolina

Joselyn Wright, MSN, RN, CMSRN, CNL
Clinical Nurse Leader
Carolinas Medical Center
Charlotte, North Carolina

Correspondence to:

Cynthia R. King, PhD, NP, MSN, CNL, FAAN
Principal & Consultant
Special Care Consultants
Dean of Nursing & Professor
Mount Aloysius College
Cresson, Pennsylvania
E-mail: cynthia.r.king@hotmail.com

Sally O'Toole Gerard, DNP, RN, CDE, CNL
Assistant Professor
CNL Track Coordinator
Fairfield University
Fairfield, Connecticut
E-mail: sgerard@fairfield.edu

1. A new graduate nurse, Jenny, approaches you and states she needs help removing a peripherally inserted central catheter (PICC). Which of the following is the best response when acting as a horizontal leader?
   A. Remove the PICC yourself
   B. Tell Jenny to find the policy and then remove the PICC
   C. Help Jenny find the policy and review it with her. Coach Jenny while she removes the PICC and provide feedback
   D. Help Jenny find the policy and refer her to a nurse with 12 years of experience for assistance
2. What organizational theory is used with rapid, unpredictable, and constant change?
   A. Systems theory
   B. Chaos theory
   C. Change theory
   D. Traditional theory
3. A 65-year-old African American male was admitted to your microsystem with hyperglycemia. The patient has a history of hypertension, gout, obesity, and smoking. The patient has a family history of diabetes and hypertension. Which statement by the patient demonstrates his understanding of modifiable risk factors for diabetes?
   A. "As I get older, my risk for diabetes increases."
   B. "I know that a family history of diabetes is a risk factor, so I will educate my children on diabetes prevention."
   C. "I will keep a record of all my blood sugars to take to my doctor's appointments."
   D. "I will attend a smoking cessation class, because I know smoking increases my risk for diabetes."
4. Your hospital is currently trialing the integration of the clinical nurse leader (CNL) role. At the end of the trial implementation period how can you, as the CNL, best illustrate the effectiveness of your role during this trial?
   A. Refer to increased patient satisfaction scores over the course of the trial
   B. Present data that demonstrates the effect of the CNL and outcomes achieved over the course of the trial
   C. Present a list of projects and tasks completed over the course of the trial
   D. Refer to your performance review over the course of the trial

5. You are a CNL on an oncology unit. Recently, there has been an increase in the number of catheter-associated urinary tract infections (CAUTIs) on your unit. After shadowing nurses and aides you observed a variety of practices, techniques, and expectations surrounding daily catheter care. Your hospital does not have a current policy or procedure regarding catheter care. As the CNL, what should you do next?
   A. Review current evidence for catheter care practice and disseminate evidence to the staff
   B. Form an interdisciplinary team meeting to evaluate current hospital catheter care policies
   C. Create a rubric for educating patients and staff on catheter care
   D. Discuss with the unit manager the clinical issue and create a set of evidence-based unit expectations and practices for the oncology unit. Evaluate the need to address this issue with a hospital-wide policy or procedure.
6. A 50-year-old woman with a history of stage 3 chronic obstructive pulmonary disease (COPD) presents to the emergency department (ED) with increased shortness of breath. Based on your lab results, what is the acid–base disorder?
   Labs as follows:
   pH 7.25 — $PaCO_2$ 50 mmHg
   HCO_3 22 mEq/L — PO_2 75
   SpO_2 88% — Na + 136
   BUN 18
   A. Uncompensated respiratory acidosis
   B. Metabolic acidosis
   C. Respiratory acidosis
   D. Uncompensated respiratory acidosis
7. A CNL evaluates a 17-year-old patient who has been a victim of rape. The patient has visible bruising and a head laceration. After the CNL's assessment, law enforcement officials have contacted the CNL requesting information regarding the attack and the visible injuries seen during the visit.
   The CNL knows she must first:
   A. Take pictures and complete the rape kit
   B. Provide law enforcement with the record as requested
   C. Call the patient's parents first
   D. Explain to the patient in order to obtain consent for release of records

8. A CNL in the neonatal intensive-care unit (NICU) is collecting data on the hours worked weekly by the staff nurses. The CNL wants to see if there is a normal distribution of hours worked. What technique is the best to display the distribution of the data collected?
   A. Run chart
   B. Fishbone chart
   C. Failure modes and effects analysis (FMEA) chart
   D. Histogram chart
9. Your pediatric oncology unit is considering the implementation of a social/activity program for child clients that would provide volunteer social interactions and age-appropriate activities to admitted clients. As the CNL for this unit, you recognize this intervention as a way to:
   A. Be helpful to the floor staff by distracting clients
   B. Be a wasteful expenditure
   C. Meet the psychosocial needs of clients
   D. Prevent poor client experience ratings on discharge surveys
10. When assessing a new microsystem, the CNL will often use a tool known as the "5 Ps." As a CNL, you recognize the "5 Ps" to include are:
    A. Purpose, patients, process, patterns, professionals
    B. Patients, providers, policies, patterns, prevention
    C. Purpose, patients, providers, patterns, prevention
    D. Patients, process, professionals, policies, patterns
11. Mr. Johnson is an 80-year-old patient who lives alone. He had fallen and was found by his neighbors. Mr. Johnson has a history of multiple falls, congestive heart failure (CHF), myocardial infarction (MI), diabetes mellitus (DM), and asthma. Mr. Johnson is admitted to the hospital with a hip fracture. Using an interdisciplinary approach, who should the CNL include in the plan of care initially?
    A. Clinical care manager, medical social worker, clinical nutritionist, CNL, and physician
    B. Clinical care manager, medical social worker, clinical nutritionist, physical therapist, registered nurse, CNL, and physician
    C. Speech therapist, clinical care manager, medical social worker, CNL, registered nurse, and nursing supervisor
    D. Clinical care manager, medical social worker, CNL, registered nurse, and nurse manager
12. As the CNL on a cardiac telemetry unit, you are performing a root cause analysis (RCA) due to the high volume of catheter-associated urinary tract infections (CAUTIs) over the last 6 months. Realizing that the

Centers for Medicare & Medicaid are on a pay-for-performance basis, you develop a CAUTI task force in an effort to reduce cost. This is an example of which of the following?

A. Implementing cost reduction and savings

B. Anticipating risk and designing plans of care to improve outcomes

C. Evaluating the effect of the healthcare financing on care access and patient outcomes

D. Applying basic business and economic principles to the microsystem

13. You notice a trend of increased central line bloodstream infection (CLBSI) on your unit. You conduct a literature search and, after critiquing and synthesizing the available evidence, you find that central line bundles have been shown to decrease CLBSI. You want to implement this bundle on your unit, and plan to evaluate the effect of this change. Which of the following best describes this process?

A. Plan-Do-Study-Act (PDSA)

B. Research

C. Process improvement

D. Evidence-based practice (EBP)

14. A CNL rounds with Dr. Camper on a Spanish-speaking patient. The CNL asks the physician to call an interpreter, but the MD states that it is not necessary because the patient's daughter speaks English. However, the CNL insists and ensures an interpreter is present. What CNL role was fulfilled?

A. Educator

B. Team manager

C. Clinician

D. Client advocate

15. During the policy formulation phase, all of the following are correct except:

A. Possible solutions are offered.

B. Political circumstances are considered.

C. A problem is identified.

D. Policy decisions are adjusted to accommodate changing circumstances or needs.

16. The unit implemented bedside reporting 6 months ago, but the change has not been sustained. As a CNL, you begin to participate in bedside reporting and provide constructive, immediate feedback to the nurses for improvement. What best describes this situation?

A. Mentoring

B. Transformational leadership

C. Coaching

D. Precepting

17. Jane, a CNL, successfully implemented an evidence-based practice (EBP) project utilizing music therapy to help with pain control in sickle cell patients on a medical–surgical unit. Jane was asked by the chief nursing officer (CNO) to implement the project within the medical division. What system will Jane be working in?

A. Mesosystem

B. Macrosystem

C. Microsystem

D. Unit system

18. Judy has a family history of type 2 diabetes. After education, Judy knows she can help to prevent diabetes by maintaining a healthy weight, healthy eating habits, and daily physical activity. Judy is exhibiting what type of prevention strategies?

A. Primary prevention

B. Secondary prevention

C. Tertiary prevention

D. Quaternary prevention

19. You are a CNL on a surgical unit. Your unit has just hired several new graduate nurses. As the CNL, what is your role in relationship to these new team members?

A. Provider of all clinical education

B. Evaluator for performance reviews

C. Coach and mentor

D. Individual with a hands-off approach to allow new nurses to develop skills independently

20. You are the CNL on a surgical unit. You have noticed that readmission rates for your orthopedic patients have increased steadily over the last several months. Upon investigation, you find that patients are reporting that they do not believe they are receiving adequate education on post-operative wound management. As the CNL, you recognize that one way you can act to promote the health of your patients is:

A. Provide direct, culturally appropriate education to all patients on your unit

B. Arrange post-op visits at the outpatient surgical clinic for all patients upon discharge

C. Educate the nursing staff regarding how they can evaluate patient health literacy, provide education at an appropriate level for each patient, and evaluate patient understanding of education provided

D. Discuss with pre-op staff beginning patient education much earlier in this hospital process

21. A mother presents to the emergency department (ED) with her 8-month-old son, who has the following symptoms: coughing, recurring respiratory infections, fatty stools, and failure to thrive. Upon examination, the infant's vitals are as follows: Temp 99.4°F, pulse 150, respirations 65, blood pressure 88/50 mmHg. A CNL in the ED receives a phone call from the laboratory stating that *Staphylococcus aureus* was found colonized in the patient's airway.

    As a CNL in the ED you know that the preceding symptoms and laboratory results are consistent with which of the following diseases?

    A. Asthma

    B. Lobar pneumonia

    C. Cystic fibrosis

    D. Croup

22. An elderly Chinese woman has just been diagnosed with terminal cancer. While discussing end-of-life care decisions with the family, patient, and CNL, the CNL notices there are conflicting viewpoints between the family and patient regarding advance directives. Which of these is the best answer regarding advance directives?

    A. In the Chinese culture, the family makes the decisions regarding end-of-life care in order not to burden the patient.

    B. It is best not to fully inform the patient of his or her condition so that he or she will remain positive.

    C. The patient has the right to enact his or her own advance directive to guide his or her medical treatments according to the Patient Self-Determination Act.

    D. The interdisciplinary team has the most information on palliative care to make the best decision.

23. A CNL in the emergency department (ED) is auditing stroke patients' charts and the administration of tissue plasminogen activator (tPA) and notices that only 83% of patients who are eligible to receive tPA are receiving it. The CNL knows that the 83% administration rate is below the national benchmark. The CNL identifies that there is a time lag in MRI. The CNL creates a stroke team to develop a guideline implementation action plan to improve the process of timing of the MRI. What is the best tool utilized by the CNL in implementing change?

A. Research study

B. Meta-analysis

C. Plan-Do-Study-Act (PDSA)

D. Standardize-Do–Study-Act (SDSA)

24. A group composed of unit-based council members was put on a task force to improve the discharge planning process because patients felt unprepared and rushed at discharge. A decision was made to create a discharge planning nurse position to educate patients the night before the discharge. Even though the new nurses did not like this solution, they deferred to the senior nurses of this group who were adamant about implementing this position. Which barrier to effective teamwork does this exemplify?

A. Physical threats

B. Groupthink

C. Team dysfunction

D. Authority gradient

25. You are a CNL on a pediatric unit. You are doing chart audits on attending physicians' daily charting and assessment notes and notice that a small number of attending physicians are not seeing patients daily. They are putting in discharge orders days prior to discharge. As a CNL, you know the hospital has a policy that attending physicians must see their patients every 24 hours. The CNL waits to see what happens during the next scheduled chart audits. What conflict resolution is demonstrated?

A. Compromise

B. Accommodate

C. Compete

D. Avoidance

26. Attending physicians have noted that on your unit nurse communication by telephone has been scattered, disjointed, lengthy, and often contains erroneous information. As the CNL, good interdisciplinary communication is a priority. To best address this issue, the CNL would:

A. Wait to see if the issue persists

B. Encourage floor nurses to provide less information when calling physicians to limit the length and complexity of their calls

C. Ask physicians to provide their feedback directly to individual nurses

D. Refamiliarize staff nurses with the use of situation background assessment recommendation (SBAR), your hospital's communication standard

27. Quality improvement (QI) is a key function of the CNL. While QI efforts can yield many benefits in healthcare, as the CNL you recognize which

of the following to be *the most important potential effect of a nursing QI effort?*

A. Increased hospital cash flow/decreased expense

B. Increased competitiveness with other facilities

C. Reduction in lawsuits/liability

D. Improvement of nursing quality indicators

28. While assisting Dr. Smith with a central line insertion you notice she did not properly execute sterile technique. What is the most appropriate way to provide feedback?

A. Stop Dr. Smith while she is talking to the patient and provide feedback

B. Ask Dr. Smith to stop the procedure so you can get her another central line insertion kit

C. Refer Dr. Smith to the policy and procedure manual and ask that she read the section on using aseptic technique

D. Debate with Dr. Smith at the bedside and tell her errors like this are the reason patients acquire hospital-acquired conditions

29. Which of the following is the best description of healthcare economics?

A. Understanding run charts

B. Competence demonstrated by knowledge and ability to articulate federal, state, and private payer system regulations and issues, as well as the impact on organizations

C. Identifying the number of patient falls per patient day

D. The number of staff assigned to work on a given shift on a given day

30. Amy, a nurse on your unit, is interested in implementing a project to improve health literacy and diabetes using follow-up phone calls. She asks the CNL for help in initiating the project. What would be her first step?

A. Identify the clinical problem

B. Implement follow-up phone calls

C. Determine outcomes of the project

D. Review literature for evidence

31. Mrs. Jones, a patient with multiple comorbidities, has been hospitalized for over 3 months due to her recent stroke. During this period, she has not progressed and has had a tracheostomy and percutaneous endoscopic gastronomy (PEG) tube placed. Two of the daughters refused to make the patient a do not resuscitate (DNR), while the son and husband want the patient to be a DNR. As a CNL, you are conflicted and want the best outcome for the patient. What is the best step for you to take?

A. Find out if the patient has an advance directive or wants to be a DNR

B. Prevent the patient from being a DNR

C. Call the physician to make the decision

D. Make the patient a DNR according to the husband's wishes

32. Team coordination skills can help avoid all of the following except:

A. Undefined team member roles

B. Poor membership involvement

C. Member conflict

D. Confusion regarding next steps

33. The CNL of the heart failure unit encourages the staff to earn advanced degrees, obtain certifications, and present and publish EBP projects. The CNL exhibits which type of leadership style?

A. Relational leadership

B. Transactional leadership

C. Situational leadership

D. Transformational leadership

34. A CNL works in an inpatient unit that provides healthcare to medical–surgical patients. This best describes which of the following?

A. Macrosystem

B. Mesosystem

C. Microsystem

D. Megasystem

35. Maureen is a 45-year-old female who is undergoing chemotherapy for ovarian cancer. Maureen complains of increased nausea, vomiting, and abdominal pain uncontrolled by medications prescribed by her oncologist. Maureen expresses that she wants to continue chemotherapy, but she is unable to eat and maintain her weight due to her symptoms. She describes the pain as unbearable and at times she is unable to get out of bed. What would be the best step for the CNL to take next?

A. Discuss code status and healthcare power of attorney with Maureen

B. Contact hospice care to arrange a meeting with Maureen

C. Call the physician and suggest a palliative care consult

D. Suggest alternative methods for pain relief such as meditation, healing touch, and aromatherapy

36. You are a CNL on a busy surgical unit. Recently, several nurses have reported confusion regarding their patients' discharge process. The nurses stated that they were often unaware of all communications between

the surgeon, discharge planners, social workers, and pharmacists. As a result, the nurses were often unaware of their patient discharge plans, status, and needs. As a CNL, how can you best improve this process?

A. Educate nurses on how to access progress notes from other providers within the current electronic health record (EHR)

B. Discuss with each healthcare team member the clinical issue regarding the discharge process and suggest the creation of a daily interdisciplinary team meeting

C. Communicate to the surgeons the nurses' concerns, and advocate for the nurses' needs for communication in their role

D. Assume responsibility for the coordination of all discharge needs for patients on the unit

37. How can the CNL best provide and educate staff on giving culturally competent care within the unit?

A. Educate staff on assessment questions/phrases in the most common secondary language present in the community or seen within the hospital

B. Educate staff on varying cultural perceptions and beliefs surrounding the concept of health

C. Provide an in-service on accessing patient education and handouts in another language

D. Ensure that nurses are assigned to the most culturally appropriate patients currently on the unit

38. A 40-year-old postpartum patient with chronic hypertension and gestational diabetes who is gravida 5 para 4 is transferred from labor and delivery to the postpartum unit with lactated Ringer's at 125 mL/hr. Upon assessment of the patient, the nurse notices the patient's fundus is three finger breaths above umbilicus and to the right of midline and her bladder is palpable. The nurse also notes moderate to heavy bleeding and a full bladder and notifies the CNL.

As a CNL, the most important nursing intervention is to:

A. Encourage the nurse to massage the fundus and heplock the patient

B. Encourage the nurse to call the physician stat to order methergine (methylergonovine maleate)

C. Encourage the nurse to monitor the patient over the next hour because there are no risk factors for a postpartum hemorrhage

D. Encourage the nurse to straight catheterize the patient to decrease the likelihood of a postpartum hemorrhage

39. A 6-year-old boy is in critical condition following a car accident. The patient has head trauma and internal bleeding. The patient's parents have stated multiple times that they are Jehovah's Witnesses and do not want their son to receive blood.

    The CNL knows that the blood transfusion is needed immediately and could save the boy's life. Which of the following statements is the best thing for the CNL to do?

    A. Listen to the parents, as U.S. minors have no legal rights and remain under parental jurisdiction

    B. Obtain a court order in the best interest of the child to receive blood, based on the avoidance of physical harm

    C. Based on religious beliefs, do not give blood

    D. Follow the physician's decision to give blood since the physician's decision overrides the parental decision

40. The group known as "Maternal Child Health" has many subunits such as pediatrics, well baby nursery, NICU, and maternity. This collection of units belongs to which system?

    A. Microsystem

    B. Mesosystem

    C. Macrosystem

    D. Megasystem

41. Which stage of Lewin's change theory involves explaining that the current situation must change?

    A. Unfreezing

    B. Adoption

    C. Evaluation

    D. Change

42. A client with complex behavior concerns is getting ready to be discharged to a skilled nursing facility. However, the client has expressed that he wishes to stay in the hospital and not be discharged. As the CNL, your best action would be to:

    A. Inform the patient and his or her family that they must go and remaining on the unit is not an option

    B. Advocate letting the client stay on the unit one extra day, then discharge tomorrow

    C. Identify the client's concerns and collaborate with the care team to see they are addressed

    D. Ask the family to help encourage the client to discharge to the skilled nursing facility

43. A healthy work environment is an important factor in supporting ongoing quality and safety. As the CNL, you recognize that the hallmarks of a healthy work environment include all of the following except:

    A. Skilled communication

    B. Upward mobility

    C. Effective decision making

    D. Appropriate staffing

44. While rounding on your cohort of patients, you are informed by one of your patients that she does not have healthcare insurance. As a CNL, you know that interdisciplinary communication is very important. What member of the team is most effective in helping with this matter?

    A. The care management team: medical social worker, clinical case manager (CCM), and medical team

    B. Pastoral care

    C. The business office of the hospital

    D. Nursing staff

45. Who can function as an important ally to the CNL in engaging frontline staff in a major initiative?

    A. Content expert

    B. Unit champion

    C. Initiative sponsor

    D. Senior leadership

46. Which of the following best utilizes the PICOT method of developing a clinical question?

    A. Will a preoperative class for coronary artery bypass graft (CABG) surgery patients decrease anxiety?

    B. What is the effect of early mobility in patients 65 years and older on length of stay?

    C. Will the implementation of quiet time and employee education of harmful effects of noise reduce peak levels and improve patient satisfaction of patients on a medical-telemetry unit over a 1-month period?

    D. Will the use of secret shoppers increase compliance with hand washing and PPE in a large hospital in the Southeast?

47. Which of the following is the best example of a CNL protecting patient autonomy?

    A. The CNL ensures the patient understands how to use an incentive spirometer.

B. The CNL ensures the patient has all information and understands the procedure for esophagogastroduodenoscopy (EGD)/colonoscopy scheduled for the morning.

C. The CNL discusses the plan of care for treatment of pneumonia with the daughter and the doctor.

D. The CNL closes the door to protect the patient's privacy when discussing her diagnosis.

48. You are a CNL on a surgical unit. Your manager has asked you to review and update the current patient skin prep procedure as needed. After reviewing the evidence, you determine the current surgical skin prep does not match current evidence suggesting a need for chlorhexidine gluconate (CHG) wipes. At your next meeting with your manager, how do you best advocate for change?

A. Provide a list of resources for the new CHG skin prep, costs, and available vendors

B. Interpret the evidence of effectiveness of the CHG wipes prep and the related patient outcomes for patients receiving this skin prep; present the findings and suggest how this could be best used to change practice on the unit

C. Present feedback from the nursing staff on the current practices on the unit

D. Alert the manager that there is a discrepancy between the current practice and evidence, and await further instructions before proceeding

49. The new hospital CNO works hard to cultivate a shared vision of leaders and followers motivating each other toward their highest potential. This is an example of which type of leadership?

A. Transformational leadership

B. Transactional leadership

C. Situational leadership

D. Hierarchical leadership

50. The CNL's role is to lead frontline staff in line with the organization's core competencies. Which of the following best describes how a CNL can promote a high-performing clinical microsystem?

A. Support an atmosphere for learning and redesign supported by continuous monitoring of care, use of benchmarking, and frequent tests of change

B. Promote a microsystem that is in silo from the community and does not cross professional boundaries

C. Encourage staff to provide opinions and feedback, though the manager will make the final decision

D. Promote engagement by sharing positive outcomes with the staff and having celebrations, but keep negative outcomes confidential in order to keep the staff from feeling defeated

51. The CNL completes a 5P assessment of the microsystem and discovers that the geriatric population has increased. Forty-three percent of the patients within the microsystem are older than 65 years. Recognizing this change, the CNL determines which of the following is an appropriate action?

A. Coordinate monthly lunch-and-learn opportunities for the staff to discuss topics related to nutrition, cognitive impairment, and mobility

B. Discuss the change with the nurse manager and order more bed alarms for the microsystem

C. Volunteer to take blood pressures and check hemoglobin A1cs at the local adult day-care center

D. Conduct a randomized control study on visual impairment in diabetic patients older than 70 years

52. Your hospital is changing to a new electronic health record (EHR) system. As a CNL, you recognize that while this change may ultimately improve workflow, during the transition there will likely be both technical issues and knowledge gaps. What are some ways you can improve the ease of transition?

A. Assess the current transition timeline, including education and practice time for the staff

B. Identify leaders on the unit who can commit to extra training on the EHR and staff support during the transition

C. Create guidelines for the nurses to use as a quick reference for locating items in the EHR

D. All of the above

53. A 16-year-old female with a history of smoking, tanning bed use, and sexual activity presents to the emergency department (ED) with a mole that is continuously bleeding and itchy. The patient is concerned that this might be a sexually transmitted disease (STD) because the mole is on her inner thigh. Upon examination, the mole is asymmetrical, 7 mm big, and has uneven borders.

As a CNL, you know these characteristics represent which of the following?

A. Genital herpes

B. Human papillomavirus

C. Basal cell carcinoma

D. Malignant melanoma

54. Marci, a surgical nurse, is reviewing the operating room schedule and sees a coworker, Angie, is having surgery that day. Marci then calls

the supervisor and manager to let them know Angie is having surgery. Marci then tells the CNL she is going to visit Angie in the postanesthesia care unit (PACU). What should the CNL do?

A. Explain to Marci that this is a violation of the Health Information Portability and Accountability Act (HIPAA) and we must protect Angie's right to privacy and confidentiality

B. Invite other nurses to visit Angie and bring her flowers

C. Nothing; since this is a coworker, this is not considered a violation of HIPAA

D. Arrange for Angie to have "VIP" treatment

55. What type of chart is used in QI and uses step-by-step symbols to plan projects and describe a process?

A. Flowchart/process mapping

B. Pareto chart

C. Control chart

D. Run chart

56. On the rehabilitation unit, the CNL notes that the stroke and amputee patients that require maximum assistance are being assigned to the float nurses. It is noted that many of these patients have had falls while being assigned to the float pool nurses. This is a patient and family dissatisfier. What type of delegation practice is in question?

A. The right circumstance

B. The right supervision

C. The right person

D. The right task

57. In recent months, there has been a marked increase in the number of intravenous (IV) infections and infiltrations on your unit. Some of these IVs were started on your unit while others were started on other units or in the emergency unit before being transferred to your unit. The nurse manager has asked you to investigate this issue. As the CNL, your best intervention would be to:

A. Call other units to make sure policies and procedures are being followed

B. Wait to see if the infection occurrences are a coincidence

C. Form a group to investigate this issue including staff nurses from your unit, representatives from IV therapy, and infection prevention services

D. Retrain all staff nurses on your unit in correct IV care procedures

58. As the CNL when engaging in a QI effort, you recognize *the first of the common steps* of the QI process to be:

A. Review literature

B. Analyze the root cause

C. Establish a clear purpose or aim

D. Select metrics

59. A Vietnamese patient is admitted with pneumonia on a medical–surgical unit. The patient appears very nervous when the medical staff enters the room. As a CNL, what is the best course of action to take in this situation?

A. Try to talk to the patient calmly and ease his fears

B. Call language services and request a Vietnamese interpreter

C. Ask your housekeeper who is from Vietnam to come in and interpret for the medical staff

D. Keep all interactions with the patient as brief as possible

60. Which of the following is not an example of healthcare finance and economics?

A. Developing and leveraging human, environmental, and material resources

B. Understanding the fiscal context in which practice occurs

C. Leading a gap analysis to create a cohesive healthcare team

D. Applying basic business and economic principles and practices

61. A nurse is trying to determine the difference between evidence-based practice (EBP) and research. She approaches her unit CNL to assist her in her dilemma. What statement best describes the appropriate response by the CNL?

A. EBP involves critiquing and synthesizing evidence, while research involves designing a study because there is a gap in knowledge.

B. EBP needs institutional review board (IRB) approval, while research does not.

C. EBP involves collecting and analyzing data, while research includes critiquing and synthesizing evidence.

D. In EBP, the first step is identifying a clinical problem, while in research identifying a clinical problem is the last step.

62. Maria, a 55-year-old Spanish-speaking patient, is scheduled for a paracentesis. You, the CNL, rounded on her with an interpreter in the morning and explained to her the procedure is scheduled for today at noon. After you mentioned this, Maria stated that she was not aware of this procedure. You noted that a consent was signed by the physician in her chart. What is the next step as a CNL?

A. Keep the consent. Utilize the teach-back method to ensure Maria understands the risk and benefits of the procedure.

B. Discard the previous consent. Explain to Maria that she needs this procedure and it is the best decision for her. Obtain a new consent.

C. Inform the physician and ensure he explains the procedure to Maria with an interpreter present and obtains a new consent.

D. Keep the consent. Leave a note for the physician and explain that the patient was unaware of the procedure.

63. The CNL completed an assessment of the community and identified a need for a public health program. Which of the following would have the potential for the greatest impact on the community?

A. Implement a small pilot program at the local hospital

B. Write a proposal to make the change and send it to the legislators to build their support for the change

C. Research and analyze public health programs in other communities

D. Write an article for the local paper discussing the need for the program

64. Lisa is a CNL who works with high-risk obstetric patients both inpatient at the hospital and outpatient in the local health clinic. Lisa follows each patient throughout his or her episodes of care, ensuring the patient receives streamlined, comprehensive care. Which critical component of lateral integration best describes what Lisa is demonstrating?

A. Coordination

B. Communication

C. Collaboration

D. Evaluation

65. From which database would the CNL collect the most useful nursing-sensitive indicator metrics?

A. National Database of Nursing Quality Indicators® (NDNQI)

B. Hospital Compare

C. The Joint Commission (TJC)

D. Nursing Quality Forum (NQF)

66. You are working with a team to reduce patient waiting time for transport to diagnostic imaging (DI). An effective goal would be to:

A. Decrease waiting time during the evening shift

B. Increase monthly patient satisfaction

C. Improve communication between the emergency department (ED) and the DI departments

D. Decrease the waiting time for DI by 5%

67. A 55-year-old male is readmitted to the hospital with hypertension four times within the past 8 months due to medication noncompliance. The patient has been given a blood pressure machine, set up with a primary

care provider, and arranged telehealth services in previous admissions. During your discussion with the patient, he states that he is taking his medication as his doctor prescribed. The patient brought his medications into the hospital, so you ask him to hand you his blood pressure medication bottle. The patient hands you the bottle labeled Neurontin. Which of the following would be the next best step for you to take as the CNL?

A. Obtain records from the patient's primary care provider

B. Coordinate a family meeting with the patient and the care team

C. Have the patient hand you the rest of the bottles, tell you what each medication is, and describe how and when he takes that medication

D. Consult with a pharmacist to determine the best medication options for the patient

68. Promotion of personal goals for professional development and continuing education is a hallmark of the CNL role. Ultimately, what is the importance of professional development?

A. Maintaining professional practice competencies

B. Fulfillment of the CNL as a lifelong learner

C. Providing an example of professional nursing to peers

D. All of the above

69. You recognize that a large proportion of your surgical patients have cultural or religious concerns about the use of blood transfusions, although the need for such transfusions are common with many of your surgeries. As the CNL at a surgical center, how can you best ensure health promotion of this population while providing culturally competent care?

A. Develop education on the importance of blood transfusions when medically necessary, and the benefits postoperatively

B. Provide resources like the other clinics in the area that may be able to perform the surgery with lowered risks of estimated blood loss

C. Evaluate evidence on alternatives to blood transfusions, such as autologous blood transfusions and alternative blood products, and present this information at an interdisciplinary team meeting

D. Educate staff on respecting client wishes and do not attempt to pressure patients into receiving transfusions

70. A 28-year-old patient with asthma is requesting the pneumococcal (PNA) vaccine. Which of the following conditions are appropriate for receiving the pneumococcal vaccine?

A. Congestive heart failure (CHF), HIV, diabetes, pregnancy

B. CHF, HIV, diabetes, sickle cell disease

C. Diabetes, chemotherapy, sickle cell disease, pregnancy

D. Pregnancy, CHF, diabetes, chemotherapy

71. A new graduate nurse expresses concern about a frenotomy of the tongue-tied newborn to the CNL. The CNL decides to accompany the new nurse to the procedure room. Upon entering the procedure room, the new nurse notices that there is no consent signed and explains to the pediatrician consent must be signed before continuing. The pediatrician hollers at the nurse and refuses to have consent signed. How should the CNL respond?

    A. The CNL hollers back that this is against hospital policy.

    B. The CNL asks the parents to sign the consent without the physician speaking to the parents.

    C. The procedure continues without consent and the CNL assures the new nurse the consent will be obtained after the procedure.

    D. The CNL and new nurse professionally explain to the physician that they will not participate in the procedure until a consent is signed and they will contact hospital administration regarding this procedural violation.

72. A CNL on a medical unit is following up with patients on warfarin therapy postdischarge and concludes that patients are not receiving adequate education on medication administration. The CNL formulates an action plan and develops a team to improve warfarin discharge education. What competency was portrayed by the CNL?

    A. Lifelong learner

    B. Delegator

    C. Lateral integration

    D. Risk anticipator

73. A small group has been formed on the medical–surgical unit to implement change. Team members also have struggles over decision making and clarity of purpose. What stage of the Tuckman and Jensen model is represented by members communicating their feelings but still viewing themselves as individuals rather than part of the team?

    A. Performing

    B. Norming

    C. Forming

    D. Storming

74. You, the CNL, have noted that many staff nurses on your unit do not use available nurse aide (NA) staff to perform routine capillary blood glucose (CBG) checks, even though they are allowed to at your hospital. When you

investigate, you discover that most nurses were unaware the NAs could perform CBG checks. You, as the CNL, share information on the tasks NAs are able to perform during the next unit staff meeting in order to:

A. Ensure each member of the care team has a clear understanding of his or her role

B. Make sure staff nurses delegate as much work as possible

C. Make sure staff are using skills and training often enough

D. Ensure the NAs have enough to do

75. Failure mode-effect analysis is best used as follows:

A. In response to a critical or sentinel event

B. Prior to a process implementation or change

C. As part of a random audit process

D. In response to malfunctioning tools or equipment

76. During your daily rounds, you are performing an advance assessment on a patient in your cohort. The patient was admitted for sepsis, appears very weak, and has a very poor appetite. The patient tells you that he has not been out of the bed for 3 days. What needs to happen to provide the best care for this patient?

A. Enter an order for physical and occupational therapy, and ask the nursing staff to perform the Egress test to assess the patient's mobility level

B. Tell the patient to get out of bed and sit up in the chair three times a day

C. Place the bed in a bed-to-chair position

D. Order an incentive spirometer for the patient

77. As you are planning a discharge for a patient in your cohort, the patient tells you that, even though she has insurance, there is a financial strain on her to pay for her medication. The patient has a history of HIV/AIDS and is currently on three antiviral medications. The patient was admitted with pneumonia on this admission and the doctor has prescribed Zyvox in addition to her other medication regimen. You investigate the cost of this medication and find out the medication will cost the patient $100 after insurance. Which of the following is the most appropriate and first action for you as the CNL?

A. Tell the patient that she should take this prescribed medication so she can get better

B. Encourage the patient to take the medication because the doctor knows best

C. Call the doctor and ask him if there is a more cost-efficient medication to treat the patient's pneumonia

D. Consult with the medical social worker to find coupons for this medication

78. A certified nursing assistant (CNA) approaches the unit CNL to discuss her frustrations in attaining appropriate equipment for patient care. The CNA explains that the clean utility room is too far and that staff constantly have to make frequent trips. The CNA wants to know what steps to take to make a change. As a CNL, what statement best describes the appropriate response?

A. "We will just have to adjust to what we have right now."

B. "Well, you have identified a problem, the next step is to review any literature that can help resolve our issue."

C. "I suggest that you and the staff take the appropriate equipment to your rooms."

D. "Well, let us implement the process that another unit is using."

79. As Jeff, a new CNL, walks into his newly assigned intensive care unit (ICU), he notices that the charge nurse assigned him as a primary care nurse for a group of a patients, like she would do for a staff nurse. Jeff discusses the role of a CNL with the charge nurse. What statement best describes the appropriate approach by Jeff?

A. Jeff asks the charge nurse if she understands the role of a CNL, and states he cannot be assigned a group of patients.

B. Jeff asks the charge nurse if she understands the role of a CNL, then explains that the CNL does not provide direct care to patients.

C. Jeff discusses that CNLs are not supposed to take patients and only coordinate care for difficult patients.

D. Jeff explains that the CNL operates in a microsystem as an advanced generalist to communicate, coordinate, and collaborate care and does not serve as a primary care nurse.

80. As a CNL, it is important to remain aware of current changes to national healthcare policies, namely from ongoing focuses from the Centers for Medicare & Medicaid Services (CMS) and law prescribed by the Affordable Care Act (ACA), both of which have set reduced reimbursement for which of the following issues?

A. Elevated readmission rates

B. Medication errors

C. Falls

D. Nurses practicing below their scope

81. How can the CNL help determine the meaningful use of the electronic health record (EHR) within his or her microsystem?

A. Identify data that should be collected and managed, and note how that data should be shared for improving client outcomes

B. Coordinate with physicians to identify which clinical information would be meaningful for the patients under their care

C. Discuss with unit leaders and stakeholders what data could provide meaningful use of the EHR within the unit

D. Review the available client data currently in the EHR and assess for meaningfulness in improving patient outcomes

82. Regarding information technology, how can the CNL improve the identification of meaningful data?

A. Clarify with nurses what vendor-related terms may be used in their documentation

B. Develop a tool to identify relevant nursing clinical data and its location within the electronic health record (EHR)

C. Advocate for standardized nursing terminology within the EHR

D. Coordinate with the informatics the best way to document care for efficient data retrieval

83. The CNL works with the interdisciplinary team and encourages all members to voice their opinion and provide feedback. What type of leadership is the CNL demonstrating?

A. Vertical leadership

B. Diagonal leadership

C. Horizontal leadership

D. Systems leadership

84. The diabetes liaison on an adult medical–surgical unit informed the team that the unit was only 45% compliant with checking blood sugars within 15 minutes after a hypoglycemic event. The team decided to implement a process change to ensure the blood sugar recheck is completed within 15 minutes. The change was implemented and there was an increase to 85% compliance of hypoglycemic rechecks. What is the next step for the team in the PDSA cycle?

A. Plan

B. Do

C. Study

D. Act

85. Isabella is a 62-year-old female who enters the community health clinic where you are employed as a CNL. The front desk staff approaches you and states that Isabella has refused to complete the standard health questionnaire form and health information release form. Isabella states

that she forgot her glasses and that she will just take the form home to complete. Which of the following would be the most appropriate response by you as the CNL?

A. Tell the front desk staff to send the forms home with Isabella and provide her with a prepaid envelope to send the forms back to the office

B. Inform Isabella that many people have difficulty understanding these forms, and ask if she would like you or someone to help her complete the forms

C. Explain the importance of completing the forms to Isabella and ensure she completes the forms prior to entering the examination room

D. Provide Isabella with a magnifying glass to allow her to read the forms more easily

86. A nurse on your unit expresses concern about her patient. The patient is an 88-year-old male on the unit due to a chronic obstructive pulmonary disease (COPD) exacerbation. He has become deconditioned and therapy is involved. The patient is due to be discharged, but still appears very weak and unsteady. During his stay, he was newly diagnosed with insulin-dependent diabetes, and although he has been educated on insulin administration, the nurse is uncertain he can properly administer the medication at home. As the CNL, how do you proceed?

A. Organize an interdisciplinary team meeting to discuss the multiple concerns over patient treatment and condition, as well as greater discharge needs

B. Place an ethics consult

C. Encourage the nurse to call the MD and relay her concerns

D. Provide tools to the nurse that can help improve the patient's functioning regarding the insulin, and advocate for the use of oxygen at home

87. Staff nurses have a clinical question regarding the effectiveness of two different surgical skin preps stocked on your unit. Both benzalkonium chloride and CHG are available, and the nurses are uncertain of the differences—particularly in terms of reducing surgical site infections. As the CNL, what is the next step to take?

A. Review research on the effectiveness of each product in reducing surgical site infections and disseminate the evidence to staff

B. Organize a study of patients on your unit, trialing the different surgical prep and tracking patient outcomes

C. Determine the most cost-effective surgical skin prep for the patient

D. Research what products are being used on other units and other hospitals within your area

88. A patient presents with severe pain in the upper right abdomen after eating a fatty meal. These symptoms lead you to suspect cholecystitis. Which assessment finding is most likely to be associated with this condition?

    A. Positive Homans' sign

    B. Positive Psoas sign

    C. Murphy's sign

    D. Aaron's sign

89. The CNL has been requested to assist with end-of-life care decision making for an elderly homeless patient who has no family; he was deemed incompetent and is now unresponsive. The best decision-making guide that the CNL could use in this situation is:

    A. Plan-Do-Study-Act (PDSA)

    B. Autonomy model

    C. Orem's self-care theory

    D. MORAL model

90. You, the CNL, are working in the ICU with a high volume of patients with prolonged Foley catheter use. What analysis tool is appropriate for the CNL to use in prevention of CAUTIs?

    A. Root cause analysis (RCA)

    B. Fishbone diagram

    C. St. Thomas risk assessment tool

    D. Failure mode-effect analysis

91. A CNL using Rogers's diffusion of innovation theory realizes while implementing a new health information management (HIM) system that when dealing with a member of the healthcare team she should:

    A. Spend a majority of time educating the laggards to become supporters of change

    B. Spend a majority of time on innovators because they will need a lot of convincing to make a change

    C. Spend a majority of time with early and late majority adopters because when they support the change it will be successful

    D. Spend very little time with the early majority adopters because they are not adaptable to change

92. A client on your unit is going home to finish rehab following a bilateral total knee replacement. You, as the CNL, would be enacting the function of lateral integrator by which of the following?

    A. Delivering the bedside discharge education

    B. Helping the client arrange transportation home

C. Making a checklist of the client's belongings to ensure nothing was left behind

D. Ensuring follow-up appointments and services, including transportation, have been scheduled

93. An RCA is best used:

A. In response to a critical or sentinel event

B. Prior to a process implementation or change

C. As part of a random audit process

D. In response to malfunctioning tools or equipment

94. You are doing a daily assessment of your patient who has transferred from the medical intensive care unit (MICU). The patient has a history of congestive heart failure (CHF), myocardial infarction, atrial fibrillation, and diabetes. During your review of the medication administration record, you notice that the warfarin has not been ordered on admission. What is your next step as the CNL?

A. Call the pharmacist and ask for the medication to be put on the medication administration record

B. Find out what dosage of the medication the patient was taking and order it

C. Notify the primary nurse and suggest that she call the physician and notify him of the near miss

D. Call your nurse manager and notify him or her of this medication error

95. As you review a patient's medical record, you notice that the patient has an order for a chest x-ray. While reviewing the chart, you realize that the patient just completed a chest x-ray several hours ago while in the emergency department (ED). CNLs understand that diagnostic tests are very expensive so you call the doctor and find that the x-ray was duplicated by mistake. Unfortunately, by the time you find this mistake you see the radiology assistant exiting the patient's room. Once the error is found, you should:

A. Perform an root cause analysis (RCA) to see why this test was duplicated

B. Notify the patient's insurance company of the additional charges

C. Notify the nurse manager of this error

D. Review the order entry

96. You, as the CNL, plan to implement the use of bed alarms and hi-low beds to prevent falls on your unit. You are completing a literature review. While doing so, you are trying to determine the strength of the articles you have obtained. What process should you use to determine the most credible evidence?

A. Plan-Do-Study-Act (PDSA)
B. Evidence-based practice
C. Melynk and Fineout-Overholt hierarchy (Level 1–7)
D. Research utilization

97. Heather, a nurse for 7 years, recently attained her MSN, CNL. She is very passionate about being involved in her local community. She volunteers frequently at a community center for underprivileged children. During her time there, she noticed that obesity is a concern with this population. What step best describes Heather's advocating for this local community center?
    A. Heather collaborates with the community center leaders to get donations from local health food corporations to ensure a healthy meal is provided for the children.
    B. Heather collaborates with another CNL and plans to do a literature review on obesity.
    C. Heather discusses her concern of obesity with the community center leaders.
    D. Heather calls other community centers for underprivileged children to inquire about obesity in their population.

98. A staff member asks you, the CNL, what is the best way to explain health policy? What statement best explains health policy?
    A. Health policy generally denotes guidelines that affect the health of the individual, families, or communities through production, provision, and financing health or healthcare services.
    B. Health policy analyzes system and outcomes datasets to anticipate individual client risk and improve quality care.
    C. Health policy evaluates the environmental healthcare outcomes.
    D. Health policy means to consult with other health professionals to design, coordinate, and evaluate client care outcomes.

99. A nurse prepares to administer a patient's morning dose of metformin. After scanning the patient and the medication, a clinical alert appears on the computer screen warning of a possible interaction between the metformin and the CT contrast dye the patient received the day before. Based on this warning, the nurse chooses to hold the metformin and alert the pharmacy that this medication should be scheduled as held for 72 hours after receiving the contrast. This is an example of a(n):
    A. Clinical decision support system
    B. Health information technology

C. Clinical alert warning system

D. Decision tree

100. The healthcare team determines that the discharge process is ineffective and must be changed. The team determines the stakeholders and utilizes a force field analysis to weigh the pros and cons of the change. This was then used to motivate other team members and encourage buy in. Utilizing Lewin's theory of change, what stage is the team in?

A. Sustaining

B. Moving

C. Refreezing

D. Unfreezing

101. Tara, a CNL on a pediatric medical–surgical unit, conducted a 5P assessment and discovered that the discharge process was fragmented and parents were not satisfied with the process. Tara created a team to develop a change in order to improve the process. What model can Tara use to rapidly implement this change and test it to determine effectiveness?

A. Plan-Do-Study-Act (PDSA)

B. Strengths, weaknesses, opportunities, and threats (SWOT) analysis

C. Fishbone diagram

D. Gap analysis

102. A Native American patient is admitted with sepsis from a urinary tract infection. The patient is very weak and unable to ambulate much further than her room. The patient tells the CNL that she is very discouraged and feels that she is not able to get better because she is unable to touch "mother earth" with her feet. The CNL gathers some dirt, grass, and flowers from outside the hospital and places it in a bucket. The CNL brings the bucket in the patient's room and helps her to stand on the dirt. Which of the following best describes what the CNL is demonstrating?

A. Cultural knowledge

B. Cultural awareness

C. Cultural skills

D. Cultural management

103. A nurse comes to you with a concern about a telephone order she received from a doctor. The doctor asked her to review a physician order for life-sustaining treatment (POLST) form with a client, then sign and place it in his chart. The nurse is uncertain if this is in her scope of practice. You advise the nurse to:

A. Complete the form as ordered by the MD

B. Review the hospital's policy and procedure manual, and handle per policy

C. Review the State Board of Nursing Scope of Practice and handle according to your scope of practice

D. All of the above

104. How can a CNL help to identify the general discharge needs of patients on his or her unit?

A. Coordinate outpatient care and follow-up appointments

B. Assess protective and predictive factors of patient health

C. Discuss with each team's doctors the anticipated discharge needs of their patients

D. Approach staff nurses about their patients' discharge needs

105. Lisa, a CNL, is educating the staff on the effects of long-term bed rest. A majority of these patients have been on bed rest with a shortened cervix since 25 weeks gestation. Which of the following statements is true?

A. Bed rest is psychologically healthy.

B. Music therapy can ease the psychological effects of bed rest.

C. Bed rest prevents deep vein thrombosis (DVTs).

D. Bed rest has been proven to prevent preterm labor.

106. Recently, several major practice changes have been implemented hospital-wide at your facility. While all of these changes are evidence based, some of the practice changes have been received by the staff on your unit with strong resistance and poor compliance. As the CNL, you recognize that the best way to approach this issue is to:

A. Have the unit manager write-up noncompliant staff

B. Advocate to have the policies altered or revoked

C. Form a task force of involved parties to identify barriers to compliance

D. Re-educate staff on the policies and their importance

107. Ongoing risk reduction and patient safety efforts are an important component of:

A. Quality improvement (QI)

B. Knowledge management

C. Change theory

D. Complexity theory

108. You are in the process of initiating a mobility team and protocol on your unit. What members of the interdisciplinary team should be considered?

A. Nursing staff, physical therapist, nurse manager, occupational therapist, CNL, clinical nurse specialist, and physician

B. Physical therapist, physician, nursing assistants, manager, and CNL

C. Medical social worker, physician, nursing staff, physical therapy staff, and CNL

D. Physical therapist, occupational therapist, nursing staff, and the discharge coordinator

109. As a CNL on a very busy medical–telemetry unit, you have noticed that nurses are not utilizing incentive spirometry for patients with acute or chronic lung conditions. To ensure that patients are given the best care, you ask the electronic order entry representative to allow incentive spirometry to be entered as a nursing task. This will be used as a reminder for the nursing staff to perform this task. What action of the CNL is this?

A. Demonstrates use of healthcare technologies to maximize healthcare outcomes

B. Understands your microsystem and uses available resources

C. Unfreezes

D. Identifies unwanted variation, rework, and waste

110. You are precepting a CNL student. She discusses her capstone project with you. She needs help determining the design of her study. She states that she will be working with diabetes patients on a medical unit. She intends to collect basic data and do a pre- and postintervention questionnaire based on the diabetes survival skills. She wants to compare the pre- and postdata to determine if her educational intervention was effective. She will not use randomization. What option best describes her study design?

A. Well-designed randomized controlled trial (RCT)

B. Quasi-experimental

C. Meta-analysis

D. Quality study

111. B.F. is a 52-year-old female recently placed with the palliative care team. The CNL makes sure that B.F. is transferred to another unit with a specific palliative care section. How is this a demonstration of advocacy?

A. Physicians understand when to transfer patients.

B. Ensures that the system meets the needs of the population.

C. Advocates for the professional nurse.

D. Applies ethics toward patient care.

112. As a CNL on your unit, you are rounding on your microsystem. Jen, a 70-year-old patient with stage IV cancer, chronic obstructive pulmonary disease (COPD), diabetes mellitus (DM), and chronic kidney

disease, is currently on an Ativan drip and morphine drip. She has a do-not-resuscitate (DNR) order and is a hospice patient. You notice she has multiple grieving family members in her room. You speak with the family and collaborate with the palliative care unit (PCU) CNL and charge nurse and decide to move the patient to a bigger room in the PCU. What CNL role was demonstrated in this scenario?

A. Advocate

B. Outcomes manager

C. Team manager

D. Risk analyst

113. With healthcare reform, the CNL recognizes that evidence-based practice (EBP) is imperative. The CNL decided that her staff should be knowledgeable about healthcare reform. She collaborated with the educator and administration team to educate the staff about healthcare reform and pay for performance. What statement best reflects the definition of pay for performance?

A. It is a voluntary program that encourages hospitals nationally to report quality measures for heart attacks, heart failure, and pneumonia.

B. It is a national program in which physicians and hospitals receive more money if their quality measures exceed certain benchmarks or if the measures improve year to year.

C. It is a process that involves the surveillance of and intervention in clinical activities of physicians for the purpose of controlling costs.

D. It is a Medicare program that began the physician quality reporting initiative.

114. A nurse on the CNL's unit asks about accessing patient education materials via the electronic health record (EHR), as well as the availability of education on Cambodia. As the CNL guides the nurse in locating these materials, she or he recognizes this as an effective use of:

A. Healthcare informatics

B. Research utilization

C. Clinical knowledge

D. Evidence-based research

115. Which of the following best demonstrates how the CNL exhibits collaboration?

A. Sets and shares clear goals for teams

B. Keeps all team members informed by e-mailing updated minutes

C. Includes all contributors to the healthcare delivery process in the team, including patients/family, and seeks consultation from all members when making decisions

D. Monitors and evaluates the use of technology and information systems

116. The CNL works in a small primary care practice and has identified that several patients have missed appointments. After investigating why the patients were not going to appointments, the CNL determines that the patients made the appointments so far in advance that they forgot them. The CNL discusses these findings with the team and they decide to implement a program with reminder calls 2 days prior to the appointment. The CNL wants to be sure to identify aspects that may positively or negatively affect the project, so the CNL suggests the team utilize which of the following?

A. 5P (persons, patients, professionals, processes, patterns) assessment

B. Plan-Do-Study-Act (PDSA) cycle

C. Strenths, weaknesses, opportunities, and threats (SWOT) analysis

D. 5S methodology

117. As the CNL is integrated into practice, what best defines his or her level of practice?

A. Unit system

B. Mesosystem

C. Microsystem

D. Macrosystem

118. Part of your hospital's pre-op admission process is to collect a urinalysis (UA), hemoglobin A1c (HgA1c), comprehensive metabolic panel (CMP), and complete blood count (CBC). You review the HgA1c results of these patients. As the CNL, how can you best work with your healthcare team to ensure health promotion of clients with elevated HgA1c results?

A. Inform patients of elevated HgA1c results, as well as implications of those results

B. Provide diabetes education to patients with elevated HgA1c results postoperatively

C. Place a consult for the diabetes educator to meet and evaluate patients with an elevated HgA1c during this admission

D. Inform the surgeons of these elevated HgA1c results and ask them to consider what the next step should be

119. Lateral integration is one of the main functions of the CNL, incorporating multiple disciplines into the care of clients and populations. Which of the following ongoing components constitute lateral integration?

A. Advocacy, assessment, clinical knowledge, evaluation

B. Collaboraion, communication, coordination, evaluation

C. Altruism, benchmarking, cost reduction, evaluation

D. Advocacy, collaboration, coordination

120. A client on your unit receives 10 times the ordered dose of an opioid, resulting in serious complications from which the patient fully recovered. In response to this occurrence, you as the CNL:

A. Reprimand the nurse who administered the medication in error to ensure it does not happen again

B. Conduct a failure mode-effect analysis

C. Conduct a root cause analysis (RCA)

D. Apologize to the client and family

121. In your cohort you work with all members of the team. You develop an effective plan of care across settings in collaboration with all disciplines, professions, and stakeholders, including patients. This would be an example of what component of lateral integration?

A. Communication

B. Coordination

C. Evaluation

D. Collaboration

122. As the CNL, you assess the needs of your unit on an ongoing basis. You notice while rounding on the nursing staff that nurses are complaining about the demands of patient care. The nurses state that the patients are requiring more help than usual. This prompts you to look at the level of intensity of care required by patients. Level of intensity of care required by patients is referred to by which of the following?

A. Volume

B. Case mix

C. Acuity

D. Staffing mix

123. You are the unit-based council chair for shared governance of a high-acuity progressive care unit. You notice that the staff is not aware of new evidence in caring for this patient population. You discuss this with the management team and the CNL to determine what can be done to increase the staff awareness and knowledge of evidence-based practice (EBP). What strategy can best be used to increase evidence into practice?

A. Start a journal club with help from CNL

B. Learn how to determine if an article is peer-reviewed

C. Encourage nurses to conduct research

D. Discuss the importance of EBP in staff meeting

124. Jennifer, a CNL student, is shadowing a CNL on a busy medical–telemetry unit. The CNL encourages Jennifer to follow up on a 24-year-old patient admitted with diabetic ketoacidosis (DKA) for the fourth time in a 2-month period. Which statement best describes the CNL student acting as a client advocate for this patient?

A. Round on the patient and consult a diabetes educator

B. Round on the patient and discuss reasons for frequent readmissions, discuss concerns with the primary nurse, order a HgA1c, and consult a diabetes educator and social worker

C. Round on the patient, and tell the primary nurse to educate the patient on diabetes

D. Discuss with the primary care nurse that the patient has been again readmitted and the patient needs more education on diabetes and preventing readmissions

125. As the CNL on a surgical unit, nurses have expressed to you their concern over conflicting orders regarding patient intravenous fluids (IVFs). Most patients have conflicting order sets for fluids and rates, as ordered by the surgeons and hospitalists. From a healthcare informatics perspective, what is the best action you can take as the CNL?

A. Coordinate with the surgical and hospitalist groups to alert them of this clinical concern

B. Instruct the nurses to discontinue the older orders per protocol to clean up the order set within the electronic health record (EHR)

C. Work with the computer specialists to create a hard stop in the system requiring physicians to verify or modify IVF orders when new orders are placed

D. Discuss with the pharmacy if there is a way to prevent more than one IVF order from being allowed in the EHR at a time

126. The CNL recognizes the importance of Hospital Consumer Assessment of Healthcare Providers and Systems (HCAHPS) scores in driving hospital reimbursement. These scores measure:

A. Core measures and patient experience

B. Core measures, patient experience, and clinical outcomes

C. Core measures, patient experience, clinical outcomes, and readmission rates

D. Patient experience, clinical outcomes, and readmission rates

127. During a unit-based council meeting, the chair states that the unit has had 10 falls this year related to bathroom needs. Frank, a staff nurse, states he conducted observations and determined these falls are likely related to a lack of purposeful hourly rounding. Judy, a nursing

assistant, states she has heard everyone is doing hourly rounding but it does not help because patients still get out of bed. Which of the following is the most appropriate response by the CNL?

A. Encourage the staff to stop hourly rounding

B. Educate the staff on the importance of utilizing evidence-based practice (EBP) like hourly rounding to prevent falls and show the evidence

C. Instruct the staff to utilize new chair alarms for all patients as these have been proven to reduce falls

D. Ask the team to search the literature for evidence related to fall prevention

128. In order to be successful while utilizing Kotter's change theory, you realize it is vital to spend time on the first step. Which of the following best represents the first step in Kotter's change theory?

A. Having celebrations for short-term wins

B. Communicating the change vision

C. Consolidating gains and producing more change

D. Obtaining buy-in and creating a sense of urgency for change

129. The primary focus of the CNL is best defined as:

A. Delivery of high-quality, evidence-based, culturally competent care at the patient's bedside

B. Educating and mentoring peers to improve clinical competence

C. Providing patient care management and leadership of the interdisciplinary team meetings

D. Evaluating and supporting evidence-based practice (EBP) decisions to ensure best possible outcomes

130. What level of prevention are you providing by performing screenings?

A. Primary

B. Secondary

C. Tertiary

D. Quaternary

131. As a CNL on a high-risk oncology unit, you recognize the need for regular access to chaplaincy services among your client population. You work with your unit and chaplaincy department to bring these services to your unit regularly. This is primarily an example of:

A. Advocacy

B. CNL role integration

C. Leadership

D. Lateral integration

132. Use of electronic health records (EHRs) can aid the CNL to conduct quality improvement (QI) efforts in which of the following ways?

A. Allow rapid access to informatics data, provide a way of ongoing monitoring, organize data into meaningful groups, and aid in the dedication of errors

B. Allow rapid access to informatics data, ensure all staff follow protocols and policies, add second checks to medication administration, and aid in the detection of errors

C. Provide a way of ongoing monitoring, add second checks to medication administration, organize data into meaningful groups, and aid in detection of errors

D. Provide a way of ongoing monitoring, ensure all staff follow protocols and policies, add second checks to medication administration, organize data into meaningful groups, and aid in the detection of errors

133. The patient confides in you and states that she does not take her medications as prescribed and does not go to her doctor's appointments due to lack of transportation. As the CNL, you discuss your findings with the CCM, and place a financial counseling consult. The CCM orders a home safety evaluation, and a medical-social worker provides bus passes and community resources. This is an example of what key element of the CNL role?

A. Ongoing evaluation

B. Communication

C. Collaboration

D. Coordination

134. The CNLs noticed that the supply room was cluttered and oftentimes supplies had expired. They created a team and conducted a 5S to organize the supply bins and reduce waste. Where will the CNLs see the cost savings with supplies reflected?

A. Capital budget

B. Cash flow budget

C. Cost-effectiveness analysis

D. Operating budget

135. A staff nurse is thinking about becoming a CNL. The unit CNL discusses with the staff nurse about the CNL's role and the importance of evidence-based practice (EBP). After further discussions, the staff nurse questions the CNL about what barriers she may face when implementing EBP. Which of the following do not describe barriers that have been recognized with initiating EBP?

A. EBP is readily available for staff and low patient loads

B. Lack of knowledge regarding EBP strategies and misperceptions about EBP

C. Lack of time and resources to search for and appraise evidence

D. Peer pressure to continue with practices that are steeped in tradition and inadequate content

136. Which statement best describes the CNL acting as a client advocate for a domestic violence victim hospitalized in her microsystem?

A. Consult a domestic violence healthcare professional (DVHP) and ensure the patient has an alias name

B. Ensure all the staff members are aware that she is a domestic violence victim

C. Consult the master of social work (MSW) and call the patient's partner to ensure that he or she will not come to the hospital

D. Consult the psychiatric physician and inform the primary care nurse

137. Recently, your unit replaced all of its current beds with air beds, designed to help prevent skin breakdown in your patients. Using informatics, what is the best way to evaluate the effectiveness of this intervention?

A. Review the electronic health record (EHR) for new pressure ulcer incidence since the new beds were utilized

B. Complete a pressure ulcer prevalence study on all currently admitted patients

C. Gather data on all patient Braden scale scores since implementation

D. Review all nurse skin integrity assessments since implementation

138. Nicole, a nurse of 5 years, comes to you with an idea for a medication administration safety zone. How can you best support Nicole with this project?

A. Guide Nicole through a literature search to determine if evidence exists to support such a change

B. Help Nicole design the medication administration safety zone

C. Set up a meeting with the manager and Nicole to discuss the project

D. Encourage Nicole to implement the project

139. The CNL works in a medical intensive care unit (MICU) at a level one trauma center. The CNL conducts a comprehensive assessment of the microsystem. All of the following are vital aspects that the CNL would need to identify within the microsystem except:

A. The rate of ventilator-associated pneumonia

B. The organization's operating budget

C. The top three diagnoses

D. The average age of patients

140. What best describes an elevator speech about the CNL's role?

A. Succinctly define, advocate, and explain the CNL's role

B. Briefly educate peers on current issues in the nursing profession

C. Summary presentation on specific measured outcomes of the CNL

D. Convince peers and stakeholders to create buy-in for the CNL

141. As the CNL on a medical floor, you recognize the importance of annual flu vaccinations, especially considering your geriatric population. How can you promote vaccination rates within your population?

A. Organize a flu clinic for staff and visitors

B. Ask a physician to order flu shots for all admitted patients, and organize a flu clinic for staff and visitors

C. Within the hospital, develop a nurse-driven protocol that allows nurses to place an order for flu shots for your population

D. Ask the physician to order flu shots for all admitted hospital patients

142. During a client's admission medication reconciliation, the admitting nurse comes to you for assistance. On review of the client's case, you discover the client has several separate opioid prescriptions from multiple different providers. When you discuss the issue with the patient, the patient tells you he or she thought each prescriber had been consulting with the others. Which function of the CNL best addresses this issue?

A. Client advocacy

B. Lateral integration

C. Injury prevention

D. Advanced clinical assessment

143. As a CNL, you recognize a sentinel event as which of the following?

A. Any unintended event that results in ANY harm, physical or psychological, to a patient

B. Any unintended event that has the POTENTIAL to result in ANY harm, physical or psychological, to a patient

C. Any unintended event that results in SIGNIFICANT harm, physical or psychological, to a patient

D. Any unintended event that has the POTENTIAL to result in SIGNIFICANT harm, physical or psychological, to a patient

144. You are a CNL on a medical–telemetry unit and orienting a new graduate nurse. Critical thinking is best demonstrated by which of the following?

A. Calling the rapid response nurse when a patient's oxygen saturation drops to 79% on 2 L of oxygen

B. Drawing scheduled hemoglobin and hematocrit

C. Delegating tasks to the nursing assistant

D. Creating a script to welcome patients to the medical–telemetry unit

145. You are a CNL working in a very busy 980-bed tertiary hospital. The hospital only has one MRI machine. This often causes delays in patient care. You write a proposal for the administrative team to advocate for more MRI scanners. If the proposal is approved, the money will come out of which budget?

A. Capital budget

B. Cash flow budget

C. Operating budget

D. Revenue

146. As a CNL, you are asked to speak to a local church group, mostly elderly, regarding the importance of annual influenza shots and pneumonia vaccines. You want to be well prepared for the talk as you know the leaders have several questions about the relationship in developing pneumonia and vaccination. You decide to develop a PICOT question and initiate a literature review. Which of the following statements best exemplifies the PICOT method?

A. For patients 65 years and older, the use of an influenza/pneumonia (PNA) vaccine will reduce the risk of developing pneumonia.

B. For patients 65 years and older, the use of an influenza/PNA vaccine will reduce the risk of developing pneumonia when compared to patients not receiving vaccination within a year.

C. For patients 65 years and older, the use of an influenza/PNA vaccine will reduce the pneumonia.

D. For patients in a church, the use of an influenza/PNA vaccine will reduce the risk of developing pneumonia in a year

147. Ranesha, a nurse on the unit, has just finished receiving bedside report on a patient, Mr. Smith, admitted with pneumonia. She told the patient his goal was to ambulate in the hallway three times that day. The CNL, Valerie, walked in the room while Ranesha discussed his goal. Valerie recognized that the goal will not work because Mr. Smith was not involved in deciding on the goal. In what way can Valerie act as a client advocate?

A. Involve the patient in setting the goal with Ranesha, to discuss the reason for setting goals, barriers, and concerns, and determine the best time for Mr. Smith to ambulate in the hallway

B. Do not discuss setting the goal and involving Mr. Smith as the nurse has already told the patient the plan for the day

C. Tell Ranesha that Mr. Smith should be in the driver's seat of his own care

D. Involve the patient by asking him what he wants to do for the day and if he replies "Nothing" then let him rest

148. The CNL knows in order to serve as a lateral integrator she or he must conduct ongoing evaluation of care delivery systems and processes. Which of the following is the best example of how the CNL demonstrates evaluation?

A. Ensures each member of the team clearly understands each member's role

B. Conducts an ongoing analysis of risk to promote patient safety

C. Synthesizes gathered information to find common goals and shares this with the team

D. Fosters open rapport across professional boundaries

149. A patient who has been diagnosed with colon cancer remarks that since his diagnosis, many people he knows have mentioned someone they know who has colon cancer. Most of these people live nearby. The patient asks you if colon cancer rates in the area have been increasing recently. The patient is asking about what type of measure?

A. Incidence

B. Prevalence

C. Mortality

D. Correlation

150. During morning report, you observe a new staff member you have been mentoring struggling to identify which of her patients she will assess first. As the CNL, you identify the priority patient as:

A. The 72-year-old patient with a chest tube to wall suction and unstable vital signs

B. The 19-year-old patient with family demanding to speak with you regarding discharge plans

C. The 57-year-old postoperative patient with patient-controlled analgesia (PCA) pump

D. The 92-year-old patient who is a high fall risk

151. You are the CNL in an outpatient pediatric clinic. The most common diagnosis for your patient population is asthma, and your patients are

frequently seen at local emergency departments (EDs) for asthma exacerbations. Which action most directly optimizes the level of function in daily life for these patients?

A. Provide or reinforce previous education to patients and families on asthma and inhaler use

B. Review discharge orders and ensure that all clients are prescribed a long- and short-acting inhaler

C. Provide an in-service at local schools to educate teachers on managing asthma exacerbations in children

D. Advocate for the development of a nurse phone triage to answer urgent patient and family asthma concerns

152. As the CNL, you recognize that leveraging technology and information systems is an important part of acting toward high-quality, patient-centered, lateral integration. Which of the following are examples of using technology and information systems to benefit patient care?

A. Use of bed alarms and use of call lights

B. TV in patient rooms with many channels, use of call lights, guest Wi-Fi Internet access, and e-readers available with e-books for patients

C. Use of bed alarms, use of call lights, remote telemetry, and bar-coded supplies and medications

D. TV in patient rooms with many channels, guest Wi-Fi Internet access, and e-readers available with e-books for patients

153. Which of the following is not a part of the National Patient Safety Guidelines (NPSG)?

A. Improve the accuracy of patient identification

B. Reduce the risk of healthcare-associated infections

C. Improve patient satisfaction

D. Prevent healthcare-associated pressure ulcers

154. During the 5P assessment, you find out that 64% of patients have Medicare, 18% have Medicaid, 16% have private insurance, and 2% have no insurance. You can conclude that the majority of your patients are what type of payer source?

A. First-party payer

B. Second-party payer

C. Fourth-party payer

D. Third-party payer

155. A staff nurse is performing a literature review on the best tool for determining health literacy for diabetic patients. When analyzing and appraising the literature, what methods can the nurse use to determine if the study is flawed?

A. Are the results of the literature reliable and critical?

B. Are the results of the literature effective and modifiable?

C. Are the results of the literature valid and reliable?

D. Are the results of the literature valid and modifiable?

156. The CNL provides integration of care by working with multiple interdependent and independent disciplines, breaking down barriers, and proactively managing care across the continuum. This describes a(n):

A. Vertical leader

B. Lateral integrator

C. Outcomes manager

D. Systems analyst

157. A nurse on your unit has a question about required documentation for a patient with a nasogastric (NG) tube to wall suction. You guide her to what resource?

A. The unit charge nurse

B. Hospital policy/procedure manual

C. The state's board of nursing scope of practice

D. The Joint Commission website

158. You are the CNL on a medical unit and recognize a frequently readmitted patient with uncontrolled diabetes. You view this patient in terms of Prochaska and DiClemente's Stages of Change model and recognize that:

A. Patients may spiral in and out of stages forward and backward.

B. Timelines for patients may vary to progress through the stages; however, they always progress forward.

C. The stages have been well studied and the timeline and progression are the same for all patients.

D. Prochaska and DiClemente's Stages of Change model does not apply to this patient.

159. Consideration of your unit's nurse workflow, specific challenges and needs of clients on your unit, staff experiences, and staff ratios are examples of which of the following important CNL function components?

A. Ongoing evaluation

B. Collaboration

C. Advanced clinical assessment

D. Knowledge management

160. Quality improvement (QI), as a function of the CNL role, is related to which core role competency of the CNL?

A. Client advocacy

B. Clinician

C. Risk anticipator

D. Team manager

161. Your hospital has just completed a study comparing outcomes in rehospitalization rates for CHF patients who received predischarge teaching from an advanced practice registered nurse (APRN) with those who received predischarge teaching from an RN. In the analysis of data, what resulting *p*-value would indicate that the intervention had a significant result?

A. <.05

B. <.8

C. <.10

D. <.22

162. A professor is discussing the difference between quantitative and qualitative research. As a CNL student, you are aware that quantitative research is related to numeric data with statistical analysis, while qualitative research focuses on nonnumeric forms of research. Which of the following is an example of a quantitative study?

A. Personal interviews

B. Randomized controlled trial

C. Ethnography

D. Phenomenology

163. Elizabeth, an 87-year-old female, is admitted to the orthopedic unit with a fractured hip. Elizabeth lives at home alone, but her retired son lives just 2 hours away and comes to visit her often. The physical therapist comes to you and states he is recommending that Elizabeth go to a rehabilitation center prior to returning home. When Elizabeth is told that she will require rehabilitation, she becomes visibly upset and states she refuses to go to a facility. Utilizing an interdisciplinary approach, you ask the social worker, case manager, physician, and physical therapist to help create a plan for Elizabeth. Which of the following is the best plan for Elizabeth?

A. Convince Elizabeth to go to a rehabilitation facility where she will receive 24-hour care and 3 hours of therapy a day

B. Keep Elizabeth in the hospital until she has fully recovered, then discharge her home

C. Discharge Elizabeth home and arrange for a physical therapist to come to her house once a week

D. Contact Elizabeth's son, inform him of Elizabeth's refusal of the rehabilitation facility, and have him help develop an alternative to the original plan for her discharge

164. A staff nurse is curious about whether emptying the nasogastric (NG) suction canister is a task that can be delegated to a CNA. You, the CNL, guide her to what resource?

A. The unit charge nurse

B. Hospital policy/procedure manual

C. The State Board of Nursing Scope of Practice

D. The Joint Commission website

165. The CNL on the unit has an idea to generate a new EBP study. He has conducted a literature review and critical appraisal. The CNL has also developed a collaborative interprofessional team to be part of the planning process. He has established a date for the research design meeting. What pertinent information should be included in his outline of the study in preparation for this meeting?

A. Form an interprofessional team

B. Perform a review of literature

C. Consult with another CNL

D. Indicate the aim of the study and research question

166. Which method of payment accounts for only 5% of the U.S. population?

A. Out-of-pocket payments

B. Employment-based private insurance

C. Government financing

D. Individual private insurance

167. What are ways in which the CNL can present his or her effectiveness and outcomes?

A. Peer-reviewed journal, conference or seminar, and TV

B. Peer-reviewed journal, conference or seminar, and Internet

C. Peer-reviewed journal and TV

D. TV and Internet

168. Judy completed an evidence-based practice (EBP) study that resulted in a 25% reduction in noise on the unit and increased patient satisfaction to 100% for patients always saying it is quiet at night. Utilizing the EBP process, what would Judy's next step be?

A. Apply for a poster presentation for a national conference

B. Compare results to a similar unit in her hospital

C. Identify stakeholders within her organization

D. Conduct a literature search and assess validity

169. The nurse manager of a regional home health services company allows the employees to determine solutions for change, and always considers their opinions, suggestions, and concerns. What type of leadership style is the manager demonstrating?

A. Autocratic

B. Laissez-faire

C. Consultative

D. Democratic

170. Patient satisfaction scores in the emergency department (ED) have shown a downward trend over the past three quarters. As a CNL in the ED, your focus is to:

A. Create a script for the triage nurse in welcoming the patient

B. Assign a volunteer to welcome patients to the hospital

C. Compare desired outcomes with national and state standards

D. Write a letter of apology to each dissatisfied patient

171. You are a CNL selected to lead a team focused on implementing a multidisciplinary clinical pathway for acute ischemic stroke and transient ischemic attack. The risk assessment tool that you have adopted identifies all of the following as independent stroke risk factors except:

A. Age

B. Systolic blood pressure

C. Liver dysfunction

D. Current smoking

E. Diabetes mellitus (DM)

172. All of the following are part of the data necessary for a CNL to fully understand and assess his or her clinical unit except:

A. The organization's budget

B. The target population and age distribution

C. The percentage of full-time equivalents (FTEs)

D. The rate of nosocomial infections and fall risks

173. A patient asks the CNL about the regulations on abortion in North Carolina. What should the CNL do?

A. Tell the patient he or she cannot answer that because it is an ethical situation

B. Let the doctor know the patient is asking about abortion

C. Inform the patient care nurse

D. Look up the regulations in North Carolina and share them with the patient

174. You are using failure mode effect and analysis (FMEA) to anticipate the risk of medication errors in the ICU related to invasive lines. You begin your FMEA analysis with:

A. The effects of each failure

B. The potential cause of each failure

C. Process mapping

D. Specific defects and delays in the medication administration process

175. Sustaining process improvement requires the use of appropriate learning principles and strategies. The CNL function that best utilizes this competency is:

A. Advocate

B. Educator

C. Clinician

D. Information manager

176. By leading which unit initiative can the CNL directly affect the financial health of the entire institution?

A. Reducing readmissions

B. Recruiting new nursing staff

C. Improving documentation compliance

D. Encouraging staff to report safety events and near-misses

177. Before beginning data collection, what is the primary key factor to determine?

A. Personnel to collect data

B. A secure database for holding data

C. Operational definitions of data

D. A user-friendly collection method

178. You are helping the nurse to care for a patient with congestive heart failure (CHF). He has just completed a transfusion of 2 units of packed red blood cells (PRBCs). Upon your entering the room, the patient complains of shortness of breath. His O_2 saturations are 85% on 2 L and he is breathing 28 respirations a minute. What drug do you anticipate administering?

A. Nitroglycerin SL

B. Lasix IV

C. Albuterol HHN

D. Prednisone PO

179. An 88-year-old woman suffers a stroke in the nursing home. She develops pneumonia and is transferred to the hospital. She continues to decline, is having trouble breathing, and becomes unconscious with little hope of recovery or quality of life. She has no family and no healthcare proxy, living will, or directions about whether she wants to be intubated or not. The physician wants to intubate the patient. The staff nurse strongly believes the patient would not want to be intubated, as the nurse had cared for the lady before she became unconscious. What is the best thing for the CNL to do first?

A. Take a vote among the staff nurses

B. Call for an ethics consultation

C. Ask the social worker to make a recommendation or decision

D. Do a literature review on quality of life of elderly patients with pneumonia

180. As the CNL on a medical–surgical unit, you have noticed a trend over the past 3 months with patients having high blood glucose before lunch and dinner. What is the best way to address this problem?

A. Investigate whether the blood glucose monitors on the unit are accurate

B. Provide an educational in-service about diabetes to the staff

C. Ensure all patients with diabetes receive a consultation with the nutritionist

D. Determine what other changes in processes have occurred on the unit in the past 3 months that could influence this trend

181. You are listening to report with a novice nurse. As part of mentoring new staff and supporting clinical decision making, you ask the new nurse which patient she should assess first. Which patient is the most important for this nurse to assess first?

A. A 46-year-old receiving IV antibiotic therapy on day 3

B. A 60-year-old 15 minutes s/p liver biopsy

C. A 56-year-old with pneumonia on day 2

D. A 72-year-old hip replacement impatiently waiting for discharge

182. A nurse on the unit comes to you and says that every shift he works day or night he finds at least one of his patients without an identification band in place. He is very concerned about patient safety and feels a harmful mistake could occur in the near future if the practice on the unit is not improved. As the CNL, how should you help this nurse?

A. Perform daily audits on all the patients and report results to management

B. Have the unit secretary make new identification bands for all the patients daily so the charge nurse can place new bands on the patients daily

C. Research a new style of patient identification bands since the current product does not stay on the patient properly

D. Provide support to the nurse on the unit who determines the problem and help him identify areas in the process to improve patient identification

183. When assessing a patient for a diagnosis of pneumonia, it is more difficult to make a proper diagnosis in the absence of the following symptom:

A. Cough

B. Cyanosis

C. Tachycardia

D. Bradycardia

184. As the CNL on a medical unit, which of the following cost-effective interventions would you support to reduce the readmission rate on your unit?

A. Keep patients one extra day to ensure they are prepared for discharge home

B. Arrange for all patients to have at least 1 week of visiting nursing postdischarge

C. Review discharge instructions with the patient and one family member

D. Begin discharge planning and teaching on the day of admission

185. A 65-year-old man with a history of chest palpitations was seen by his cardiologist for new onset palpitations. He was put on a beta-blocker and told to return for a follow-up in 1 week after taking a stress test. The beta-blocker's action includes:

A. Increasing the consistency of the heart rate

B. Decreasing the ability of the heart muscle to contract

C. Decreasing the chance of dysrhythmia

D. Increasing contractility and decreasing heart rate

186. To demonstrate active listening, the CNL would exhibit which behavior?

A. Avoid making any facial expressions

B. Preserve at least 3 ft between the parties

C. Lean slightly forward

D. Fold hands in the lap

187. To confirm a scope of practice question, the CNL should consult which administrative body guidelines?

A. The Joint Commission

B. Centers for Medicare & Medicaid Services

C. Hospital Policy and Procedure Manual

D. State Nursing Practice Act

188. Which of the following is not part of the PDSA change model?

A. Plan

B. Assess

C. Do

D. Study

189. In order to generate ideas aimed at designing an implementation plan, a team reviews the topic and members verbalize solution ideas in a random fashion. This is an example of which of the following strategies?

A. Multivoting

B. Process mapping

C. Brainstorming

D. Nominal group technique

190. You have been charged with examining the heart failure 30-day readmission rate of your unit. In doing so, it is important for you to examine data from what other sources?

A. National and state readmission rates

B. National benchmarks

C. Readmissions to other units in your hospital

D. All of the above

191. You have done some research and found a new fall prevention tool that you would like to trial on your unit. The tool was recently developed and tested at a large city hospital with a population of open heart patients. You are not sure that this tool can be effectively implemented in your small community hospital. You are questioning the tool's:

A. Relative risk

B. External validity

C. Transportability

D. Causal association

192. A nurse approaches you and expresses her knowledge deficit regarding the difference between signs and symptoms of left- and right-sided heart failure. You explain the physiology between the two types of heart failure and identify that which of the following has a primary symptom of right-sided heart failure?

A. Shortness of breath on exertion

B. Heart murmur and distended veins

C. Peripheral edema

D. Cool extremities and weak peripheral pulses

193. Vaccinations are considered what level of prevention?

A. Primary

B. Secondary

C. Tertiary

D. None of these

194. Medicaid covers which population?

A. Employed

B. Underinsured

C. Unemployed

D. Poor and disabled

195. While being admitted to the unit after a car accident, the patient informs you that she has been off her psychiatric medications Seroquel and Celexa due to the cost and no longer has a doctor. As an advocate, you would talk with the physician in hopes of obtaining what two consults?

A. Medicine and clinical case manager (CCM)

B. Psychiatry and social worker

C. CCM and social worker

D. Medicine and psychiatry

196. D.M. is 80 years old and admitted for a hip fracture, caused by a fall from standing. As a CNL, you would know a fracture obtained this way is typically found from what?

A. Osteomyelitis

B. Osteoporosis

C. Anemia

D. Rheumatoid arthritis

197. You are caring for Sara, a 76-year-old grandmother recovering from heart failure. You know that she is ready to go home because:

A. Her ECG is normal, her pulse oximetry is normal, and she has a supportive family to help care for her at home.

B. She tells you she is ready to go home.

C. You observe her ambulating in the hallway, free from dyspnea.

D. She says she is free from dyspnea and fatigue, she has a follow-up appointment set up for the following Monday morning, and her daughter said she can drive her to the appointment

198. You are working with your team to modify the unit's budget. You know that the best way to create a budget is:

A. Looking at the previous budget's variance

B. Requesting a large capital budget

C. Being in line with your budget goal

D. Utilizing a case mix

199. A new health policy is being voted on in Congress. Your professional organization supports this policy and is recruiting nurses to go to Washington, DC, to help promote their view and to have a bigger voice. You do not support this policy. Your manager wants you to go as a leader and represent your unit. What should you do?

A. You should go, as you need to stick together with your professional organization and yield to your manager.

B. You should learn more about the policy and why your organization supports it.

C. You should politely decline, as you do not agree with the policy.

D. You should go, but rally against the policy since you do not agree with it. This is America and you are exercising your freedom of speech.

200. You want to do some research for a potential policy change. All of the following are excellent resources except:

A. Centers for Disease Control

B. Wikipedia

C. American Diabetes Association

D. Institute for Healthcare Improvement

Case Study 1

Michael is a CNL on an adult medical–surgical unit in a large urban hospital. Michael conducted a 5P (persons, patients, professionals, processes, patterns) assessment of the unit and noticed a large amount of pneumonia patients were being readmitted within 30 days. Michael would like to form a team to investigate the readmissions further and come up with a plan on how to reduce the readmission rate.

1. Utilizing an interdisciplinary approach, who should Michael include in the team?

   A. Nurse, hospitalist, physical therapist, and dietician

   B. Respiratory therapist, nurse, pulmonologist, and case manager

   C. Nurse, gerontologist, case manager, and physical therapist

   D. Respiratory therapist, pulmonologist, case manager, and dietician

The team investigates the readmissions and discovered that most of the patients were 65 years and older and were discharged home alone. The team also notices inconsistencies in the plan of care. Some patients received incentive spirometers and education from respiratory therapists, while others did not. Everyone understands that there is a need for change in order to prevent readmissions.

2. The team is unsure how to approach this change, so what should Michael suggest as the next step?

   A. Conduct a literature review to determine evidence-based practice (EBP) on caring for pneumonia patients

   B. Review the intensive care unit's plan of care for pneumonia patients

   C. Investigate the pneumonia readmissions from last year to determine if the same trends exist

   D. Determine the respiratory therapists' role in caring for patients with pneumonia

The team has a vision and a strategy on how to approach this process change. They decide to create a pneumonia pathway with a comprehensive, streamlined plan of care including evidence-based nursing tasks, education from respiratory therapy, and discharge follow-up home health visits. The team shares the plan with the unit through presentations and e-mails. The staff expresses enthusiasm about the new changes.

3. Utilizing Kotter's theory of change, what step is the team demonstrating now?

   A. Anchor new approaches in the culture

   B. Generate short-term wins

   C. Consolidate gains and produce more change

   D. Communicate the change vision

The team wants to implement the process change and observe what happens, but they are unsure what method to use.

4. What method should Michael suggest?
   A. 5S
   B. 5P
   C. Failure mode effect and analysis (FMEA)
   D. Plan-Do-Study-Act (PDSA)

Jonathan, a 67-year-old Caucasian male, is admitted to Michael's unit. Michael decides to round on Jonathan to see how the new pneumonia pathway is progressing. Michael asks Jonathan how he likes the education sessions with the respiratory therapist. Jonathan states he is learning a lot and really enjoys the opportunity to ask questions. Jonathan then states that he has asked the nurse for an incentive spirometer, but he never received one. Michael apologizes to Jonathan.

5. What should Michael do next?
   A. Obtain an incentive spirometer and teach Jonathan how to properly use it
   B. Coach the nurse on utilizing the evidence-based pneumonia pathway
   C. Notify the unit manager that the pathway is not being followed
   D. Follow up with Jonathan tomorrow to ensure he received an incentive spirometer

Case Study 2

You are a new CNL on a unit that is not familiar with the role. Recently, your unit has had a breakdown in the discharge process leading to poor patient outcomes. The problem appears to be a lack of coordination between the interdisciplinary team; patients are being discharged before PT/OT has fully cleared them, before pharmacy can review their home meds and education, and often without patient-specific dressing orders and supplies. There is uncertainty about why this issue has arisen in recent months. As a CNL, you would like to try and address these issues.

1. How can you quickly explain the concept of the CNL and its potential in regards to this situation to your manager and other leaders or stakeholders on your unit?
   A. A root cause analysis (RCA)
   B. A summary presentation
   C. An elevator speech
   D. A situation background assessment recommendation (SBAR)

Your unit's leadership is initially uncertain on how the focus of the CNL differs from other APRN.

2. You explain:
   A. The main focus of the CNL is on evidence-based practice (EBP) and clinical outcomes.
   B. The main focus of the CNL is on coordination of care and discharge planning.
   C. The main focus of the CNL is on the specific needs of a cohort of patients and RCA.
   D. The main focus of the CNL is on anticipating needs of patients and RCA.

You are given permission and allowed to implement the CNL role on a trial basis with the discharge process.

3. How do you best proceed with investigating the lapse in the discharge process?
   A. Interview each member of the interdisciplinary team to identify his or her opinions of the discharge process
   B. Create an interdisciplinary team meeting to discuss the discharge process and known issues
   C. Begin leading a new discharge process on your unit and act as a care coordinator on your unit
   D. Continue the current discharge process

One issue identified through your investigation is that surgeons have not been entering home wound care instructions, with the consequence that nurses are not triggered to educate the patient with anything specific on the discharge paperwork. The surgeons wonder if nurses can identify the wound care needs of each patient, place a nursing order for wound care, and then educate the patient on discharge.

4. As the CNL, you investigate whether this is an appropriate nursing task and within the nursing scope of practice by reviewing:
   A. The Joint Commission
   B. Centers for Medicare & Medicaid standards
   C. Your state's Nurse Practice Act
   D. Your hospital's policy and procedure manual

After this process, the discharge issues on your unit have improved.

5. As a trial CNL, whose buy-in will be the most important in fully implementing the CNL role in the hospital?

A. The chief nursing officer (CNO)

B. The unit manager

C. The members of the interdisciplinary team

D. The staff affected by your outcomes

Case Study 3

A 36-year-old Hispanic woman is pregnant with her third child. She has had one live birth and one stillbirth. She is 5'2" tall and weighs 220 lb., and her BMI is 40.2. Her current blood pressure is 140/80 mmHg. Her past obstetrical history includes a cesarean section for a 9 lb. 5 oz. live female at 38 weeks gestation. She also had a vaginal stillborn birth at 36 weeks gestation weighing 7 lb. 2 oz. Both of these births were in Honduras. This patient presents to the clinic after recently arriving in the United States at 32 weeks gestation with complaints of headache, blurred vision, lethargy, and diaphoresis. The patient arrives with no record of her prenatal care. The following lab results are from today's visit: urine dipstick 3+ glycosuria and no proteinuria, fasting blood sugar of 58 mg/dL, and a biophysical profile of 8/10. An oral glucose tolerance test (OGTT) was also done today with a result of 150 mg/dL.

1. Which of the following interventions is appropriate for the nurse to tell the CNL?

   A. The patient is experiencing hyperglycemia and should be given a protein snack.

   B. The patient is experiencing hyperglycemia and should be given insulin and 1 cup of milk.

   C. The patient is experiencing hypoglycemia and should be given insulin and 1 cup of orange juice.

   D. The patient is experiencing hypoglycemia and should be given 1 cup of skim milk.

2. The patient's blood sugar should be repeated after the snack at what interval?

   A. 1 hour

   B. 15 minutes

   C. 30 minutes

   D. 2 hours

3. What does the result of the 150 mg/dL from the OGTT signify?

   A. Based on a value greater than 140 mg/dL, the patient should have 3-hour 100-g OGTT within 1 week.

B. The results are within normal limits and do not meet the threshold for the diagnosis of gestational diabetes.

C. A fasting blood sugar should be checked as soon as possible.

D. Based on this abnormal value, the 3-hour OGTT is not required.

4. What are the risk factors for this patient developing gestational diabetes?

A. Obesity, advanced maternal age

B. Previous infant with birth weight greater than 9 lb., stillbirth, hypertension, and proteinuria

C. Obesity, advanced maternal age, Hispanic/Latina, previous infant with birth weight greater than 9 lb., and stillbirth

D. Hispanic/Latina, stillbirth, and proteinuria

Case Study 4

You are informed by your nurse manager about a large clinical issue involving a patient that has occurred on another unit. In your role as the CNL, hospital leadership has asked for you to temporarily work on a new unit to investigate the issue and offer solutions to improve practice. The clinical incident involved a postoperative patient on patient-controlled anesthesia (PCA) with a low-dose continuous infusion who became extremely oversedated during the night. When the nurse discovered the patient, he had a respiratory rate of 5, oxygen saturations in the 60s, and appeared grossly cyanotic.

1. How do you begin orienting to this new unit and the situation?

A. Perform a 5P (persons, patients, professionals, processes, patterns) assessment of the unit

B. Review hospital policy and procedures related to PCA use

C. Perform a root cause analysis (RCA)

D. Create an interdisciplinary team to address this issue

2. As you begin to investigate the issue, what is one way you can present *a graphical* representation of the different factors that contributed to the issue?

A. An RCA

B. A fishbone diagram

C. A concept map

D. A clinical decision tree

3. What process do you use to fully investigate the clinical incident?

A. Plan-Do-Study-Act (PDSA)

B. 5P assessment

C. Root cause analysis

D. Clinical decision tree

Through your analysis, you identify that this patient also had a diagnosis of obstructive sleep apnea (OSA). The patient was not placed on a continuous pulse oximeter. The nurse had last rounded on the patient approximately 1 hour prior to discovery.

4. You question the appropriateness of the PCA orders given the risks and patient's comorbidities. What information do you gather next?

   A. Discuss with the surgeons their rationale behind the order

   B. Review the current evidence on PCA use and oversedation

   C. Contact a peer in the sleep center to discuss risks and benefits of OSA and PCA use

   D. Examine the current hospital policy and procedure manual

Your analysis indicates a need to change the hospital's current policy on PCA use, increase education on opioid use in conjunction with an OSA diagnosis, and improve the hospital policy regarding patient PCA monitoring.

5. What is one system the CNL can use to implement these changes?

   A. PDSA

   B. RCA

   C. Clinical decision tree

   D. Concept map

Case Study 5

Ms. Jones is a 35-year-old patient admitted to your microsystem. The patient has a history of obesity, hypertension, obstructive sleep apnea (OSA), type 2 diabetes, tracheostomy, and is on a ventilator at night. Ms. Jones is currently unemployed and waiting on her disability approval. The patient was living in an apartment with her 18-year-old daughter and three grandchildren. The 35-year-old mother was admitted into the hospital because of a power outage in her two-bedroom apartment.

1. As a CNL, what key stakeholders would you include to provide this patient with the best outcomes?

   A. Medical social worker, clinical case manager (CCM), primary nurse, clinical nutritionist, CNL, respiratory therapist, and physician

   B. Physical therapist, occupational therapist, CNL, primary nurse, medical social worker, and laboratory technician

C. Clinical care manager, primary nurse, medical social worker, and respiratory therapist

D. Pharmacist, clinical care manager, medical social worker, occupational therapist, and physical therapist

While reviewing your patient's chart, you notice that the patient has a 13.5 hemoglobin A1c. During rounds, you notice that the family brought the patient pasta with Alfredo sauce from home.

2. What would be the most appropriate next step as a CNL?

   A. Discuss the importance of following a diabetic diet with the patient and her family

   B. Ask the physician to consult the diabetes educator and clinical nutritionist, and discuss the risk of diabetes with the patient and her family

   C. Take the food out of the room and tell the patient that she needs to lose weight to be there for her grandchildren

   D. Ask the patient if she has been taking her insulin appropriately

While you are discussing discharge planning with Ms. Jones, you find out that she does not have the means to pay for the electrical work at her home. You ask Ms. Jones if she has any family to stay with her while she resolves the electrical issues and she says that there is no one available to help her.

3. What is the best statement from the CNL at this time?

   A. "Would you consider a short-term stay at a nursing facility until this problem is resolved?"

   B. "We cannot keep you in the hospital forever, Ms. Jones. It costs too much."

   C. "I will discuss this with the director for case management and see if she will pay for your electrical work."

   D. "Let me refer you to the social worker and CCM."

Ms. Jones has now been in the hospital for 2 months, and she develops shortness of breath and pain in her right leg. Your patient has developed a pulmonary embolus, which requires an admission to the intensive care unit.

4. As a CNL, what would be the most appropriate intervention after assuring quality care is provided for this patient?

   A. Form a multidisciplinary team to review the patient's plan of care and gather whether anything can be done to prevent this from occurring

   B. Perform a root cause analysis (RCA)

   C. Review this case with your nurse manager

   D. Review the chart to see if Ms. Jones was mobile during her hospital stay

Ms. Jones is better now and is ready for discharge. She will be going home on Lovenox injections twice a day and transitioning to Coumadin.

5. To ensure that Ms. Jones has the best possible outcomes, what key member of the team should the CNL consult with for follow-up?
   A. Home health nurse for lab draws, family, physician, diabetes telehealth, and medical social worker
   B. Nursing assistant, home health nurse, family, physician, physical therapy, and CNL
   C. Diabetes telehealth, CNL, medical social worker, and occupational therapy
   D. Home health nurse for lab draws, CNL, and family

Case Study 6

You are a CNL student contemplating a topic for your capstone project. You believe that patients transferred from the medical intensive care unit (MICU) to your medical unit are frequently transferred back to the intensive care unit (ICU) due to multiple rapid response team (RRT) calls.

1. You want to look further into whether this is truly a concern for your unit. What first step should you take as a CNL student?
   A. Assess the current rate of RRTs and transfers back; collect data to see how many patients are transfer-backs to the MICU
   B. Implement a process to reduce transfers back to the MICU
   C. Perform a literature review on RRTs and transfers back
   D. Design a study to decrease RRTs and transfers back to MICU

After assessing your unit population, you find that the rate of RRTs and transfers back to the ICU is higher than the national mean.

2. What should be your next step?
   A. Design a study and implement the best practice
   B. Perform a literature review and create a team
   C. Design a study and perform a literature review
   D. Identify the problem and create a PICOT question

When performing a literature review, you stumble upon several articles from various websites. You are trying to determine the most reliable source to use for the literature review.

3. Which resource is the best choice for you to use to perform a literature review?
   A. Google
   B. Mayo Clinic
   C. Cumulative Index Nursing and Allied Health (CINAHL)
   D. Wikipedia

You created a PICOT question: "Will the use of a CNL assessing potential patients to be transferred from the MICU to the medical unit prevent transfers-back and decrease RRTs within a 6-month period?" After performing a literature review, you found several results on your topic.

4. Which of the following demonstrates the strongest level of evidence?
   A. A well-designed randomized control trial study about using an ICU rounding nurse to decrease RRT calls
   B. An article discussing a quasi-experimental study that reduced the frequency of RRTs utilizing an educational intervention
   C. A meta-analysis of randomized control trial studies that demonstrated a significant improvement in reducing the number of bounce backs and RRTs to ICUs
   D. A descriptive study about the challenges of a medical unit using RRTs

After synthesizing the data, you decide that the best practice is to perform an educational intervention for nurses about RRTs and transfers-back and assess patients prior to transferring them to a medical unit.

5. Prior to the implementation process, what is the best step for you to take next?
   A. Form a team of stakeholders
   B. Develop a comparison group
   C. Talk to the manager
   D. Start the implementation process

23

Answers and Rationales

1. A new graduate nurse, Jenny, approaches you and states she needs help removing a peripherally inserted central catheter (PICC). Which of the following is the best response when acting as a horizontal leader?

   A. Remove the PICC yourself

   B. Tell Jenny to find the policy and then remove the PICC

   C. Help Jenny find the policy and review it with her. Coach Jenny while she removes the PICC and provide feedback

   D. Help Jenny find the policy and refer her to a nurse with 12 years of experience for assistance

Answer C—Rationale: The clinical nurse leader (CNL) acts as a horizontal leader by helping the new graduate nurse to learn through sharing knowledge and coaching, rather than doing the task for the nurse.

2. What organizational theory is used with rapid, unpredictable, and constant change?

   A. Systems theory

   B. Chaos theory

   C. Change theory

   D. Traditional theory

Answer B—Rationale: Chaos theory is used to understand rapidly changing, unpredictable healthcare environments.

3. A 65-year-old African American male was admitted to your microsystem with hyperglycemia. The patient has a history of hypertension, gout, obesity, and smoking. The patient has a family history of diabetes and

hypertension. Which statement by the patient demonstrates his understanding of modifiable risk factors for diabetes?

A. "As I get older, my risk for diabetes increases."

B. "I know that a family history of diabetes is a risk factor, so I will educate my children on diabetes prevention."

C. "I will keep a record of all my blood sugars to take to my doctor's appointments."

D. "I will attend a smoking cessation class, because I know smoking increases my risk for diabetes."

Answer D—Rationale: Modifiable risk factors are lifestyle factors that a person can alter in order to prevent disease. Smoking cessation class is an intervention for modifying the risk factor of smoking.

4. Your hospital is currently trialing the integration of the clinical nurse leader (CNL) role. At the end of the trial implementation period how can you, as the CNL, best illustrate the effectiveness of your role during this trial?

A. Refer to increased patient satisfaction scores over the course of the trial

B. Present data that demonstrates the effect of the CNL and outcomes achieved over the course of the trial

C. Present a list of projects and tasks completed over the course of the trial

D. Refer to your performance review over the course of the trial

Answer B—Rationale: The CNL should present the effect and outcomes to illustrate the importance of the integration of his or her role. Increased patient satisfaction is not necessarily directly related to the CNL. Presentation of projects and tasks completed does not address measurable outcomes. Performance review of the individual does not indicate outcomes were affected.

5. You are a CNL on an oncology unit. Recently, there has been an increase in the number of catheter-associated urinary tract infections (CAUTIs) on your unit. After shadowing nurses and aides you observed a variety of practices, techniques, and expectations surrounding daily catheter care. Your hospital does not have a current policy or procedure regarding catheter care. As the CNL, what should you do next?

A. Review current evidence for catheter care practice and disseminate evidence to the staff

B. Form an interdisciplinary team meeting to evaluate current hospital catheter care policies

C. Create a rubric for educating patients and staff on catheter care

D. Discuss with the unit manager the clinical issue and create a set of evidence-based unit expectations and practices for the oncology unit. Evaluate the need to address this issue with a hospital-wide policy or procedure

Answer D—Rationale: CNLs should gather and disseminate evidence to solve clinical problems; however, that should not be the initial step. Further review of hospital practices and policies may come after this issue is addressed. Creation of a rubric for educating patients and staff on catheter care may come after reviewing evidence. The CNL should act to solve the clinical issue in the short term, and evaluate the need for a larger policy to address gaps in practice hospital-wide.

6. A 50-year-old woman with a history of stage 3 chronic obstructive pulmonary disease (COPD) presents to the emergency department (ED) with increased shortness of breath. Based on your lab results, what is the acid–base disorder?

   Labs as follows:

pH 7.25	$PaCO_2$ 50 mmHg
HCO_3 22 mEq/L	PO_2 75
SpO_2 88%	Na + 136
BUN 18	

   A. Uncompensated respiratory acidosis

   B. Metabolic acidosis

   C. Respiratory acidosis

   D. Uncompensated respiratory acidosis

Answer A—Rationale: Based on the clinical scenario, the pH is decreased (less than 7.35); therefore, the patient has acidosis. The $PaCO_2$ is elevated (more than 45 mmHg), which is also consistent with the pH. The HCO_3 is within normal limits, which suggests the kidneys are not compensating. COPD is commonly associated with respiratory acidosis.

7. A CNL evaluates a 17-year-old patient who has been a victim of rape. The patient has visible bruising and a head laceration. After the CNL's assessment, law enforcement officials have contacted the CNL requesting information regarding the attack and the visible injuries seen during the visit.

   The CNL knows she must first:

   A. Take pictures and complete the rape kit

   B. Provide law enforcement with a record as requested

C. Call the patient's parents first

D. Explain to the patient in order to obtain consent for release of records

Answer D—Rationale: Legally, there must be consent from the patient to share information with law enforcement and to abide by Health Insurance Portability and Accountability Act (HIPAA) regulations.

8. A CNL in the neonatal intensive care unit (NICU) is collecting data on the hours worked weekly by the staff nurses. The CNL wants to see if there is a normal distribution of hours worked. What technique is the best to display the distribution of the data collected?

A. Run chart

B. Fishbone chart

C. Failure modes and effects analysis (FMEA) chart

D. Histogram chart

Answer D—Rationale: Histogram is a graphical representation, showing a visual impression of the distribution of data.

9. Your pediatric oncology unit is considering the implementation of a social/activity program for child clients that would provide volunteer social interactions and age-appropriate activities to admitted clients. As the CNL for this unit, you recognize this intervention as a way to:

A. Be helpful to the floor staff by distracting clients

B. Be a wasteful expenditure

C. Meet the psychosocial needs of clients

D. Prevent poor client experience ratings on discharge surveys

Answer C—Rationale: While social interaction and activities may provide distraction to clients and prevent poor client experiences, such a program would most importantly meet the holistic needs of young clients that may otherwise be neglected during a lengthy hospital stay. They also act to integrate such services with the medical care being delivered, meeting the CNL's call to develop and integrate services across settings in a holistic manner.

10. When assessing a new microsystem, the CNL will often use a tool known as the "5 Ps." As a CNL, you recognize the "5 Ps" to include are:

A. **Purpose, patients, process, patterns, professionals**

B. Patients, providers, policies, patterns, prevention

C. Purpose, patients, providers, patterns, prevention

D. Patients, process, professionals, policies, patterns

Answer A—Rationale: These answers make up the 5 Ps; the others are components of other aspects of the CNL's functions or tools.

11. Mr. Johnson is an 80-year-old patient who lives alone. He had fallen and was found by his neighbors. Mr. Johnson has a history of multiple falls, congestive heart failure (CHF), myocardial infarction (MI), diabetes mellitus (DM), and asthma. Mr. Johnson is admitted to the hospital with a hip fracture. Using an interdisciplinary approach, who should the CNL include in the plan of care initially?

    A. Clinical care manager, medical social worker, clinical nutritionist, CNL, and physician

    B. Clinical care manager, medical social worker, clinical nutritionist, physical therapist, **registered nurse, CNL, and physician**

    C. Speech therapist, clinical care manager, medical social worker, CNL, registered nurse, and nursing supervisor

    D. Clinical care manager, medical social worker, CNL, registered nurse, and nurse manager

Answer B—Rationale: An interdisciplinary team is composed of many disciplines who work together toward a patient's and family's common goals, such as safe discharge coordination. Learning to advocate for clients occurs by communicating effectively with other interdisciplinary team members, including nurses in other settings. The opportunity to learn and work in an interdisciplinary team will provide the best opportunity to give patients the best outcome.

12. As the CNL on a cardiac telemetry unit, you are performing a root cause analysis (RCA) due to the high volume of catheter-associated urinary tract infections (CAUTIs) over the last 6 months. Realizing that the Centers for Medicare & Medicaid are on a pay-for-performance basis, you develop a CAUTI task force in an effort to reduce costs. This is an example of which of the following?

    A. Implementing cost reduction and savings

    B. Anticipating risk and designing plans of care to improve outcomes

    C. Evaluating the effect of the healthcare financing on care access and patient outcomes

    D. Applying basic business and economic principles to the microsystem

Answer B—Rationale: CNLs must have the ability to critically evaluate and anticipate risks to client safety; this is a critical component role.

13. You notice a trend of increased central line bloodstream infection (CLBSI) on your unit. You conduct a literature search and, after critiquing and synthesizing the available evidence, you find that central line bundles have been shown to decrease CLBSI. You want to

implement this bundle on your unit, and plan to evaluate the effect of this change. Which of the following best describes this process?

A. Plan-Do-Study-Act (PDSA)

B. Research

C. Process improvement

D. Evidence-based practice (EBP)

Answer D—Rationale: EBP involves applying the best available research evidence, clinical expertise, and patient preferences to improve a clinical outcome.

14. A CNL rounds with Dr. Camper on a Spanish-speaking patient. The CNL asks the physician to call an interpreter, but the MD states that it is not necessary because the patient's daughter speaks English. However, the CNL insists and ensures an interpreter is present. What CNL role was fulfilled?

A. Educator

B. Team manager

C. Clinician

D. Client advocate

Answer D—Rationale: Client advocacy is a hallmark of the CNL's role. As a client advocate, the CNL assumes accountability for the delivery of high-quality care, including the evaluation of care outcomes and provision of leadership in improving care. Historically, the nursing role has emphasized partnership with clients—whether individuals, families, groups, or communities—in order to foster and support active participation in determining healthcare decisions. In addition, the CNL advocates for improvement in the institution or healthcare system and the nursing profession.

15. During the policy formulation phase, all of the following are correct except:

A. Possible solutions are offered.

B. Political circumstances are considered.

C. A problem is identified.

D. Policy decisions are adjusted to accommodate changing circumstances or needs.

Answer D—Rationale: Policy formulation is the development of effective and acceptable courses of action in order to address what has been placed on the policy agenda. This should include the following characteristics: (a) The problem is identified, (b) possible solutions are offered, (c) political circumstances are considered, and (d) policy makers, stakeholders, and legislative staff are involved.

16. The unit implemented bedside reporting 6 months ago, but the change has not been sustained. As a CNL, you begin to participate in bedside reporting and provide constructive, immediate feedback to the nurses for improvement. What best describes this situation?

    A. Mentoring

    B. Transformational leadership

    C. Coaching

    D. Precepting

Answer C—Rationale: The CNL coaches by evaluating team members and providing constructive feedback. Mentoring is a long-term relationship between two individuals focused on clinical advancement.

17. Jane, a CNL, successfully implemented an evidence-based practice (EBP) project utilizing music therapy to help with pain control in sickle cell patients on a medical–surgical unit. Jane was asked by the chief nursing officer (CNO) to implement the project within the medical division. What system will Jane be working in?

    A. Mesosystem

    B. Macrosystem

    C. Microsystem

    D. Unit system

Answer A—Rationale: The mesosystem encompasses multiple microsystems, such as a medical division within a hospital.

18. Judy has a family history of type 2 diabetes. After education, Judy knows she can help to prevent diabetes by maintaining a healthy weight, healthy eating habits, and daily physical activity. Judy is exhibiting what type of prevention strategies?

    A. Primary prevention

    B. Secondary prevention

    C. Tertiary prevention

    D. Quaternary prevention

Answer A—Rationale: The purpose of primary prevention is to prevent the onset of chronic illness, focusing on healthy lifestyle habits and behaviors.

19. You are a CNL on a surgical unit. Your unit has just hired several new graduate nurses. As the CNL, what is your role in relationship to these new team members?

    A. Provider of all clinical education

    B. Evaluator for performance reviews

    C. Coach and mentor

    D. Individual with a hands-off approach to allow new nurses to develop skills independently

Answer C—Rationale: The role of the CNL is to mentor and support all nurses on the unit, especially new nurses. Although the CNL may act as an educator, he or she does not guide the education and training of nurses on the unit. The CNL is not a member of management and does not complete employee performance reviews. While the CNL may take a hands-off approach, he or she should still offer support and mentorship to his or her peers.

20. You are the CNL on a surgical unit. You have noticed that readmission rates for your orthopedic patients have increased steadily over the last several months. Upon investigation, you find that patients are reporting that they do not believe they are receiving adequate education on post-operative wound management. As the CNL, you recognize that one way you can act to promote the health of your patients is:

    A. Provide direct, culturally appropriate education to all patients on your unit

    B. Arrange post-op visits at the outpatient surgical clinic for all patients upon discharge

    C. Educate the nursing staff regarding how they can evaluate patient health literacy, provide education at an appropriate level for each patient, and evaluate patient understanding of education provided

    D. Discuss with pre-op staff beginning patient education much earlier in this hospital process

Answer C—Rationale: Although the CNL may do direct patient teaching, it may not be possible to coordinate the discharge education for all patients on the unit; this would depend upon the patient's nurse. Post-op visits are important follow-ups for patients, but do not need to be scheduled by the CNL. Valuable teaching may occur preoperatively; however, demonstration of wound care and dressings cannot occur until after the surgery. CNLs should educate nurses on how to best provide education to their patients, and ensure that nurses understand how to evaluate health literacy.

21. A mother presents to the emergency department (ED) with her 8-month-old son, who has the following symptoms: coughing, recurring respiratory infections, fatty stools, and failure to thrive. Upon examination, the infant's vitals are as follows: Temp 99.4°F, pulse 150, respirations 65, blood pressure 88/50 mmHg. A CNL in the ED receives a phone call from the laboratory stating that *Staphylococcus aureus* was found colonized in the patient's airway.

    As a CNL in the ED, you know that the preceding symptoms and laboratory results are consistent with which of the following diseases?

    A. Asthma

    B. Lobar pneumonia

    C. Cystic fibrosis

    D. Croup

Answer C—Rationale: Cough, recurring respiratory infections, fatty stool, and failure to thrive are all symptoms of cystic fibrosis. Many children with cystic fibrosis have colonizing *Staphylococcus aureus* in their airways.

22. An elderly Chinese woman has just been diagnosed with terminal cancer. While discussing end-of-life care decisions with the family, patient, and CNL, the CNL notices there are conflicting viewpoints between the family and patient regarding advance directives. Which of these is the best answer regarding advance directives?

    A. In the Chinese culture, the family makes the decisions regarding end-of-life care in order not to burden the patient.

    B. It is best not to fully inform the patient of his or her condition so that he or she will remain positive.

    C. The patient has the right to enact his or her own advance directive to guide his or her medical treatments according to the Patient Self-Determination Act.

    D. The interdisciplinary team has the most information on palliative care to make the best decision.

Answer C—Rationale: The Patient Self-Determination Act explains the patient's right to accept or the right to refuse medical or surgical treatment. The patient is also entitled to receive information about the right to create his or her own advance directive.

23. A CNL in the emergency department (ED) is auditing stroke patients' charts and the administration of tissue plasminogen activator (tPA) and notices that only 83% of patients who are eligible to receive tPA are receiving it. The CNL knows that the 83% administration rate is below the national benchmark. The CNL identifies that there is a time lag in MRI.

The CNL creates a stroke team to develop a guideline implementation action plan to improve the process of timing of the MRI. What is the best tool utilized by the CNL in implementing change?

A. Research study

B. Meta-analysis

C. Plan-Do-Study-Act (PDSA)

D. Standardize-Do-Study-Act

Answer C—Rationale: PDSA is a model for quickly and easily testing ideas that could lead to improvement, based on existing ideas, research, feedback, theory, reviews, audits, or evidence of what has worked elsewhere.

24. A group composed of unit-based council members was put on a task force to improve the discharge planning process because patients felt unprepared and rushed at discharge. A decision was made to create a discharge planning nurse position to educate patients the night before the discharge. Even though the new nurses did not like this solution, they deferred to the senior nurses of this group who were adamant about implementing this position. Which barrier to effective teamwork does this exemplify?

A. Physical threats

B. Groupthink

C. Team dysfunction

D. Authority gradient

Answer B—Rationale: Groupthink is a phenomenon that occurs when group members try to minimize conflict and reach consensus too early without fully vetting all ideas and consequences.

25. You are a CNL on a pediatric unit. You are doing chart audits on attending physicians' daily charting and assessment notes and notice that a small number of attending physicians are not seeing patients daily. They are putting in discharge orders days prior to discharge. As a CNL, you know the hospital has a policy that attending physicians must see their patients every 24 hours. The CNL waits to see what happens during the next scheduled chart audits. What conflict resolution is demonstrated?

A. Compromise

B. Accommodate

C. Compete

D. Avoidance

Answer D—Rationale: Avoidance is characterized by behaviors that either ignore or refuse to engage in the conflict.

26. Attending physicians have noted that on your unit nurse communication by telephone has been scattered, disjointed, lengthy, and often contains erroneous information. As the CNL, good interdisciplinary communication is a priority. To best address this issue, the CNL would:

   A. Wait to see if the issue persists

   B. Encourage floor nurses to provide less information when calling physicians to limit the length and complexity of their calls

   C. Ask physicians to provide their feedback directly to individual nurses

   D. Refamiliarize staff nurses with the use of situation background assessment recommendation (SBAR), your hospital's communication standard

Answer D—Rationale: While professionals should provide direct feedback to each other in a meaningful, constructive manner and limiting communication to key information is an important aspect of clear communication, the use of a standardized tool, already a standard at this hospital, would most readily help to guide nurses to communicate in a clear, concise, efficient manner to ensure high-quality communication between care team members.

27. Quality improvement (QI) is a key function of the CNL. While QI efforts can yield many benefits in healthcare, as the CNL you recognize which of the following to be *the most important potential effect of a nursing QI effort*?

   A. Increased hospital cash flow/decreased expense

   B. Increased competitiveness with other facilities

   C. Reduction in lawsuits/liability

   D. Improvement of nursing quality indicators

Answer D—Rationale: While a QI effort may yield any of these potential answers, only the improvement of nursing quality indicators is patient centered.

28. While assisting Dr. Smith with a central line insertion you notice she did not properly execute sterile technique. What is the most appropriate way to provide feedback?

   A. Stop Dr. Smith while she is talking to the patient and provide feedback

   B. Ask Dr. Smith to stop the procedure so you can get her another central line insertion kit

   C. Refer Dr. Smith to the policy and procedure manual and ask that she read the section on using aseptic technique

   D. Debate with Dr. Smith at the bedside and tell her errors like this are the reason patients acquire hospital-acquired conditions

Answer B—Rationale: The most important action is to protect the patient by providing another sterile central line insertion kit.

29. Which of the following is the best description of healthcare economics?
    A. Understanding run charts
    B. Competence demonstrated by knowledge and ability to articulate federal, state, and private payer system regulations and issues, as well as the impact on organizations
    C. Identifying the number of patient falls per patient day
    D. The number of staff assigned to work on a given shift on a given day

Answer B—Rationale: The CNL has a very powerful role to fill when it comes to economics and healthcare finance. The CNL must understand finance to make the most appropriate decisions in regard to services provided, by whom, and for the length of time.

30. Amy, a nurse on your unit, is interested in implementing a project to improve health literacy and diabetes using follow-up phone calls. She asks the CNL for help in initiating the project. What would be her first step?
    A. Identify the clinical problem
    B. Implement follow-up phone calls
    C. Determine outcomes of the project
    D. Review literature for evidence

Answer A—Rationale: According to the EBP process, identifying the clinical problem is the first step.

31. Mrs. Jones, a patient with multiple comorbidities, has been hospitalized for over 3 months due to her recent stroke. During this period, she has not progressed and has had a tracheostomy and percutaneous endoscopic gastronomy (PEG) tube placed. Two of the daughters refused to make the patient a do not resuscitate (DNR), while the son and husband want the patient to be a DNR. As a CNL, you are conflicted and want the best outcome for the patient. What is the best step for you to take?
    A. Find out if the patient has an advance directive or wants to be a DNR
    B. Prevent the patient from being a DNR
    C. Call the physician to make the decision
    D. Make the patient a DNR according to the husband's wishes

Answer A—Rationale: You, as the CNL, are acting as a client advocate. You are taking the next step to ensure appropriate care is provided for the patient. You assume accountability for the delivery of high-quality care, including the evaluation of care outcomes and provision of leadership in improving care.

32. Team coordination skills can help avoid all of the following except:

    A. Undefined team member roles

    B. Poor membership involvement

    C. Member conflict

    D. Confusion regarding next steps

Answer C—Rationale: In most working groups, conflict arises at some point. In addition to sound team coordination skills, the CNL must also possess effective conflict management skills.

33. The CNL of the heart failure unit encourages the staff to earn advanced degrees, obtain certifications, and present and publish EBP projects. The CNL exhibits which type of leadership style?

    A. Relational leadership

    B. Transactional leadership

    C. Situational leadership

    D. Transformational leadership

Answer D—Rationale: A transformational leader motivates others to higher performance.

34. A CNL works in an inpatient unit that provides healthcare to medical–surgical patients. This best describes which of the following?

    A. Macrosystem

    B. Mesosystem

    C. Microsystem

    D. Megasystem

Answer C—Rationale: The microsystem is used to describe the small, functional, frontline unit that provides the most healthcare to the most people.

35. Maureen is a 45-year-old female who is undergoing chemotherapy for ovarian cancer. Maureen complains of increased nausea, vomiting, and abdominal pain uncontrolled by medications prescribed by her oncologist. Maureen expresses that she wants to continue chemotherapy, but she is unable to eat and maintain her weight due to her symptoms. She describes the pain as unbearable and at times she is unable to get out of bed. What would be the best step for the CNL to take next?

    A. Discuss code status and healthcare power of attorney with Maureen

    B. Contact hospice care to arrange a meeting with Maureen

C. Call the physician and suggest a palliative care consult

D. Suggest alternative methods for pain relief such as meditation, healing touch, and aromatherapy

Answer C—Rationale: Palliative care focuses on improving the quality of life for individuals by concentrating on pain and symptom management, communication, and coordinated care. Palliative care would help Maureen control symptoms of nausea, vomiting, and pain while she continues treatment.

36. You are a CNL on a busy surgical unit. Recently, several nurses have reported confusion regarding their patients' discharge process. The nurses stated that they were often unaware of all communications between the surgeon, discharge planners, social workers, and pharmacists. As a result, the nurses were often unaware of their patient discharge plans, status, and needs. As a CNL, how can you best improve this process?

   A. Educate nurses on how to access progress notes from other providers within the current electronic health record (EHR)

   B. Discuss with each healthcare team member the clinical issue regarding the discharge process and suggest the creation of a daily interdisciplinary team meeting

   C. Communicate to the surgeons the nurses' concerns, and advocate for the nurses' needs for communication in their role

   D. Assume responsibility for the coordination of all discharge needs for patients on the unit

Answer B—Rationale: CNLs should advocate for the role of the professional nurse as an equal part of the interdisciplinary team. Education for nurses on accessing progress notes does not address the issue of nurses not being communicated with as part of the team. Communication to surgeons may improve communication to the nurse, but does not necessarily improve communication between each provider equally. The CNL should not assume all of the responsibility of patient discharge planning.

37. How can the CNL best provide and educate staff on giving culturally competent care within the unit?

   A. Educate staff on assessment questions/phrases in the most common secondary language present in the community or seen within the hospital

   B. Educate staff on varying cultural perceptions and beliefs surrounding the concept of health

C. Provide an in-service on accessing patient education and handouts in another language

D. Ensure that nurses are assigned to the most culturally appropriate patients currently on the unit

Answer B—Rationale: Nurses should never attempt to use a family member or their own limited ability for conversation in another language; a certified medical interpreter should be used. An in-service on accessing education in multiple languages would likely be very useful to staff, but is not as good an intervention as education on cultural differences. Staffing and patient assignment should not be based on only cultural associations; individual preferences may also need to be considered.

38. A 40-year-old postpartum patient with chronic hypertension and gestational diabetes who is gravida 5 para 4 is transferred from labor and delivery to the postpartum unit with lactated Ringer's at 125 mL/hr. Upon assessment of the patient, the nurse notices the patient's fundus is three finger breaths above umbilicus and to the right of midline and her bladder is palpable. The nurse also notes moderate to heavy bleeding and a full bladder and notifies the CNL.

    As a CNL, the most important nursing intervention is to:

    A. Encourage the nurse to massage the fundus and heplock the patient

    B. Encourage the nurse to call the physician stat to order Methergine (methylergonovine maleate)

    C. Encourage the nurse to monitor the patient over the next hour because there are no risk factors for a postpartum hemorrhage

    D. Encourage the nurse to straight catherize the patient to decrease the likelihood of a postpartum hemorrhage

Answer D—Rationale: The patient is at risk for a hemorrhage due to being a multipara and having a full bladder. Methergine is contraindicated in patients with hypertension.

39. A 6-year-old boy is in critical condition following a car accident. The patient has head trauma and internal bleeding. The patient's parents have stated multiple times that they are Jehovah's Witnesses and do not want their son to receive blood.

    The CNL knows that the blood transfusion is needed immediately and could save the boy's life. Which of the following statements is the best thing for the CNL to do?

    A. Listen to the parents, as U.S. minors have no legal rights and remain under parental jurisdiction

    B. Obtain a court order in the best interest of the child to receive blood, based on the avoidance of physical harm

C. Based on religious beliefs, do not give blood

D. Follow the physician's decision to give blood since the physician's decision overrides the parental decision

Answer B—Rationale: The child's interests as well as the state policies outweigh the parental rights to refuse medical treatment for a minor. A court order is needed to enforce this.

40. The group known as "Maternal Child Health" has many subunits such as pediatrics, well baby nursery, NICU, and maternity. This collection of units belongs to which system?

A. Microsystem

B. Mesosystem

C. Macrosystem

D. Megasystem

Answer B—Rationale: A mesosystem is a collection of other microsystems that facilitate processes.

41. Which stage of Lewin's change theory involves explaining that the current situation must change?

A. Unfreezing

B. Adoption

C. Evaluation

D. Change

Answer A—Rationale: Unfreezing is a process that involves finding a method of making it possible for people to let go of an old pattern that was counterproductive in some way.

42. A client with complex behavior concerns is getting ready to be discharged to a skilled nursing facility. However, the client has expressed that he wishes to stay in the hospital and not be discharged. As the CNL, your best action would be to:

A. Inform the patient and his or her family that they must go and remaining on the unit is not an option

B. Advocate letting the client stay on the unit one extra day, then discharge tomorrow

C. Identify the client's concerns and collaborate with the care team to see they are addressed

D. Ask the family to help encourage the client to discharge to the skilled nursing facility

Answer C—Rationale: Clients can often experience apprehension when changing care settings. Identifying specific concerns and working rapidly to ensure they are addressed in collaboration with other members of the care team can greatly reduce a client's hesitation. Additionally, such collaboration ensures other members of the care team are aware of the clients' concerns, possibly providing additional information and insight regarding the clients and their care needs.

43. A healthy work environment is an important factor in supporting ongoing quality and safety. As the CNL, you recognize that the hallmarks of a healthy work environment include all of the following except:

A. Skilled communication

B. Upward mobility

C. Effective decision making

D. Appropriate staffing

Answer B—Rationale: Upward mobility is not a hallmark of a healthy work environment or area of focus for the CNL.

44. While rounding on your cohort of patients, you are informed by one of your patients that she does not have healthcare insurance. As a CNL, you know that interdisciplinary communication is very important. What member of the team is most effective in helping with this matter?

A. The care management team: medical social worker, clinical case manager (CCM), and medical team

B. Pastoral care

C. The business office of the hospital

D. Nursing staff

Answer A—Rationale: The case management team works closely with the medical team to ensure that patients have the means to pay for their medication.

45. Who can function as an important ally to the CNL in engaging frontline staff in a major initiative?

A. Content expert

B. Unit champion

C. Initiative sponsor

D. Senior leadership

Answer B—Rationale: B is the best answer because as a CNL implementing a major initiative, you want individuals who will help advocate and support your initiative. A champion is someone who fights or speaks publicly in support of a person, belief, cause, or initiative.

46. Which of the following best utilizes the PICOT method of developing a clinical question?

   A. Will a preoperative class for coronary artery bypass graft (CABG) surgery patients decrease anxiety?

   B. What is the effect of early mobility in patients 65 years and older on length of stay?

   C. Will the implementation of quiet time and employee education of harmful effects of noise reduce peak levels and improve patient satisfaction of patients on a medical–telemetry unit over a 1-month period?

   D. Will the use of secret shoppers increase compliance with hand washing and PPE in a large hospital in the Southeast?

Answer C—Rationale: C is the best choice as it addresses the population, intervention, outcome, and time period.

47. Which of the following is the best example of a CNL protecting patient autonomy?

   A. The CNL ensures the patient understands how to use an incentive spirometer.

   B. The CNL ensures the patient has all information and understands the procedure for esophagogastroduodenoscopy (EGD)/colonoscopy scheduled for the morning.

   C. The CNL discusses the plan of care for treatment of pneumonia with the daughter and the doctor.

   D. The CNL closes the door to protect the patient's privacy when discussing her diagnosis.

Answer B—Rationale: The CNL protects patients' autonomy by keeping them well informed and ensuring they understand their decision about their plan of care.

48. You are a CNL on a surgical unit. Your manager has asked you to review and update the current patient skin prep procedure as needed. After reviewing the evidence, you determine the current surgical skin prep does not match current evidence suggesting a need for chlorhexidine gluconate (CHG) wipes. At your next meeting with your manager, how do you best advocate for change?

   A. Provide a list of resources for the new CHG skin prep, costs, and available vendors

   B. Interpret the evidence of effectiveness of the CHG wipes prep and the related patient outcomes for patients receiving this skin prep; present the findings and suggest how this could be best used to change practice on the unit

C. Present feedback from the nursing staff on the current practices on the unit

D. Alert the manager that there is a discrepancy between the current practice and evidence, and await further instructions before proceeding

Answer B—Rationale: As the CNL, you should assess evidence, interpret research for policy makers or stakeholders, and offer suggestions for improvement to practice. Providing a list of resources to the manager does not create buy-in for the change. Feedback from nurses does not address evidence. CNLs should always provide suggestions for practice improvement.

49. The new hospital CNO works hard to cultivate a shared vision of leaders and followers motivating each other toward their highest potential. This is an example of which type of leadership?

A. Transformational leadership

B. Transactional leadership

C. Situational leadership

D. Hierarchical leadership

Answer A—Rationale: A transformational leader believes that leaders and followers motivate each other toward the end goal of developing followers into leaders. This is accomplished by leading and motivating by example.

50. The CNL's role is to lead frontline staff in line with the organization's core competencies. Which of the following best describes how a CNL can promote a high-performing clinical microsystem?

A. Support an atmosphere for learning and redesign supported by continuous monitoring of care, use of benchmarking, and frequent tests of change

B. Promote a microsystem that is in silo from the community and does not cross professional boundaries

C. Encourage staff to provide opinions and feedback, though the manager will make the final decision

D. Promote engagement by sharing positive outcomes with the staff and having celebrations, but keep negative outcomes confidential in order to keep the staff from feeling defeated

Answer A—Rationale: The CNL can promote high quality in high-performing clinical microsystems by providing a supportive atmosphere for continuous process improvement.

51. The CNL completes a 5P assessment of the microsystem and discovers that the geriatric population has increased. Forty-three percent of the

patients within the microsystem are older than 65 years. Recognizing this change, the CNL determines which of the following is an appropriate action?

A. Coordinate monthly lunch-and-learn opportunities for the staff to discuss topics related to nutrition, cognitive impairment, and mobility

B. Discuss the change with the nurse manager and order more bed alarms for the microsystem

C. Volunteer to take blood pressures and check hemoglobin A1cs at the local adult day-care center

D. Conduct a randomized control study on visual impairment in diabetic patients older than 70 years

Answer A—Rationale: The CNL recognizes it is important for the staff to be well prepared to care for the patient population. Malnutrition, cognitive impairment, and immobility are common geriatric problems. Educational opportunities will help inform the staff, allowing them to provide evidence-based care.

52. Your hospital is changing to a new electronic health record (EHR) system. As a CNL, you recognize that while this change may ultimately improve workflow, during the transition there will likely be both technical issues and knowledge gaps. What are some ways you can improve the ease of transition?

A. Assess the current transition timeline, including education and practice time for the staff

B. Identify leaders on the unit who can commit to extra training on the EHR and staff support during the transition

C. Create guidelines for the nurses to use as a quick reference for locating items in the EHR

D. All of the above

Answer D—Rationale: The CNL should consider the timeline for any education or training implemented occurring on their unit. Advocating for nurses during this time allows them to focus on the change. Identification of leaders who can act as peer educators supports the staff. The CNL should create tools to help increase or support workflow.

53. A 16-year-old female with a history of smoking, tanning bed use, and sexual activity presents to the emergency department (ED) with a mole that is continuously bleeding and itchy. The patient is concerned that this might be a sexually transmitted disease (STD) because the mole is on her inner thigh. Upon examination, the mole is asymmetrical, 7 mm big, and has uneven borders.

As a CNL, you know these characteristics represent which of the following?

A. Genital herpes

B. Human papillomavirus

C. Basal cell carcinoma

D. Malignant melanoma

Answer D—Rationale: The ABCDE's of malignant melanoma include asymmetrical; uneven borders; variety of colors; large diameter greater than 6 mm; and evolving.

54. Marci, a surgical nurse, is reviewing the operating room schedule and sees a coworker, Angie, is having surgery that day. Marci then calls the supervisor and manager to let them know Angie is having surgery. Marci then tells the CNL she is going to visit Angie in the postanesthesia care unit (PACU). What should the CNL do?

A. Explain to Marci that this is a violation of the Health Information Portability and Accountability Act (HIPAA) and we must protect Angie's right to privacy and confidentiality

B. Invite other nurses to visit Angie and bring her flowers

C. Nothing; since this is a coworker, this is not considered a violation of HIPAA

D. Arrange for Angie to have "VIP" treatment

Answer A—Rationale: As a CNL, you should be a guardian of information and educator to the nurses on the unit regarding HIPAA.

55. What type of chart is used in QI and uses step-by-step symbols to plan projects and describe a process?

A. Flowchart/process mapping

B. Pareto chart

C. Control chart

D. Run chart

Answer A—Rationale: Flowchart/process mapping is a graphic illustration of the steps in a process.

56. On the rehabilitation unit, the CNL notes that the stroke and amputee patients that require maximum assistance are being assigned to the float nurses. It is noted that many of these patients have had falls while being assigned to the float nurses. This is a patient and family dissatisfier. What type of delegation practice is in question?

A. The right circumstance

B. The right supervision

C. The right person

D. The right task

Answer C—Rationale: The licensed nurse delegating the task must ensure that the delegatee possesses and has demonstrated the knowledge base and appropriate skills and resources to perform the task and provide adequate supervision and evaluation to ensure the patient's safety and appropriate outcome.

57. In recent months, there has been a marked increase in the number of intravenous (IV) infections and infiltrations on your unit. Some of these IVs were started on your unit while others were started on other units or in the emergency unit before being transferred to your unit. The nurse manager has asked you to investigate this issue. As the CNL, your best intervention would be to:

A. Call other units to make sure policies and procedures are being followed

B. Wait to see if the infection occurrences are a coincidence

C. Form a group to investigate this issue including staff nurses from your unit, representatives from IV therapy, and infection prevention services

D. Retrain all staff nurses on your unit in correct IV care procedures

Answer C—Rationale: Because this issue involves shared responsibility and is a serious concern, it should also be addressed with collaboration, shared investigation, and decision making that occurs in a robust, focused workgroup.

58. As the CNL when engaging in a QI effort, you recognize *the first of the common steps* of the QI process to be:

A. Review literature

B. Analyze the root cause

C. Establish a clear purpose or aim

D. Select metrics

Answer C—Rationale: Establishing a clear aim or purpose for a QI effort is foundational to all other pieces. While other steps may occur first and trigger a QI effort, such as a sentinel resulting in an RCA that then becomes part of a QI effort, when the actual QI portion starts it is important to provide a clear, explicit purpose to provide focus and mission to participating players.

59. A Vietnamese patient is admitted with pneumonia on a medical–surgical unit. The patient appears very nervous when the medical staff enters the room. As a CNL, what is the best course of action to take in this situation?

A. Try to talk to the patient calmly and ease his fears

B. Call language services and request a Vietnamese interpreter

C. Ask your housekeeper who is from Vietnam to come in and interpret for the medical staff

D. Keep all interactions with the patient as brief as possible

Answer B—Rationale: The CNL bridges cultural and linguistic barriers by being an advocate for the patient and his or her family. An interpreter should be present anytime there is a language barrier.

60. Which of the following is not an example of healthcare finance and economics?

A. Developing and leveraging human, environmental, and material resources

B. Understanding the fiscal context in which practice occurs

C. Leading a gap analysis to create a cohesive healthcare team

D. Applying basic business and economic principles and practices

Answer C—Rationale: A gap analysis is a method of assessing the differences in performance between a business information system or application to determine whether the system requirements are being met and, if not, the step needed to do so. It is not an example of healthcare finance and economics.

61. A nurse is trying to determine the difference between evidence-based practice (EBP) and research. She approaches her unit CNL to assist her in her dilemma. What statement best describes the appropriate response by the CNL?

A. EBP involves critiquing and synthesizing evidence, while research involves designing a study because there is a gap in knowledge.

B. EBP needs institutional review board (IRB) approval, while research does not.

C. EBP involves collecting and analyzing data, while research includes critiquing and synthesizing evidence.

D. In EBP, the first step is identifying a clinical problem, while in research identifying a clinical problem is the last step.

Answer A—Rationale: The EBP process involves these steps: identify clinical problem, review literature/search for evidence, critique evidence, synthesize evidence and patient view, implement evidence-based change, evaluate outcomes, and present or publish findings. Both EBP and research can require IRB approval. The research process is done for a gap in knowledge: identify the clinical problem, review literature/search for evidence, design a study, write a research proposal, collect and analyze data, and present or publish the findings.

62. Maria, a 55-year-old Spanish-speaking patient, is scheduled for a paracentesis. You, the CNL, rounded on her with an interpreter in the morning and explained to her the procedure is scheduled for today at noon. After you mentioned this, Maria stated that she was not aware of this procedure. You noted that a consent was signed by the physician in her chart. What is the next step as a CNL?

    A. Keep the consent. Utilize the teach-back method to ensure Maria understands the risk and benefits of the procedure.

    B. Discard the previous consent. Explain to Maria that she needs this procedure and it is the best decision for her. Obtain a new consent.

    C. Inform the physician and ensure he explains the procedure to Maria with an interpreter present and obtains a new consent.

    D. Keep the consent. Leave a note for the physician and explain that the patient was unaware of the procedure.

Answer C—Rationale: The CNL protects patients' autonomy by keeping them well informed and ensuring they understand their decision about their plan of care. The CNL addresses the language barrier, ensuring an interpreter is present to assist in understanding, and a new consent is signed.

63. The CNL completed an assessment of the community and identified a need for a public health program. Which of the following would have the potential for the greatest impact on the community?

    A. Implement a small pilot program at the local hospital

    B. Write a proposal to make the change and send it to the legislators to build their support for the change

    C. Research and analyze public health programs in other communities

    D. Write an article for the local paper discussing the need for the program

Answer B—Rationale: The CNL is responsible for influencing regulatory, legislative, and public policy to promote and preserve healthy communities. The CNL is advocating for a healthy community by writing to legislators.

64. Lisa is a CNL who works with high-risk obstetric patients both inpatient at the hospital and outpatient in the local health clinic. Lisa follows each patient throughout his or her episodes of care, ensuring the patient receives streamlined, comprehensive care. Which critical component of lateral integration best describes what Lisa is demonstrating?

A. Coordination

B. Communication

C. Collaboration

D. Evaluation

Answer A—Rationale: The CNL coordinates care by managing the care of clients across settings and episodes of care. Coordination is not to be confused with collaboration. Collaboration is defined as an interdisciplinary process of problem solving that involves shared responsibility for decision making and execution of plans of care.

65. From which database would the CNL collect the most useful nursing-sensitive indicator metrics?

A. National Database of Nursing Quality Indicators® (NDNQI)

B. Hospital Compare

C. The Joint Commission (TJC)

D. Nursing Quality Forum (NQF)

Answer A—Rationale: The NDNQI evaluates unit and hospital-specific nursing-sensitive data. NDNQI also provides benchmarks that can be used for comparison.

66. You are working with a team to reduce patient waiting time for transport to diagnostic imaging (DI). An effective goal would be to:

A. Decrease waiting time during the evening shift

B. Increase monthly patient satisfaction

C. Improve communication between the emergency department (ED) and the DI departments

D. Decrease the waiting time for DI by 5%

Answer D—Rationale: Improvement goals must be specific and measurable. The team must have clear, measurable results to indicate whether an implementation resulted in improvement.

67. A 55-year-old male is readmitted to the hospital with hypertension four times within the past 8 months due to medication noncompliance. The patient has been given a blood pressure machine, set up with a primary care provider, and arranged telehealth services in previous admissions. During your discussion with the patient, he states that he is taking his medication as his doctor prescribed. The patient brought his medications into the hospital, so you ask him to hand you his blood pressure medication bottle. The patient hands you the bottle labeled Neurontin. Which of the following would be the next best step for you to take as the CNL?

A. Obtain records from the patient's primary care provider

B. Coordinate a family meeting with the patient and the care team

C. Have the patient hand you the rest of the bottles, tell you what each medication is, and describe how and when he takes that medication

D. Consult with a pharmacist to determine the best medication options for the patient

Answer C—Rationale: Oftentimes, patients develop coping skills to help with limited literacy, leading healthcare providers to misjudge their ability to comprehend patient teaching. By having the patient explain how and when he takes medications, the CNL can assess the patient's ability to understand his regimen. The patient may have difficulty reading and may need an alternative method for understanding his regimen such as color coding bottles rather than reading labels.

68. Promotion of personal goals for professional development and continuing education is a hallmark of the CNL role. Ultimately, what is the importance of professional development?

A. Maintaining professional practice competencies

B. Fulfillment of the CNL as a lifelong learner

C. Providing an example of professional nursing to peers

D. All of the above

Answer D—Rationale: The development of goals and continuing education maintains the CNL's competencies, illustrates the CNL is a lifelong learner, and provides an example to their peers.

69. You recognize that a large proportion of your surgical patients have cultural or religious concerns about the use of blood transfusions, although the need for such transfusions are common with many of your surgeries. As the CNL at a surgical center, how can you best ensure health promotion of this population while providing culturally competent care?

A. Develop education on the importance of blood transfusions when medically necessary, and the benefits postoperatively

B. Provide resources like the other clinics in the area that may be able to perform the surgery with lowered risks of estimated blood loss

C. Evaluate evidence on alternatives to blood transfusions, such as autologous blood transfusions and alternative blood products, and present this information at an interdisciplinary team meeting

D. Educate staff on respecting client wishes and do not attempt to pressure patients into receiving transfusions

Answer C—Rationale: Although still debated, many communities believe that autologous blood transfusions are acceptable and the blood is still from "self." Education on transfusions and benefits may be useful but does not truly address the patients' concerns. Providing resources on where else to seek care is not appropriate.

70. A 28-year-old patient with asthma is requesting the pneumococcal vaccine. Which of the following conditions are appropriate for receiving the pneumococcal vaccine?

A. Congestive heart failure (CHF), HIV, diabetes, pregnancy

B. CHF, HIV, diabetes, sickle cell disease

C. Diabetes, chemotherapy, sickle cell disease, pregnancy

D. Pregnancy, CHF, diabetes, chemotherapy

Answer B—Rationale: All of these medical conditions require a patient to receive the pneumococcal vaccination.

71. A new graduate nurse expresses concern about a frenotomy of the tongue-tied newborn to the CNL. The CNL decides to accompany the new nurse to the procedure room. Upon entering the procedure room, the new nurse notices that there is no consent signed and explains to the pediatrician consent must be signed before continuing. The pediatrician hollers at the nurse and refuses to have consent signed. How should the CNL respond?

A. The CNL hollers back that this is against hospital policy.

B. The CNL asks the parents to sign the consent without the physician speaking to the parents.

C.The procedure continues without consent and the CNL assures the new nurse the consent will be obtained after the procedure.

D. The CNL and new nurse professionally explain to the physician that they will not participate in the procedure until a consent is signed and they will contact hospital administration regarding this procedural violation.

Answer D—Rationale: Part of the CNL's duties is to discuss difficult situations in which the nurse must advocate for her patients. Consent must always be signed for a procedure with a physician present and a nurse as a witness.

72. A CNL on a medical unit is following up with patients on warfarin therapy postdischarge and concludes that patients are not receiving adequate education on medication administration. The CNL formulates an action plan and develops a team to improve warfarin discharge education. What competency was portrayed by the CNL?

A. Lifelong learner

B. Delegator

C. Lateral integration

D. Risk anticipator

Answer D—Rationale: Risk anticipation is the ability to critically evaluate and anticipate risks to client safety; this is a critical component to the CNL role.

73. A small group has been formed on the medical–surgical unit to implement change. Team members also have struggles over decision making and clarity of purpose. What stage of the Tuckman and Jensen's model is represented by members communicating their feelings but still viewing themselves as individuals rather than part of the team?

A. Performing

B. Norming

C. Forming

D. Storming

Answer D—Rationale: The storming phase is where competition and conflict are at their highest.

74. You, the CNL, have noted that many staff nurses on your unit do not use available nurse aide (NA) staff to perform routine capillary blood glucose (CBG) checks, even though they are allowed to at your hospital. When you investigate, you discover that most nurses were unaware the NAs could perform CBG checks. You, as the CNL, share information on the tasks NAs are able to perform during the next unit staff meeting in order to:

A. Ensure each member of the care team has a clear understanding of his or her role

B. Make sure staff nurses delegate as much work as possible

C. Make sure staff are using skills and training often enough

D. Ensure the NAs have enough to do

Answer A—Rationale: Ensuring mutual understanding of roles among care team members is a key component of the coordination piece of lateral integration.

75. Failure mode-effect analysis is best used as follows:

A. In response to a critical or sentinel event

B. Prior to a process implementation or change

C. As part of a random audit process

D. In response to malfunctioning tools or equipment

Answer B—Rationale: The purpose of a failure mode-effect analysis is to anticipate potential problems; by virtue, this is best conducted prior to a process implementation.

76. During your daily rounds, you are performing an advance assessment on a patient in your cohort. The patient was admitted for sepsis and appears very weak, and has a very poor appetite. The patient tells you that he has not been out of the bed for 3 days. What needs to happen to provide the best care for this patient?

    A. Enter an order for physical and occupational therapist, and ask the nursing staff to perform the Egress test to assess the patient's mobility level

    B. Tell the patient to get out of bed and sit up in the chair three times a day

    C. Place the bed in a bed-to-chair position

    D. Order an incentive spirometer for the patient

Answer A—Rationale: The CNL understands the role of the interdisciplinary team members including PT and OT. Bedside nurses and CNLs are at the frontline caring for patients, assessing interventions, and listening to patient concerns, and are the best advocates for patients receiving care from other team members.

77. As you are planning a discharge for a patient in your cohort, the patient tells you that, even though she has insurance, there is a financial strain on her to pay for her medication. The patient has a history of HIV/AIDS and is currently on three antiviral medications. The patient was admitted with pneumonia on this admission and the doctor has prescribed Zyvox in addition to her other medication regimen. You investigate the cost of this medication and find out the medication will cost the patient $100 after insurance. Which of the following is the most appropriate and first action for you as the CNL?

    A. Tell the patient that she should take this prescribed medication so she can get better

    B. Encourage the patient to take the medication because the doctor knows best

    C. Call the doctor and ask him if there is a more cost-efficient medication to treat the patient's pneumonia

    D. Consult with the medical social worker to find coupons for this medication

Answer C—Rationale: The CNL uses her knowledge and collaboration skills to reduce cost of care delivery and increase compliance.

78. A certified nursing assistant (CNA) approaches the unit CNL to discuss her frustrations in attaining appropriate equipment for patient care. The CNA explains that the clean utility room is too far and that staff constantly have to make frequent trips. The CNA wants to know what steps to take to make a change. As a CNL, what statement best describes the appropriate response?

    A. "We will just have to adjust to what we have right now."

    B. "Well, you have identified a problem, the next step is to review any literature that can help resolve our issue."

    C. "I suggest that you and the staff take the appropriate equipment to your rooms."

    D. "Well, let us implement the process that another unit is using."

Answer B—Rationale: The CNA already identified a problem, the first step of EBP. The second step of the EBP process is to review the literature.

79. As Jeff, a new CNL, walks into his newly assigned intensive care unit (ICU), he notices that the charge nurse assigned him as a primary care nurse for a group of a patients, like she would do for a staff nurse. Jeff discusses the role of a CNL with the charge nurse. What statement best describes the appropriate approach by Jeff?

    A. Jeff asks the charge nurse if she understands the role of a CNL, and states he cannot be assigned a group of patients.

    B. Jeff asks the charge nurse if she understands the role of a CNL, then explains that the CNL does not provide direct care to patients.

    C. Jeff discusses that CNLs are not supposed to take patients and only coordinate care for difficult patients.

    D. Jeff explains that the CNL operates in a microsystem as an advanced generalist to communicate, coordinate, and collaborate care and does not serve as a primary care nurse.

Answer D—Rationale: The CNL operates in a microsystem as an advanced generalist who communicates, coordinates, and collaborates care with major stakeholders. The CNL is a leader in the nursing profession. The CNL in this scenario is protecting the CNL role by advocating for the appropriate use of a CNL.

80. As a CNL, it is important to remain aware of current changes to national healthcare policies, namely from ongoing focuses from the Centers for Medicare & Medicaid Services (CMS) and law prescribed by the Affordable Care Act (ACA), both of which have set reduced reimbursement for which of the following issues?

    A. Elevated readmission rates

    B. Medication errors

C. Falls

D. Nurses practicing below their scope

Answer A—Rationale: While each item is an important focus for the CNL, and B and C can result in nonreimbursed costs, the ACA via the CMS has set reducing hospital readmission rates as a key priority, and decreases reimbursements for hospitals with frequent readmissions.

81. How can the CNL help determine the meaningful use of the EHR within his or her microsystem?

A. Identify data that should be collected and managed, and note how that data should be shared for improving client outcomes

B. Coordinate with physicians to identify which clinical information would be meaningful for the patients under their care

C. Discuss with unit leaders and stakeholders what data could provide meaningful use of the EHR within the unit

D. Review the available client data currently in the EHR and assess for meaningfulness in improving patient outcomes

Answer A—Rationale: The CNL should be able to identify meaningful data, as well as its collection and management, and use that data to improve clinical outcomes on the unit.

82. Regarding information technology, how can the CNL improve the identification of meaningful data?

A. Clarify with nurses what vendor-related terms may be used in their documentation

B. Develop a tool to identify relevant nursing clinical data and its location within the electronic health record (EHR)

C. Advocate for standardized nursing terminology within the EHR

D. Coordinate with the informatics the best way to document care for efficient data retrieval

Answer C—Rationale: The most important way the CNL can improve the identification of meaningful data is through the standardization of nursing technology within the EHR, away from the use of any vendor-related terms.

83. The CNL works with the interdisciplinary team and encourages all members to voice their opinion and provide feedback. What type of leadership is the CNL demonstrating?

A. Vertical leadership

B. Diagonal leadership

C. Horizontal leadership

D. Systems leadership

Answer C—Rationale: Horizontal leadership focuses more on collaboration and equality within the group. Vertical leadership is a top-down style of leadership with one team leader driving down change.

84. The diabetes liaison on an adult medical–surgical unit informed the team that the unit was only 45% compliant with checking blood sugars within 15 minutes after a hypoglycemic event. The team decided to implement a process change to ensure the blood sugar recheck is completed within 15 minutes. The change was implemented and there was an increase to 85% compliance of hypoglycemic rechecks. What is the next step for the team in the PDSA cycle?

    A. Plan

    B. Do

    C. Study

    D. Act

Answer D—Rationale: After analysis of the results of the trial (also known as study), the team will then act by devising the next steps based on the analysis.

85. Isabella is a 62-year-old female who enters the community health clinic where you are employed as a CNL. The front desk staff approaches you and states that Isabella has refused to complete the standard health questionnaire form and health information release form. Isabella states that she forgot her glasses and that she will just take the form home to complete. Which of the following would be the most appropriate response by you as the CNL?

    A. Tell the front desk staff to send the forms home with Isabella and provide her with a prepaid envelope to send the forms back to the office

    B. Inform Isabella that many people have difficulty understanding these forms, and ask if she would like you or someone to help her complete the forms

    C. Explain the importance of completing the forms to Isabella and ensure she completes the forms prior to entering the examination room

    D. Provide Isabella with a magnifying glass to allow her to read the forms more easily

Answer B—Rationale: Patients will frequently hide issues with health literacy due to feelings of embarrassment and shame. Healthcare providers may pick up on behavioral clues such as patients that provide incomplete forms, make excuses such as they forgot their glasses, or state they will complete the paperwork at home.

86. A nurse on your unit expresses concern about her patient. The patient is an 88-year-old male on the unit due to a chronic obstructive pulmonary disease (COPD) exacerbation. He has become deconditioned and therapy is involved. The patient is due to be discharged, but still appears very weak and unsteady. During his stay he was newly diagnosed with insulin-dependent diabetes, and although he has been educated on insulin administration, the nurse is uncertain he can properly administer the medication at home. As the CNL, how do you proceed?

    A. Organize an interdisciplinary team meeting to discuss the multiple concerns over patient treatment and condition, as well as greater discharge needs

    B. Place an ethics consult

    C. Encourage the nurse to call the MD and relay her concerns

    D. Provide tools to the nurse that can help improve the patient's functioning regarding the insulin, and advocate for the use of oxygen at home

Answer A—Rationale: When multiple healthcare team members are involved in a patient's care and coordination of their healthcare needs, the interdisciplinary team meeting can best coordinate needs.

87. Staff nurses have a clinical question regarding the effectiveness of two different surgical skin preps stocked on your unit. Both benzalkonium chloride and CHG are available, and the nurses are uncertain of the differences—particularly in terms of reducing surgical site infections. As the CNL, what is the next step to take?

    A. Review research on the effectiveness of each product in reducing surgical site infections and disseminate the evidence to staff

    B. Organize a study of patients on your unit, trialing the different surgical prep and tracking patient outcomes

    C. Determine the most cost-effective surgical skin prep for the patient

    D. Research what products are being used on other units and other hospitals within your area

Answer A—Rationale: CNLs should act to review evidence to answer clinical questions. Organizing a study to evaluate the greater trends of one skin prep versus another may be a lengthy process when evidence is already available.

88. A patient presents with severe pain in the upper right abdomen after eating a fatty meal. These symptoms lead you to suspect cholecystitis. Which assessment finding is most likely to be associated with this condition?

A. Positive Homans sign

B. Positive Psoas sign

C. Murphy's sign

D. Aaron's sign

Answer C—Rationale: A positive Murphy's sign is identified when the patient inhales and feels pain due to the inflamed gallbladder pushing into the palpating hand.

89. The CNL has been requested to assist with end-of-life care decision making for an elderly homeless patient who has no family; he was deemed incompetent and is now unresponsive. The best decision-making guide that the CNL could use in this situation is:

 A. Plan-Do-Study-Act (PDSA)

 B. Autonomy model

 C. Orem's self-care theory

 D. MORAL model

Answer D—Rationale: This is a model that addresses ethical issues and guides an objective, orderly, and systematic decision.

90. You, the CNL, are working in the ICU with a high volume of patients with prolonged Foley catheter use. What analysis tool is appropriate for the CNL to use in prevention of CAUTIs?

 A. Root cause analysis (RCA)

 B. Fishbone diagram

 C. St. Thomas risk assessment tool

 D. Failure mode-effect analysis

Answer D—Rationale: The failure mode-effect analysis tool is a proactive risk assessment of high-risk or high-vulnerability areas that identifies and improves steps in a process, with a focus on failure prevention, not detection.

91. A CNL using Rogers's diffusion of innovation theory realizes while implementing a new health information management (HIM) system that when dealing with a member of the healthcare team she should:

 A. Spend a majority of time educating the laggards to become supporters of change

 B. Spend a majority of time on innovators because they will need a lot of convincing to make a change

C. Spend a majority of time with early and late majority adopters because when they support the change it will be successful

D. Spend very little time with the early majority adopters because they are not adaptable to change

Answer C—Rationale: Looking at Rogers's diffusion of innovation theory's bell curve, 2.5% of people are innovators. Following them are the early adopters (13.5%) and then the early majority (34%), consumers who make their moves through the market more carefully, but tend to adopt a new product more quickly than most. At the hump of the bell curve are the late majority (34%), consumers who adopt a new product only after the majority has weighed in on its value. Finally, sloping downward are laggards (16%), the critics, curmudgeons, and haters who do their best to resist adoption but will eventually do so.

92. A client on your unit is going home to finish rehab following a bilateral total knee replacement. You, as the CNL, would be enacting the function of lateral integrator by which of the following?

A. Delivering the bedside discharge education

B. Helping the client arrange transportation home

C. Making a checklist of the client's belongings to ensure nothing was left behind

D. Ensuring follow-up appointments and services, including transportation, have been scheduled

Answer D—Rationale: While the CNL might be useful in any of these areas, ensuring proper scheduling of follow-up care with other providers is a function of coordination, a key component of the CNL's role as a lateral integrator.

93. An RCA is best used:

A. In response to a critical or sentinel event

B. Prior to a process implementation or change

C. As part of a random audit process

D. In response to malfunctioning tools or equipment

Answer A—Rationale: An RCA is meant to respond to a critical event or critical "near-miss" event to understand how it occurred and is intended as a retrospective tool.

94. You are doing a daily assessment of your patient who has transferred from the medical intensive care unit (MICU). The patient has a history of congestive heart failure (CHF), myocardial infarction, atrial fibrillation, and diabetes. During your review of the medication

administration record, you notice that the warfarin has not been ordered on admission. What is your next step as the CNL?

A. Call the pharmacist and ask for the medication to be put on the medication administration record

B. Find out what dosage of the medication the patient was taking and order it

C. Notify the primary nurse and suggest that she call the physician and notify him of the near miss

D. Call your nurse manager and notify him or her of this medication error

Answer C—Rationale: The CNL assesses patients' needs, is a risk anticipator, and communicates effectively with team members to prevent patients from having an adverse event.

95. As you review a patient's medical record, you notice that the patient has an order for a chest x-ray. While reviewing the chart, you realize that the patient just completed a chest x-ray several hours ago while in the emergency department (ED). CNLs understand that diagnostic tests are very expensive so you call the doctor and find that the x-ray was duplicated by mistake. Unfortunately, by the time you find this mistake you see the radiology assistant exiting the patient's room. Once the error is found, you should:

A. Perform a root cause analysis (RCA) to see why this test was duplicated

B. Notify the patient's insurance company of the additional charges

C. Notify the nurse manager of this error

D. Review the order entry

Answer A—Rationale: Identifying processes that yield errors and negative outcomes for patients is a critical duty of the CNL. This is done through RCA. It is the job of the CNL to identify and help reduce cost to the patient.

96. You, as the CNL, plan to implement the use of bed alarms and hi-low beds to prevent falls on your unit. You are completing a literature review. While doing so, you are trying to determine the strength of the articles you have obtained. What process should you use to determine the most credible evidence?

A. Plan-Do-Study-Act (PDSA)

B. Evidence-based practice

C. Melynk and Fineout-Overholt hierarchy (Level 1–7)

D. Research utilization

Answer C—Rationale: The Melynk and Fineout-Overholt hierarchy includes seven levels based on the design (Level 1: systematic review or meta-analysis of randomized controlled trials [RCTs] and evidence-based clinical practice guidelines to Level 7: expert opinion and/or expert committee reports).

97. Heather, a nurse for 7 years, recently attained her MSN-CNL. She is very passionate about being involved in her local community. She volunteers frequently at a community center for underprivileged children. During her time there, she noticed that obesity is a concern with this population. What step best describes Heather's advocating for this local community center?

    A. Heather collaborates with the community center leaders to get donations from local health food corporations to ensure a healthy meal is provided for the children.

    B. Heather collaborates with another CNL and plans to do a literature review on obesity.

    C. Heather discusses her concern of obesity with the community center leaders.

    D. Heather calls other community centers for underprivileged children to inquire about obesity in their population.

Answer A—Rationale: The CNL advocates by building partnerships with community organizations to identify and address health disparities.

98. A staff member asks you, the CNL, what is the best way to explain health policy? What statement best explains health policy?

    A. Health policy generally denotes guidelines that affect the health of the individual, families, or communities through production, provision, and financing health or healthcare services.

    B. Health policy analyzes system and outcomes datasets to anticipate individual client risk and improve quality care.

    C. Health policy evaluates the environmental healthcare outcomes.

    D. Health policy means to consult with other health professionals to design, coordinate, and evaluate client care outcomes.

Answer A—Rationale: Answers B–D are all related to QI, risk reduction, and patient safety rather than health policy.

99. A nurse prepares to administer a patient's morning dose of metformin. After scanning the patient and the medication, a clinical alert appears on the computer screen warning of a possible interaction between the metformin and the CT contrast dye the patient received the day before. Based on this warning, the nurse chooses to hold the metformin and

alert the pharmacy that this medication should be scheduled as held for 72 hours after receiving the contrast. This is an example of a:

A. Clinical decision support system

B. Health information technology

C. Clinical alert warning system

D. Decision tree

Answer A—Rationale: Automated warnings within the EHR are an example of a clinical decision support system. The EHR itself is health information technology. While this was a clinical alert it also aided in guiding the nurse to action.

100. The healthcare team determines that the discharge process is ineffective and must be changed. The team determines the stakeholders and utilizes a force field analysis to weigh the pros and cons of the change. This was then used to motivate other team members and encourage buy in. Utilizing Lewin's theory of change, what stage is the team in?

A. Sustaining

B. Moving

C. Refreezing

D. Unfreezing

Answer D—Rationale: The first step of Lewin's theory of change is the unfreezing stage. In order to battle the resistance of change, the leader must assess readiness for change and motivate others to see the reason for change.

101. Tara, a CNL on a pediatric medical–surgical unit, conducted a 5P assessment and discovered that the discharge process was fragmented and parents were not satisfied with the process. Tara created a team to develop a change in order to improve the process. What model can Tara use to rapidly implement this change and test it to determine effectiveness?

A. Plan-Do-Study-Act (PDSA)

B. Strengths, weaknesses, opportunities, and threats (SWOT) analysis

C. Fishbone diagram

D. Gap analysis

Answer A—Rationale: PDSA is a model used to conduct rapid cyclical review of a process change to encourage continuous and ongoing efforts to improve.

102. A Native American patient is admitted with sepsis from a urinary tract infection. The patient is very weak and unable to ambulate much

further than her room. The patient tells the CNL that she is very discouraged and feels that she is not able to get better because she is unable to touch "mother earth" with her feet. The CNL gathers some dirt, grass, and flowers from outside the hospital and places it in a bucket. The CNL brings the bucket in the patient's room and helps her to stand on the dirt. Which of the following best describes what the CNL is demonstrating?

A. Cultural knowledge

B. Cultural awareness

C. Cultural skills

D. Cultural management

Answer C—Rationale: Cultural skills are described as the ability to identify, assess, and incorporate the values, beliefs, and cultural customs of an individual.

103. A nurse comes to you with a concern about a telephone order she received from a doctor. The doctor asked her to review a physician order for life-sustaining treatment (POLST) form with a client, then sign and place it in his chart. The nurse is uncertain if this is in her scope of practice. You advise the nurse to:

A. Complete the form as ordered by the MD

B. Review the hospital's policy and procedure manual, and handle per policy

C. Review the State Board of Nursing Scope of Practice and handle according to your scope of practice

D. All of the above

Answer C—Rationale: The CNL should identify the State Board of Nursing as the correct source of any scope of practice questions, and advise the nurse that it is not within her scope.

104. How can a CNL help to identify the general discharge needs of patients on his or her unit?

A. Coordinate outpatient care and follow-up appointments

B. Assess protective and predictive factors of patient health

C. Discuss with each team's doctors the anticipated discharge needs of their patients

D. Approach staff nurses about their patients' discharge needs

Answer B—Rationale: Assessing protective and predictive factors of patient health is the best way a CNL can identify potential needs or issues with patient discharges.

105. Lisa, a CNL, is educating the staff on the effects of long-term bed rest. A majority of these patients have been on bed rest with a shortened cervix since 25 weeks gestation. Which of the following statements is true?

A. Bed rest is psychologically healthy.

B. Music therapy can ease the psychological effects of bed rest.

C. Bed rest prevents deep vein thrombosis (DVT).

D. Bed rest has been proven to prevent preterm labor.

Answer B—Rationale: Bed rest can be detrimental to a mother's psychological well-being, because there is separation between the patient and her family. The patient can also experience financial burdens, which put a strain on the family. Currently, there is no evidence that bed rest prevents preterm labor.

106. Recently, several major practice changes have been implemented hospital-wide at your facility. While all of these changes are evidence based, some of the practice changes have been received by the staff on your unit with strong resistance and poor compliance. As the CNL, you recognize that the best way to approach this issue is to:

A. Have the unit manager write-up noncompliant staff

B. Advocate to have the policies altered or revoked

C. Form a task force of involved parties to identify barriers to compliance

D. Re-educate staff on the policies and their importance

Answer C—Rationale: While any of these interventions may be appropriate, when addressing any issue, especially issues with strong opinions and various stakeholders, it is critical that the CNL solicit input from all invested players.

107. Ongoing risk reduction and patient safety efforts are an important component of:

A. Quality improvement (QI)

B. Knowledge management

C. Change theory

D. Complexity theory

Answer A—Rationale: Ongoing risk reduction and patient safety monitoring are components of QI.

108. You are in the process of initiating a mobility team and protocol on your unit. What members of the interdisciplinary team should be considered?

A. Nursing staff, physical therapist, nurse manager, occupational therapist, CNL, clinical nurse specialist, and physician

B. Physical therapist, physician, nursing assistants, manager, and CNL

C. Medical social worker, physician, nursing staff, physical therapy staff, and CNL

D. Physical therapist, occupational therapist, nursing staff, and the discharge coordinator

Answer A—Rationale: An interdisciplinary team must include all key stakeholders so that patients can have the best outcomes.

109. As a CNL on a very busy medical–telemetry unit, you have noticed that nurses are not utilizing incentive spirometry for patients with acute or chronic lung conditions. To ensure that patients are given the best care, you ask the electronic order entry representative to allow incentive spirometry to be entered as a nursing task. This will be used as a reminder for the nursing staff to perform this task. What action of the CNL is this?

A. Demonstrates use of healthcare technologies to maximize healthcare outcomes

B. Understands your microsystem and uses available resources

C. Unfreezes

D. Identifies unwanted variation, rework, and waste

Answer A—Rationale: The CNL is on the frontline at the point of care delivery, making recommendations to management and other providers about disease management and use of standardized protocols, ensuring that all charges incurred are assessed and tracked to the appropriate cost center. The CNL should be involved in healthcare technologies and informatics.

110. You are precepting a CNL student. She discusses her capstone project with you. She needs help determining the design of her study. She states that she will be working with diabetes patients on a medical unit. She intends to collect basic data and do a pre- and postintervention questionnaire based on the diabetes survival skills. She wants to compare the pre- and postdata to determine if her educational intervention was effective. She will not use randomization. What option best describes her study design?

A. Well-designed randomized controlled trial (RCT)

B. Quasi-experimental

C. Meta-analysis

D. Quality study

Answer B—Rationale: A quasi-experiment is not a true experiment. A quasi-experiment does not have randomly assigned groups, but would include pre- and postmeasures.

111. B.F. is a 52-year-old female recently placed with the palliative care team. The CNL makes sure that B.F. is transferred to another unit with a specific palliative care section. How is this a demonstration of advocacy?

A. Physicians understand when to transfer patients.

B. It ensures that the system meets the needs of the population.

C. It advocates for the professional nurse.

D. It applies ethics toward patient care.

Answer B—Rationale: Make sure the patient is placed where the most optimal outcomes and palliative care can be delivered.

112. As a CNL on your unit, you are rounding on your microsystem. Jen, a 70-year-old patient with stage IV cancer, chronic obstructive pulmonary disease (COPD), diabetes mellitus (DM), and chronic kidney disease, is currently on an Ativan drip and morphine drip. She has a do-not-resuscitate (DNR) order and is a hospice patient. You notice she has multiple grieving family members in her room. You speak with the family and collaborate with the palliative care unit (PCU) CNL and charge nurse and decide to move the patient to a bigger room in the PCU. What CNL role was demonstrated in this scenario?

A. Advocate

B. Outcomes manager

C. Team manager

D. Risk analyst

Answer A—Rationale: The CNL acted as a client advocate to ensure the best situation for the patient and family by coordination of care through the use of resources and services.

113. With healthcare reform, the CNL recognizes that evidence-based practice (EBP) is imperative. The CNL decided that her staff should be knowledgeable about healthcare reform. She collaborated with the educator and administration team to educate the staff about healthcare reform and pay for performance. What statement best reflects the definition of pay for performance?

A. It is a voluntary program that encourages hospitals nationally to report quality measures for heart attacks, heart failure, and pneumonia.

B. It is a national program in which physicians and hospitals receive more money if their quality measures exceed certain benchmarks or if the measures improve year to year.

C. It is a process that involves the surveillance of and intervention in clinical activities of physicians for the purpose of controlling costs.

D. It is a Medicare program that began the physician quality reporting initiative.

Answer B—Rationale: Pay for performance gained widespread acceptance in healthcare; it goes one step above pay for reporting, as it requires physicians or hospitals to report quality measures, in which they receive more money if their quality measures exceed certain benchmarks or if the measures improve year to year.

114. A nurse on the CNL's unit asks about accessing patient education materials via the electronic health record (EHR), as well as the availability of education on Cambodia. As the CNL guides the nurse in locating these materials, she or he recognizes this as an effective use of:

A. Healthcare informatics

B. Research utilization

C. Clinical knowledge

D. Evidence-based research

Answer A—Rationale: Accessing appropriate education in patients' native language is culturally competent; however, the ability to locate and provide these materials is effective use of healthcare informatics.

115. Which of the following best demonstrates how the CNL exhibits collaboration?

A. Sets and shares clear goals for teams

B. Keeps all team members informed by e-mailing updated minutes

C. Includes all contributors to the healthcare delivery process in the team, including patients/family, and seeks consultation from all members when making decisions

D. Monitors and evaluates the use of technology and information systems

Answer C—Rationale: The CNL seeks collaboration and consultation with all contributors to the healthcare delivery process, including the patient and family.

116. The CNL works in a small primary care practice and has identified that several patients have missed appointments. After investigating why the patients were not going to appointments, the CNL determines that the patients made the appointments so far in advance

that they forgot them. The CNL discusses these findings with the team and they decide to implement a program with reminder calls 2 days prior to the appointment. The CNL wants to be sure to identify aspects that may positively or negatively affect the project, so the CNL suggests the team utilize which of the following?

A. 5P (persons, patients, professionals, processes, patterns) assessment

B. Plan-Do-Study-Act (PDSA) cycle

C. Strengths, weaknesses, opportunities, and threats (SWOT) analysis

D. 5S methodology

Answer C—Rationale: A SWOT analysis is a vital assessment for successful planning and implementation of a change. A SWOT analysis is used to determine strengths, weaknesses, opportunities, and threats that may affect the project.

117. As the CNL is integrated into practice, what best defines his or her level of practice?

A. Unit system

B. Mesosystem

C. **Microsystem**

D. Macrosystem

Answer C—Rationale: The CNL works on the microsystem level.

118. Part of your hospital's pre-op admission process is to collect a urinalysis (UA), hemoglobin A1c (HgA1c), comprehensive metabolic panel (CMP), and complete blood count (CBC). You review the HgA1c results of these patients. As the CNL, how can you best work with your healthcare team to ensure health promotion of clients with elevated HgA1c results?

A. Inform patients of elevated HgA1c results, as well as implications of those results

B. Provide diabetes education to patients with elevated HgA1c results postoperatively

C. Place a consult for the diabetes educator to meet and evaluate patients with an elevated HgA1c during this admission

D. Inform the surgeons of these elevated HgA1c results and ask them to consider what the next step should be

Answer C—Rationale: CNLs should work to incorporate other members of the interdisciplinary team in the patient's care when needed and appropriate.

119. Lateral integration is one of the main functions of the CNL, incorporating multiple disciplines into the care of clients and populations.

Which of the following ongoing components constitute lateral integration?

A. Advocacy, assessment, clinical knowledge, evaluation

B. Collaboration, communication, coordination, evaluation

C. Altruism, benchmarking, cost reduction, evaluation

D. Advocacy, collaboration, coordination

Answer B—Rationale: Communication, collaboration, coordination, and evaluation—while all the components listed make up important aspects of different CNL roles, only these four address lateral integration.

120. A client on your unit receives 10 times the ordered dose of an opioid, resulting in serious complications from which the patient fully recovered. In response to this occurrence, you as the CNL:

A. Reprimand the nurse who administered the medication in error to ensure it does not happen again

B. Conduct a failure mode-effect analysis

C. Conduct a root cause analysis (RCA)

D. Apologize to the client and family

Answer C—Rationale: The priority is to conduct an RCA, which would include investigating what occurred with the nurse who administered the opioid and identify any issues in personal or unit process that may have affected the error, to prevent not only the individual nurse from making the same mistake again, but the whole unit from making a similar mistake. Errors should be met with investigation, not with punishment. If there is a performance issue, then it should be addressed by management.

121. In your cohort you work with all members of the team. You develop an effective plan of care across settings in collaboration with all disciplines, professions, and stakeholders, including patients. This would be an example of what component of lateral integration?

A. Communication

B. Coordination

C. Evaluation

D. Collaboration

Answer D—Rationale: Collaboration is defined as the interdisciplinary process of problem solving that involves shared responsibility for decision making as well as the execution of specific plans of care while working toward a common goal. The CNL promotes collaboration and consultation with all contributors to the healthcare delivery process, including the patient and his or her family.

122. As the CNL, you assess the needs of your unit on an ongoing basis. You notice while rounding on the nursing staff that nurses are complaining about the demands of patient care. The nurses state that the patients are requiring more help than usual. This prompts you to look at the level of intensity of care required by patients. Level of intensity of care required by patients is referred to by, which of the following?

A. Volume

B. Case mix

C. Acuity

D. Staffing mix

Answer C—Rationale: Acuity is the level of intensity of care required by patients.

123. You are the unit-based council chair for shared governance of a high-acuity progressive care unit. You notice that the staff is not aware of new evidence in caring for this patient population. Youdiscuss this with the management team and the CNL to determine what can be done to increase the staff awareness and knowledge of EBP. What strategy can best be used to increase evidence into practice?

A. Start a journal club with help from CNL

B. Learn how to determine if an article is peer-reviewed

C. Encourage nurses to conduct research

D. Discuss the importance of EBP in staff meeting

Answer A—Rationale: Strategies to increase evidence into practice include ensure policies/procedures are based upon the latest literature, journal club, nursing grand rounds, update staff on latest evidence in short gatherings, link quality indicators in EBP, and mentor staff to complete EBP activities for school and clinical ladder.

124. Jennifer, a CNL student, is shadowing a CNL on a busy medical–telemetry unit. The CNL encourages Jennifer to follow up on a 24-year-old patient admitted with diabetic ketoacidosis (DKA) for the fourth time in a 2-month period. Which statement best describes the CNL student acting as a client advocate for this patient?

A. Round on the patient and consult a diabetes educator

B. Round on the patient and discuss reasons for frequent readmissions, discuss concerns with the primary nurse, order a HgA1c, and consult a diabetes educator and social worker

C. Round on the patient, and tell the primary nurse to educate the patient on diabetes

D. Discuss with the primary care nurse that the patient has been again readmitted and the patient needs more education on diabetes and preventing readmissions

Answer B—Rationale: The CNL demonstrates advocacy for the patient by involving the patient and discussing possible reasons for readmission and taking an interdisciplinary approach to address patient concern.

125. As the CNL on a surgical unit, nurses have expressed to you their concern over conflicting orders regarding patient intravenous fluids (IVFs). Most patients have conflicting order sets for fluids and rates, as ordered by the surgeons and hospitalists. From a healthcare informatics perspective, what is the best action you can take as the CNL?

A. Coordinate with the surgical and hospitalist groups to alert them of this clinical concern

B. Instruct the nurses to discontinue the older orders per protocol to clean up the order set within the electronic health record (EHR)

C. Work with the computer specialists to create a hard stop in the system requiring physicians to verify or modify IVF orders when new orders are placed

D. Discuss with the pharmacy if there is a way to prevent more than one IV fluid order from being allowed in the EHR at a time

Answer C—Rationale: From the healthcare informatics perspective, creating a hard stop that requires doctors to evaluate the current orders would be most beneficial. There are times when multiple fluid orders may be clinically appropriate, and changes to the system to not allow more than one order under any circumstance would not be beneficial.

126. The CNL recognizes the importance of Hospital Consumer Assessment of Healthcare Providers and Systems (HCAHPS) scores in driving hospital reimbursement. These scores measure:

A. Core measures and patient experience

B. Core measures, patient experience, and clinical outcomes

C. Core measures, patient experience, clinical outcomes, and readmission rates

D. Patient experience, clinical outcomes, and readmission rates

Answer A—Rationale: HCAHPS measure core measures and the patient experience, but do not assess actual clinical outcomes, patient mortality, or readmission rates.

127. During a unit-based council meeting, the chair states that the unit has had 10 falls this year related to bathroom needs. Frank, a staff nurse, states he conducted observations and determined these falls are likely related to a lack of purposeful hourly rounding. Judy, a nursing assistant, states she has heard everyone is doing hourly rounding but it does not help because patients still get out of bed. Which of the following is the most appropriate response by the CNL?

    A. Encourage the staff to stop hourly rounding

    B. Educate the staff on the importance of utilizing evidence-based practice (EBP) like hourly rounding to prevent falls and show the evidence

    C. Instruct the staff to utilize new chair alarms for all patients as these have been proven to reduce falls

    D. Ask the team to search the literature for evidence related to fall prevention

Answer B—Rationale: The CNL coaches and leads teams to sustain a culture of safety by utilizing EBPs.

128. In order to be successful while utilizing Kotter's change theory, you realize it is vital to spend time on the first step. Which of the following best represents the first step in Kotter's change theory?

    A. Having celebrations for short-term wins

    B. Communicating the change vision

    C. Consolidating gains and producing more change

    D. Obtaining buy-in and creating a sense of urgency for change

Answer D—Rationale: Kotter's change theory emphasizes that adequate time be placed on the first step of change, which is establishing a sense of urgency in order to have adequate buy-in from stakeholders.

129. The primary focus of the CNL is best defined as:

    A. Delivery of high quality, evidence-based, culturally competent care at the patient's bedside

    B. Educating and mentoring peers to improve clinical competence

    C. Providing patient care management and leadership of the interdisciplinary team meetings

    D. Evaluating and supporting evidence-based practice (EBP) decisions to ensure best possible outcomes

Answer D—Rationale: The focus of the CNL is on ensuring outcomes, and the CNL does so by evaluating and implementing evidence-based research.

130. What level of prevention are you providing by performing screenings?

A. Primary

B. Secondary

C. Tertiary

D. Quaternary

Answer B—Rationale: Secondary prevention involves activities that help increase early identification of disease.

131. As a CNL on a high-risk oncology unit, you recognize the need for regular access to chaplaincy services among your client population. You work with your unit and chaplaincy department to bring these services to your unit regularly. This is primarily an example of:

A. Advocacy

B. CNL role integration

C. Leadership

D. Lateral integration

Answer D—Rationale: Accessing resources across disciplines to meet the needs of a client population in a patient-centered manner addresses specifically lateral integration.

132. Use of electronic health records (EHRs) can aid the CNL to conduct quality improvement (QI) efforts in which of the following ways?

A. Allow rapid access to informatics data, provide a way of ongoing monitoring, organize data into meaningful groups, and aid in the dedication of errors

B. Allow rapid access to informatics data, ensure all staff follow protocols and policies, add second checks to medication administration, and aid in the detection of errors

C. Provide a way of ongoing monitoring, add second checks to medication administration, organize data into meaningful groups, and aid in detection of errors

D. Provide a way of ongoing monitoring, ensure all staff follow protocols and policies, add second checks to medication administration, organize data into meaningful groups, and aid in the detection of errors

Answer A—Rationale: Many EHR products can achieve each of these functions; however, not all are a part of QI efforts. Also, an EHR cannot ensure people act within established policies and procedures. Additionally, while an EHR can provide additional safeguards to medication administration and may improve safety, it does not help the CNL conduct QI efforts.

133. The patient confides in you and states that she does not take her medications as prescribed and does not go to her doctor's appointments due to lack of transportation. As the CNL, you discuss your findings with the CCM, and place a financial counseling consult. The CCM orders a home safety evaluation, and a medical-social worker provides bus passes and community resources. This is an example of what key element of the CNL role?

A. Ongoing evaluation

B. Communication

C. Collaboration

D. Coordination

Answer D—Rationale: Coordination requires intentional planning and direction. The CNL is responsible for coordinating the flow of communication, activities of the team members, and the services provided to the patients.

134. The CNLs noticed that the supply room was cluttered and oftentimes supplies had expired. They created a team and conducted a 5S to organize the supply bins and reduce waste. Where will the CNLs see the cost savings with supplies reflected?

A. Capital budget

B. Cash flow budget

C. Cost-effectiveness analysis

D. Operating budget

Answer D—Rationale: The operating budget is the day-to-day operations of the unit, including revenue, volume, and expenses. Cost savings related to supplies would be in the operating budget.

135. A staff nurse is thinking about becoming a CNL. The unit CNL discusses with the staff nurse about the CNL's role and the importance of evidence-based practice (EBP). After further discussions, the staff nurse questions the CNL about what barriers she may face when implementing EBP. Which of the following do not describe barriers that have been recognized with initiating EBP?

A. EBP is readily available for staff and low patient loads

B. Lack of knowledge regarding EBP strategies and misperceptions about EBP

C. Lack of time and resources to search for and appraise evidence

D. Peer pressure to continue with practices that are steeped in tradition and inadequate content

Answer A—Rationale: Nurses, physicians, and other health professionals cite a number of barriers to EBP including: lack of knowledge regarding EBP strategies, misperceptions or negative views about research and evidence-based care, lack of belief EBP will result in more positive outcomes than traditional care, voluminous amounts of information in professional journals, lack of time and resources to search for and appraise evidence, overwhelming patient loads, organizational constraints, demands from patients for a certain type of treatment, peer pressure to continue with practices that are steeped in tradition, and adequate content and behavioral skills regarding EBP in educational programs.

136. Which statement best describes the CNL acting as a client advocate for a domestic violence victim hospitalized in her microsystem?

A. Consult domestic violence healthcare professional (DVHP) and ensure the patient has an alias name

B. Ensure all the staff members are aware that she is a domestic violence victim

C. Consult the master of social work (MSW) and call the patient's partner to ensure that he or she will not come to the hospital

D. Consult the psychiatric physician and inform the primary care nurse

Answer A—Rationale: Consulting DVHP and ensuring the patient has an alias name is the best approach in providing patient advocacy. The CNL is advocating for patient safety.

137. Recently, your unit replaced all of its current beds with air beds, designed to help prevent skin breakdown in your patients. Using informatics, what is the best way to evaluate the effectiveness of this intervention?

A. Review the electronic health record (EHR) for new pressure ulcer incidence since the new beds were utilized

B. Complete a pressure ulcer prevalence study on all currently admitted patients

C. Gather data on all patient Braden scale scores since implementation

D. Review all nurse skin integrity assessments since implementation

Answer A—Rationale: The best way to evaluate the effectiveness of the implementation of air beds is to review the incidence of new pressure ulcers. A prevalence study only assesses pressure ulcers at the current time. The Braden scale does not necessarily indicate effectiveness of preventing skin breakdown. Reviewing all assessments is unneeded, as the data regarding pressure ulcers is the only meaningful data.

138. Nicole, a nurse of 5 years, comes to you with an idea for a medication administration safety zone. How can you best support Nicole with this project?

A. Guide Nicole through a literature search to determine if evidence exists to support such a change

B. Help Nicole design the medication administration safety zone

C. Set up a meeting with the manager and Nicole to discuss the project

D. Encourage Nicole to implement the project

Answer A—Rationale: The CNL serves as a horizontal leader by assisting nursing staff in using EBP principles to design care for individuals. The CNL helps Nicole to search for the best evidence by conducting a literature review.

139. The CNL works in a medical intensive care unit (MICU) at a level one trauma center. The CNL conducts a comprehensive assessment of the microsystem. All of the following are vital aspects that the CNL would need to identify within the microsystem except:

A. The rate of ventilator-associated pneumonia

B. The organization's operating budget

C. The top three diagnoses

D. The average age of patients

Answer B—Rationale: The assessment of the microsystem focuses on the small, frontline unit, which does not include the organization's operating budget. The rate of nosocomial infections, top diagnoses, and age of patients within the microsystem are vital information for the CNL.

140. What best describes an elevator speech about the CNL's role?

A. Succinctly define, advocate, and explain the CNL's role

B. Briefly educate peers on current issues in the nursing profession

C. Provide a summary presentation on specific measured outcomes of the CNL

D. Convince peers and stakeholders to create buy-in for the CNL

Answer A—Rationale: The elevator speech should define, advocate, and explain the CNL role. A summary of the specific outcomes does not address the role itself. While the elevator speech may work to create buy-in, it should do so by defining and explaining the role.

141. As the CNL on a medical floor, you recognize the importance of annual flu vaccinations, especially considering your geriatric population. How can you promote vaccination rates within your population?

A. Organize a flu clinic for staff and visitors

B. Ask a physician to order flu shots for all admitted patients, and organize a flu clinic for staff and visitors

C. Within the hospital, develop a nurse-driven protocol that allows nurses to place an order for flu shots for your population

D. Ask the physician to order flu shots for all admitted hospital patients

Answer C—Rationale: Nurse-driven protocols are an excellent way to ensure that the population receives vaccinations. Flu shots may not be appropriate for all hospitalized patients, based on personal beliefs or current treatment, and should not be mass ordered.

142. During a client's admission medication reconciliation, the admitting nurse comes to you for assistance. On review of the client's case, you discover the client has several separate opioid prescriptions from multiple different providers. When you discuss the issue with the patient, the patient tells you he or she thought each prescriber had been consulting with the others. Which function of the CNL best addresses this issue?

A. Client advocacy

B. Lateral integration

C. Injury prevention

D. Advanced clinical assessment

Answer B—Rationale: While aspects of each of these functions could be used to address parts of this issue, only lateral integration addresses coordinating multiple players across multiple disciplines, collaboratively, toward the common goal of proper, safe management of pain for this complex patient through improved communication among these stakeholders and with the client, as well as collaboration for proper ongoing monitoring and evaluation of the client.

143. As a CNL, you recognize a sentinel event as which of the following?

A. Any unintended event that results in ANY harm, physical or psychological, to a patient

B. Any unintended event that has the POTENTIAL to result in ANY harm, physical or psychological, to a patient

C. Any unintended event that results in SIGNIFICANT harm, physical or psychological, to a patient

D. Any unintended event that has the POTENTIAL to result in SIGNIFICANT harm, physical or psychological, to a patient

Answer C—Rationale: A sentinel event only occurs if the event reaches and significantly harms a patient.

144. You are a CNL on a medical–telemetry unit and orienting a new graduate nurse. Critical thinking is best demonstrated by which of the following?

A. Calling the rapid response nurse when a patient's oxygen saturation drops to 79% on 2L of oxygen

B. Drawing scheduled hemoglobin and hematocrit

C. Delegating tasks to the nursing assistant

D. Creating a script to welcome patients to the medical–telemetry unit

Answer A—Rationale: Critical thinking underlies independent and interdependent decision making. Critical thinking includes questioning, analysis, synthesis, interpretation, interference, inductive and deductive reasoning, intuition, application, and creativity.

145. You are a CNL working in a very busy 980-bed tertiary hospital. The hospital only has one MRI machine. This often causes delays in patient care. You write a proposal for the administrative team to advocate for more MRI scanners. If the proposal is approved, the money will come out of which budget?

A. Capital budget

B. Cash flow budget

C. Operating budget

D. Revenue

Answer A—Rationale: Capital budget involves large dollar amounts and long-term investments like equipment.

146. As a CNL, you are asked to speak to a local church group, mostly elderly, regarding the importance of annual influenza shots and pneumonia vaccines. You want to be well prepared for the talk as you know the leaders have several questions about the relationship in developing pneumonia and vaccination. You decide to develop a PICOT question and initiate a literature review. Which of the following statements best exemplifies the PICOT method?

A. For patients 65 years and older, the use of an influenza/pneumonia (PNA) vaccine vaccine will reduce the risk of developing pneumonia.

B. For patients 65 years and older, the use of an influenza/PNA vaccine will reduce the risk of developing pneumonia when compared to patients not receiving vaccination within a year.

C. For patients 65 years and older, the use of an influenza/PNA vaccine will reduce the pneumonia.

D. For patients in a church, the use of an influenza/PNA vaccine will reduce the risk of developing pneumonia in a year

Answer B—Rationale: PICOT is a process in which clinical questions are phrased to reveal the most relevant information (P = patient population; I = intervention, C = comparison; O = outcome).

147. Ranesha, a nurse on the unit, has just finished receiving bedside report on a patient, Mr. Smith, admitted with pneumonia. She told the patient his goal was to ambulate in the hallway three times that day. The CNL, Valerie, walked in the room while Ranesha discussed his goal. Valerie recognized that the goal will not work because Mr. Smith was not involved in deciding on the goal. In what way can Valerie act as a client advocate?

A. Involve the patient in setting the goal with Ranesha, to discuss the reason for setting goals, barriers, and concerns, and determine the best time for Mr. Smith to ambulate in the hallway

B. Do not discuss setting the goal and involving Mr. Smith as the nurse has already told the patient the plan for the day

C. Tell Ranesha that Mr. Smith should be in the driver's seat of his own care

D. Involve the patient by asking him what he wants to do for the day and if he replies "Nothing" then let him rest

Answer A—Rationale: The CNL keeps the patient informed and ensures he understands the reason for setting goals and involves him in making healthcare decisions.

148. The CNL knows in order to serve as a lateral integrator she or he must conduct ongoing evaluation of care delivery systems and processes. Which of the following is the best example of how the CNL demonstrates evaluation?

A. Ensures each member of the team clearly understands each member's role

B. Conducts an ongoing analysis of risk to promote patient safety

C. Synthesizes gathered information to find common goals and shares this with the team

D. Fosters open rapport across professional boundaries

Answer B—Rationale: The CNL monitors not only the final outcomes of care, but also the implementation and ongoing progression of care. By analyzing and evaluating risk, adjustments can be made to improve the overall outcomes while promoting patient safety.

149. A patient who has been diagnosed with colon cancer remarks that since his diagnosis, many people he knows have mentioned someone they know who has colon cancer. Most of these people live nearby. The patient asks you if colon cancer rates in the area have been increasing recently. The patient is asking about what type of measure?

A. Incidence

B. Prevalence

C. Mortality

D. Correlation

Answer A—Rationale: This would measure the number of new cases of colon cancer in the area during a specific period.

150. During morning report, you observe a new staff member you have been mentoring struggling to identify which of her patients she will assess first. As the CNL, you identify the priority patient as:

A. The 72-year-old patient with a chest tube to wall suction and unstable vital signs

B. The 19-year-old patient with family demanding to speak with you regarding discharge plans

C. The 57-year-old postoperative patient with patient-controlled analgesia (PCA) pump

D. The 92-year-old patient who is a high-fall risk

Answer A—Rationale: The priority assessment is the patient with a chest tube to ensure both patency of the tube and adequate airway.

151. You are the CNL in an outpatient pediatric clinic. The most common diagnosis for your patient population is asthma, and your patients are frequently seen at local emergency departments (EDs) for asthma exacerbations. Which action most directly optimizes the level of function in daily life for these patients?

A. Provide or reinforce previous education to patients and families on asthma and inhaler use

B. Review discharge orders and ensure that all clients are prescribed a long- and short-acting inhaler

C. Provide an in-service at local schools to educate teachers on managing asthma exacerbations in children

D. Advocate for the development of a nurse phone triage to answer urgent patient and family asthma concerns

Answer B—Rationale: Many of these interventions can help promote knowledge on what to do in the event of an asthma exacerbation; however, ensuring that each patient has the proper inhalers best optimizes the daily level of function.

152. As the CNL, you recognize that leveraging technology and information systems is an important part of acting toward high quality, patient-centered, lateral integration. Which of the following are examples of using technology and information systems to benefit patient care?

A. Use of bed alarms and use of call lights

B. TV in patient rooms with many channels, use of call lights, guest Wi-Fi Internet access, and e-readers available with e-books for patients

C. Use of bed alarms, use of call lights, remote telemetry, and bar-coded supplies, and medications

D. TV in patient rooms with many channels, guest Wi-Fi Internet access, and e-readers available with e-books for patients

Answer C—Rationale: This answer addresses technology used in patient care while the others address technology used in patient experience and satisfaction.

153. Which of the following is not a part of the National Patient Safety Guidelines (NPSG)?

A. Improve the accuracy of patient identification

B. Reduce the risk of healthcare-associated infections

C. Improve patient satisfaction

D. Prevent healthcare-associated pressure ulcers

Answer C—Rationale: While a part of the NPSGs, improving patient satisfaction it is not, by itself, an NPSG.

154. During the 5P assessment, you find out that 64% of patients have Medicare, 18% have Medicaid, 16% have private insurance, and 2% have no insurance. You can conclude that the majority of your patients are what type of payer source?

A. First-party payer

B. Second-party payer

C. Fourth-party payer

D. Third-party payer

Answer D—Rationale: Third-party payers include government and private insurance entities.

155. A staff nurse is performing a literature review on the best tool for determining health literacy for diabetic patients. When analyzing and appraising the literature, what methods can the nurse use to determine if the study is flawed?

A. Are the results of the literature reliable and critical?

B. Are the results of the literature effective and modifiable?

C. Are the results of the literature valid and reliable?

D. Are the results of the literature valid and modifiable?

Answer C—Rationale: Three questions to consider when appraising any study: Are the results for the study valid? Are the results reliable? Will the results be applicable to study?

156. The CNL provides integration of care by working with multiple interdependent and independent disciplines, breaking down barriers, and proactively managing care across the continuum. This describes a(n):

A. Vertical leader

B. Lateral integrator

C. Outcomes manager

D. Systems analyst

Answer B—Rationale: Lateral integration of care involves the delivering and coordination of care using a multidisciplinary approach. The CNL can oversee care provided by the healthcare team, identify barriers, and work with the team to proactively manage potential problems.

157. A nurse on your unit has a question about required documentation for a patient with a nasogastric (NG) tube to wall suction. You guide her to what resource?

A. The unit charge nurse

B. **Hospital policy/procedure manual**

C. The States Board of Nursing Scope of Practice

D. The Joint Commission website

Answer B—Rationale: The most reliable resource is the hospital policy and procedure manual. While the charge nurse may be a source of knowledge, it is not the best or official source.

158. You are the CNL on a medical unit and recognize a frequently readmitted patient with uncontrolled diabetes. You view this patient in terms of Prochaska and DiClemente's Stages of Change model and recognize that:

A. Patients may spiral in and out of stages forward and backward.

B. Timelines for patients may vary to progress through the stages; however, they always progress forward.

C. The stages have been well studied and the timeline and progression are the same for all patients.

D. Prochaska and DiClemente's Stages of Change model does not apply to this patient.

Answer A—Rationale: Prochaska and DiClemente's Stages of Change model states that each patient may experience each phase at different speeds, and may move forward or backward repeatedly through the stages.

159. Consideration of your unit's nurse workflow, specific challenges and needs of clients on your unit, staff experiences, and staff ratios are examples of which of the following important CNL function components?

A. Ongoing evaluation

B. Collaboration

C. Advanced clinical assessment

D. Knowledge management

Answer A—Rationale: These are examples of a CNL continuing to assess and reassess important aspects of the care delivery system and used processes. including the monitoring not only of patient outcomes but experiences at each step of the care process, which embodies the ongoing evaluation aspect of the CNL as a lateral integrator.

160. Quality improvement (QI), as a function of the CNL role, is related to which core role competency of the CNL?

A. Client advocacy

B. Clinician

C. Risk anticipator

D. Team manager

Answer C—Rationale: QI is a direct function of risk anticipation.

161. Your hospital has just completed a study comparing outcomes in rehospitalization rates for CHF patients who received predischarge teaching from an advanced practice registered nurse (APRN) with those who received predischarge teaching from an RN. In the analysis of data, what resulting *p*-value would indicate that the intervention had a significant result?

A. <.05

B. <.8

C. <.10

D. <.22

Answer A—Rationale: A value less than 0.05 is a significant statistical finding in research.

162. A professor is discussing the difference between quantitative and qualitative research. As a CNL student, you are aware that quantitative research is related to numeric data with statistical analysis, while qualitative research focuses on non-numeric forms of research. Which of the following is an example of a quantitative study?

A. Personal interviews

B. Randomized controlled trial (RCT)

C. Ethnography

D. Phenomenology

Answer B—Rationale: RCT is a quantitative research process that is a true experiment; it is the strongest design to support cause-and-effect relationships, in which subjects are randomly selected.

163. Elizabeth, an 87-year-old female, is admitted to the orthopedic unit with a fractured hip. Elizabeth lives at home alone, but her retired son lives just 2 hours away and comes to visit her often. The physical therapist comes to you and states he is recommending that Elizabeth go to a rehabilitation center prior to returning home. When Elizabeth is told that she will require rehabilitation, she becomes visibly upset and states she refuses to go to a facility. Utilizing an interdisciplinary approach, you ask the social worker, case manager, physician, and physical therapist to help create a plan for Elizabeth. Which of the following is the best plan for Elizabeth?

A. Convince Elizabeth to go to a rehabilitation facility where she will receive 24-hour care and 3 hours of therapy a day

B. Keep Elizabeth in the hospital until she has fully recovered, then discharge her home

C. Discharge Elizabeth home and arrange for a physical therapist to come to her house once a week

D. Contact Elizabeth's son, inform him of Elizabeth's refusal of the rehabilitation facility, and have him help develop an alternative to the original plan for her discharge

Answer D—Rationale: The CNL generally needs to involve multiple disciplines in the plan for discharge, but the CNL must also encourage the patient and family to participate. Elizabeth was not willing to go to a rehabilitation center, so the best option would be for her to go home with her son where she can be safe and monitored, while receiving home health services.

164. A staff nurse is curious about whether emptying the nasogastric (NG) suction canister is a task that can be delegated to a CNA. You, the CNL, guide her to what resource?

A. The unit charge nurse

B. Hospital policy/procedure manual

C. The State Board of Nursing Scope of Practice

D. The Joint Commission website

Answer C—Rationale: The most reliable source for what tasks may be delegated is the individual state's scope of practice.

165. The CNL on the unit has an idea to generate a new EBP study. He has conducted a literature review and critical appraisal. The CNL has also developed a collaborative interprofessional team to be part of the planning process. He has established a date for the research design meeting. What pertinent information should be included in his outline of the study in preparation for this meeting?

A. Form an interprofessional team

B. Perform a review of literature

C. Consult with another CNL

D. Indicate the aim of the study and research question

Answer D—Rationale: When developing a study outline for a meeting, questions related to the study that should be answered include: Is this idea feasible and clinically important? What is the aim of the study, along with the research question or hypothesis to be tested? What are the potential sources of data? Are there valid and reliable instruments to measure the desired outcomes? What should be the inclusion and exclusion criteria for the potential study participants? What are the essential elements of the intervention, if applicable?

166. Which method of payment accounts for only 5% of the U.S. population?

A. Out-of-pocket payments

B. Employment-based private insurance

C. Government financing

D. Individual private insurance

Answer D—Rationale: This information is available in health policy books.

167. What are ways in which the CNL can present his or her effectiveness and outcomes?

A. Peer-reviewed journal, conference or seminar, and TV

B. Peer-reviewed journal, conference or seminar, and Internet

C. Peer-reviewed journal and TV

D. TV and Internet

Answer B—Rationale: All are valid ways in which the CNL can disseminate his or her effectiveness and outcomes (journal articles, conference, and Internet).

168. Judy completed an evidence-based practice (EBP) study that resulted in a 25% reduction in noise on the unit and increased patient satisfaction to 100% for patients always saying it is quiet at night. Utilizing the EBP process, what would Judy's next step be?

A. Apply for a poster presentation for a national conference

B. Compare results to a similar unit in her hospital

C. Identify stakeholders within her organization

D. Conduct a literature search and assess validity

Answer A—Rationale: The final step of the EBP process is to disseminate findings via presentations or publications.

169. The nurse manager of a regional home health services company allows the employees to determine solutions for change, and always considers their opinions, suggestions, and concerns. What type of leadership style is the manager demonstrating?

A. Autocratic

B. Laissez-faire

C. Consultative

D. Democratic

Answer D—Rationale: Democratic leadership involves the whole group in the decision-making process.

170. Patient satisfaction scores in the ED have shown a downward trend over the past three quarters. As a CNL in the emergency department (ED), your focus is to:

A. Create a script for the triage nurse in welcoming the patient

B. Assign a volunteer to welcome patients to the hospital

C. Compare desired outcomes with national and state standards

D. Write a letter of apology to each dissatisfied patient

Answer C—Rationale: Patient satisfaction is an important client care outcome. And client care outcomes are a measure of quality practice. CNLs must know how to compare desired outcomes that will improve safety, effectiveness, timeliness, efficiency, quality, and the degree to which they are client centered.

171. You are a CNL selected to lead a team focused on implementing a multidisciplinary clinical pathway for acute ischemic stroke and transient ischemic attack. The risk assessment tool that you have adopted identifies all of the following as independent stroke risk factors except:

A. Age
B. Systolic blood pressure
C. Liver dysfunction
D. Current smoking
E. Diabetes mellitus (DM)

Answer C—Rationale: Independent stroke predictors include age, systolic blood pressure, hypertension, DM, current smoking, established cardiovascular disease (any one of MI, angina or coronary insufficiency, CHF, or intermittent claudication), atrial fibrillation, and left ventricular hypertrophy on electrocardiogram (ECG).

172. All of the following are part of the data necessary for a CNL to fully understand and assess his or her clinical unit except:

A. The organization's budget
B. The target population and age distribution
C. The percentage of full-time equivalents (FTEs)
D. The rate of nosocomial infections and fall risks

Answer A—Rationale: A comprehensive assessment of the clinical unit is a foundation for the work of the CNL but does not include the financial statement of the organization. The financial statement or budget has to do with the macrosystem and not the microsystem.

173. A patient asks the CNL about the regulations on abortion in North Carolina. What should the CNL do?

A. Tell the patient he or she cannot answer that because it is an ethical situation
B. Let the doctor know the patient is asking about abortion
C. Inform the patient care nurse
D. Look up the regulations in North Carolina and share them with the patient

Answer D—Rationale: Being able to look up policies and regulations is an important role of the CNL, along with educating patients. Giving the policy does not cross any ethical barriers; it is only providing facts.

174. You are using failure mode effect and analysis (FMEA) to anticipate the risk of medication errors in the ICU related to invasive lines. You begin your FMEA analysis with:

A. The effects of each failure
B. The potential cause of each failure

C. Process mapping

D. Specific defects and delays in the medication administration process

Answer C—Rationale: Utilizing tools for process improvement can provide new insights into routine practices.

175. Sustaining process improvement requires the use of appropriate learning principles and strategies. The CNL function that best utilizes this competency is:

A. Advocate

B. Educator

C. Clinician

D. Information manager

Answer B—Rationale: CNL competencies are described in the AACN white paper. Nursing education involves using appropriate learning principles and strategies.

176. By leading which unit initiative can the CNL directly affect the financial health of the entire institution?

A. Reducing readmissions

B. Recruitment of new nursing staff

C. Improving documentation compliance

D. Encouraging staff to report safety events and near-misses

Answer A—Rationale: Medicare reimbursement rates include a penalty to those healthcare institutions with 30-day readmission rates that are higher than national benchmarks. Thus, the CNL may greaty affect finances by reducing readmissions.

177. Before beginning data collection, what is the primary key factor to determine?

A. Personnel to collect data

B. A secure database for holding data

C. Operational definitions of data

D. A user-friendly collection method

Answer C—Rationale: Operational definitions clearly define what is to be collected and helps avoid confusion for those collecting the data; this should be the first step. Clear operational definitions also help those who are interpreting the data. Failure to determine operational definitions may result in data that are inaccurate.

178. You are helping the nurse to care for a patient with congestive heart failure (CHF). He has just completed a transfusion of 2 units of packed red blood cells (PRBCs). Upon your entering the room, the

patient complains of shortness of breath. His O_2 saturations are 85% on 2 L and he is breathing 28 respirations a minute. What drug do you anticipate administering?

A. Nitroglycerin SL

B. Lasix IV

C. Albuterol HHN

D. Prednisone PO

Answer B—Rationale: The patient is most likely in pulmonary edema. Lasix is a loop diuretic.

179. An 88-year-old woman suffers a stroke in the nursing home. She develops pneumonia and is transferred to the hospital. She continues to decline, is having trouble breathing, and becomes unconscious with little hope of recovery or quality of life. She has no family and no healthcare proxy, living will, or directions about whether she wants to be intubated or not. The physician wants to intubate the patient. The staff nurse strongly believes the patient would not want to be intubated, as the nurse had cared for the lady before she became unconscious. What is the best thing for the CNL to do first?

A. Take a vote among the staff nurses

B. Call for an ethics consultation

C. Ask the social worker to make a recommendation or decision

D. Do a literature review on quality of life of elderly patients with pneumonia

Answer B—Rationale: When a patient has not declared his or her wishes and there is no family or documentation and there is a dispute, then there is an ethical issue and the best choice is to ask for an ethics consultation.

180. As the CNL on a medical–surgical unit, you have noticed a trend over the past 3 months with patients having high blood glucose before lunch and dinner. What is the best way to address this problem?

A. Investigate whether the blood glucose monitors on the unit are accurate

B. Provide an educational in-service about diabetes to the staff

C. Ensure all patients with diabetes receive a consultation with the nutritionist

D. Determine what other changes in processes have occurred on the unit in the past 3 months that could influence this trend

Answer D—Rationale: While checking the accuracy of blood glucose meters, providing education to staff and patients is important. However, other processes on the unit that have changed need to be further evaluated to determine their influence on patient outcomes.

181. You are listening to report with a novice nurse. As part of mentoring new staff and supporting clinical decision making, you ask the new nurse which patient she should assess first. Which patient is the most important for this nurse to assess first?

   A. A 46-year-old receiving IV antibiotic therapy on day 3

   B. A 60-year-old 15 minutes s/p liver biopsy

   C. A 56-year-old with pneumonia on day 2

   D. A 72-year-old hip replacement impatiently waiting for discharge

Answer B—Rationale: Post-op liver biopsy patients have an increased risk of bleeding and need close monitoring after the procedure. The question does not indicate how recently the biopsy was done; therefore, this is the best choice based on the information provided.

182. A nurse on the unit comes to you and says that every shift he works day or night he finds at least one of his patients without an identification band in place. He is very concerned about patient safety and feels a harmful mistake could occur in the near future if the practice on the unit is not improved. As the CNL, how should you help this nurse?

   A. Perform daily audits on all the patients and report results to management

   B. Have the unit secretary make new identification bands for all the patients daily so the charge nurse can place new bands on the patients daily

   C. Research a new style of patient identification bands since the current product does not stay on the patient properly

   D. Provide support to the nurse on the unit who determines the problem and help him identify areas in the process to improve patient identification

Answer D—Rationale: Part of the CNL's role is to provide staff with education, support, and the tools needed to improve practice. This nurse is already concerned about improving a process. As a CNL, it is important to foster leadership and ownership instead of providing solutions to problems.

183. When assessing a patient for a diagnosis of pneumonia, it is more difficult to make a proper diagnosis in the absence of the following symptom:

   A. Cough

   B. Cyanosis

C. Tachycardia

D. Bradycardia

Answer A—Rationale: Cough is one of the paramount symptoms used to help diagnose pneumonia.

184. As the CNL on a medical unit, which of the following cost-effective interventions would you support to reduce the readmission rate on your unit?

A. patients one extra day to ensure they are prepared for discharge home

B. Arrange for all patients to have at least 1 week of visiting nursing postdischarge

C. Review discharge instructions with the patient and one family member

D. Begin discharge planning and teaching on the day of admission

Answer D—Rationale: Using every opportunity to communicate to and educate the patient and family on their care and planning for discharge will better prepare the patient and family for returning home in a cost-effective manner.

185. A 65-year-old man with a history of chest palpitations was seen by his cardiologist for new onset palpitations. He was put on a beta-blocker and told to return for a follow-up in 1 week after taking a stress test. The beta-blocker's action includes:

A. Increasing the consistency of the heart rate

B. Decreasing the ability of the heart muscle to contract

C. Decreasing the chance of dysrhythmia

D. Increasing contractility and decreasing heart rate

Answer D—Rationale: This is the mechanism of action of all beta-blocker medications.

186. To demonstrate active listening, the CNL would exhibit which behavior?

A. Avoid making any facial expressions

B. Preserve at least 3 ft between the parties

C. Lean slightly forward

D. Fold hands in the lap

Answer C—Rationale: Leaning slightly forward indicates desire to concentrate on the interaction at hand and relays openness and attention to the talker.

187. To confirm a scope of practice question, the CNL should consult which administrative body guidelines?

   A. The Joint Commission

   B. Centers for Medicare & Medicaid Services

   C. Hospital Policy and Procedure Manual

   D. State Nursing Practice Act

Answer D—Rationale: Scope of practice is defined according to each individual state. The CNL must have a full understanding of licensure standards of practice according to role before delegation of tasks.

188. Which of the following is not part of the PDSA change model?

   A. Plan

   B. Assess

   C. Do

   D. Study

Answer B—Rationale: The PDSA change model consists of plan, do, study, and act.

189. In order to generate ideas aimed at designing an implementation plan, a team reviews the topic and members verbalize solution ideas in a random fashion. This is an example of which of the following strategies?

   A. Multivoting

   B. Process mapping

   C. **Brainstorming**

   D. Nominal group technique

Answer C—Rationale: Brainstorming is creative, interactive, and unstructured, as team members suggest possible ideas in a free-flow format without regard to the details of the suggested solutions.

190. You have been charged with examining the heart failure 30-day readmission rate of your unit. In doing so, it is important for you to examine data from what other sources?

   A. National and state readmission rates

   B. National benchmarks

   C. Readmissions to other units in your hospital

   D. All of the above

Answer D—Rationale: The 30-day readmission rates are a key factor in CMS reimbursement rates to hospitals. A CNL should have a broad perspective of readmission rates across multiple settings. The CNL can then resource share with other areas to gain insight into best practices and pre-existing initiatives at the microsystem, hospital, state, and national levels.

191. You have done some research and found a new fall prevention tool that you would like to trial on your unit. The tool was recently developed and tested at a large city hospital with a population of open heart patients. You are not sure that this tool can be effectively implemented in your small community hospital. You are questioning the tool's:

A. Relative risk

B. External validity

C. Transportability

D. Causal association

Answer B—Rationale: External validity is the degree to which the results of the original study are applicable to a population other than the one initially targeted.

192. A nurse approaches you and expresses her knowledge deficit regarding the difference between signs and symptoms of left- and right-sided heart failure. You explain the physiology between the two types of heart failure and identify which of the following has a primary symptom of right-sided heart failure?

A. Shortness of breath on exertion

B. Heart murmur and distended veins

C. Peripheral edema

D. Cool extremities and weak peripheral pulses

Answer C—Rationale: Right-sided heart failure leads to congestion of systemic capillaries. This generates excess fluid accumulation in the body and usually affects the dependent parts of the body first.

193. Vaccinations are considered what level of prevention?

A. Primary

B. Secondary

C. Tertiary

D. None of these

Answer A—Rationale: Vaccinations are preventative and therefore considered a primary level of prevention.

194. Medicaid covers which population?

A. Employed

B. Underinsured

C. Unemployed

D. Poor and disabled

Answer D—Rationale: Medicaid is a publicly funded insurance provided to the poor and disabled in each state.

195. While being admitted to the unit after a car accident, the patient informs you that she has been off her psychiatric medications Seroquel and Celexa due to the cost and no longer has a doctor. As an advocate, you would talk with the physician in hopes of obtaining what two consults?

A. Medicine and clinical case manager (CCM)

B. Psychiatry and social worker

C. CCM and social worker

D. Medicine and psychiatry

Answer B—Rationale: Without a physician to monitor the results of the patient withdrawing herself from these two medicines, the result could be detrimental. This consult can also help get the patient back with a psychiatrist upon discharge. The social worker would assist with any social issues upon discharge, such as affording medications.

196. D.M. is 80 years old and admitted for a hip fracture, caused by a fall from standing. As a CNL, you would know a fracture obtained this way is typically found from what?

A. Osteomyelitis

B. Osteoporosis

C. Anemia

D. Rheumatoid arthritis

Answer B—Rationale: A fracture of the hip from a fall that occurs from standing is indicative of osteoporosis. It is imperative for CNLs to identify such patterns to help the patient get a holistic plan of care.

197. You are caring for Sara, a 76-year-old grandmother recovering from heart failure. You know that she is ready to go home because:

A. Her ECG is normal, her pulse oximetry is normal, and she has a supportive family to help care for her at home.

B. She tells you she is ready to go home.

C. You observe her ambulating in the hallway, free from dyspnea.

D. She says she is free from dyspnea and fatigue, she has a follow-up appointment set up for the following Monday morning, and her daughter said she can drive her to the appointment.

Answer C—Rationale: HF symptoms are often not well evaluated, as clients remain relatively inactive while in the hospital. Activities such as walking in the hall provide an opportunity for objective evaluation of dyspnea, fatigue, and gait issues.

198. You are working with your team to modify the unit's budget. You know that the best way to create a budget is:

   A. Looking at the previous budget's variance

   B. Requesting a large capital budget

   C. Being in line with your budget goal

   D. Utilizing a case mix

Answer D—Rationale: Case mix is the best way to create a budget. It looks at human and material costs and environmental resources.

199. A new health policy is being voted on in Congress. Your professional organization supports this policy and is recruiting nurses to go to Washington, DC, to help promote their view and to have a bigger voice. You do not support this policy. Your manager wants you to go as a leader and represent your unit. What should you do?

   A. You should go, as you need to stick together with your professional organization and yield to your manager.

   B. You should learn more about the policy and why your organization supports it.

   C. You should politely decline, as you do not agree with the policy.

   D. You should go, but rally against the policy since you do not agree with it. This is America and you are exercising your freedom of speech.

Answer B—Rationale: You should know how your professional organization stands—we need to support each other and have one voice as nurses.

200. You want to do some research for a potential policy change. All of the following are excellent resources, except:

   A. Centers for Disease Control

   B. Wikipedia

   C. American Diabetes Association

   D. Institute for Healthcare Improvement

Answer B—Rationale: Wikipedia is NOT a valid or credible site—anyone can post to this site.

Case Study 1

Michael is a CNL on an adult medical–surgical unit in a large urban hospital. Michael conducted a 5P (persons, patients, professionals, processes, patterns) assessment of the unit and noticed a large amount of pneumonia patients were being readmitted within 30 days. Michael would like to form a team to investigate the readmissions further and come up with a plan on how to reduce the readmission rate.

1. Utilizing an interdisciplinary approach, who should Michael include in the team?

   A. Nurse, hospitalist, physical therapist, and dietician

   B. Respiratory therapist, nurse, pulmonologist, and case manager

   C. Nurse, gerontologist, case manager, and physical therapist

   D. Respiratory therapist, pulmonologist, case manager, and dietician

Answer B—Rationale: The CNL works as a lateral integrator to communicate, collaborate, and coordinate a variety of disciplines that will participate in a plan of care. In order to create the best team to approach pneumonia readmissions, Michael must include a nurse, respiratory therapist, and a case manager. A physician should also be included, and in this case the pulmonologist is an excellent choice for pneumonia patients.

The team investigates the readmissions and discovered that most of the patients were 65 years and older and were discharged home alone. The team also notices inconsistencies in the plan of care. Some patients received incentive spirometers and education from respiratory therapists, while others did not. Everyone understands that there is a need for change in order to prevent readmissions.

2. The team is unsure how to approach this change, so what should Michael suggest as the next step?

   A. Conduct a literature review to determine evidence-based practice (EBP) on caring for pneumonia patients

   B. Review the intensive care unit's plan of care for pneumonia patients

   C. Investigate the pneumonia readmissions from last year to determine if the same trends exist

   D. Determine the respiratory therapists' role in caring for patients with pneumonia

Answer A—Rationale: The CNL promotes the use of EBP when designing care for patients. After identifying a clear aim, the team must search the evidence to determine best practices for pneumonia patients.

The team has a vision and a strategy on how to approach this process change. They decide to create a pneumonia pathway with a comprehensive, streamlined plan of care including evidence-based nursing tasks, education from respiratory therapist, and discharge follow-up home health visits. The team shares the plan with the unit through presentations and e-mails. The staff expresses enthusiasm about the new changes.

3. Utilizing Kotter's theory of change, what step is the team demonstrating now?

   A. Anchor new approaches in the culture

   B. Generate short-term wins

   C. Consolidate gains and produce more change

   D. Communicate the change vision

Answer D—Rationale: The team is communicating the change vision to the unit by telling them the plan and how the process change will be implemented.

The team wants to implement the process change and observe what happens, but they are unsure what method to use.

4. What method should Michael suggest?

   A. 5S

   B. 5P

   C. Failure mode effect and analysis (FMEA)

   D. Plan-Do-Study-Act (PDSA)

Answer D—Rationale: The PDSA would be the best method because it is a rapid cycle review that includes comprehensive planning, implementing change while observing, analysis of data, and devising next steps based on outcomes. This approach is best used for encouraging continuous, ongoing efforts to improve outcomes.

Jonathan, a 67-year-old Caucasian male, is admitted to Michael's unit. Michael decides to round on Jonathan to see how the new pneumonia pathway is progressing. Michael asks Jonathan how he likes the education sessions with the respiratory therapist. Jonathan states he is learning a lot and really enjoys the opportunity to ask questions. Jonathan then states that he has asked the nurse for an incentive spirometer, but he never received one. Michael apologizes to Jonathan.

5. What should Michael do next?

   A. Obtain an incentive spirometer and teach Jonathan how to properly use it

   B. Coach the nurse on utilizing the evidence-based pneumonia pathway

C. Notify the unit manager that the pathway is not being followed

D. Follow up with Jonathan tomorrow to ensure he received an incentive spirometer

Answer B—Rationale: Michael should provide immediate feedback to the nurse, and coach the nurse on following EBP.

Case Study 2

You are a new CNL on a unit that is not familiar with the role. Recently, your unit has had a breakdown in the discharge process leading to poor patient outcomes. The problem appears to be a lack of coordination between the interdisciplinary team; patients are being discharged before PT/OT has fully cleared them, before pharmacy can review their home meds and education, and often without patient-specific dressing orders and supplies. There is uncertainty about why this issue has arisen in recent months. As a CNL, you would like to try and address these issues.

1. How can you quickly explain the concept of the CNL and its potential in regards to this situation to your manager and other leaders or stakeholders on your unit?

   A. A root cause analysis (RCA)

   B. A summary presentation

   C. An elevator speech

   D. A situation background assessment recommendation (SBAR)

Answer C—Rationale: An elevator speech is a short precise detailed way to explain the CNL role and how it can help in this situation.

Your unit's leadership is initially uncertain on how the focus of the CNL differs from other APRNs.

2. You explain:

   A. The main focus of the CNL is on evidence-based practice (EBP) and clinical outcomes

   B. The main focus of the CNL is on coordination of care and discharge planning

   C. The main focus of the CNL is on the specific needs of a cohort of patients and RCA

   D. The main focus of the CNL is on anticipating needs of patients and RCA

Answer A—Rationale: From the white paper, the CNL is a generalist that focuses on EBP and outcomes. Although RCA and discharge planning are important, they are not the main focus of the CNL role.

You are given permission and allowed to implement the CNL role on a trial basis with the discharge process.

3. How do you best proceed with investigating the lapse in the discharge process?
   A. Interview each member of the interdisciplinary team to identify his or her opinions of the discharge process
   B. Create an interdisciplinary team meeting to discuss the discharge process and known issues
   C. Begin leading a new discharge process on your unit and act as a care coordinator on your unit
   D. Continue the current discharge process

Answer B—Rationale: The next step is to create an interdisciplinary team and have a meeting to discuss how to address the issues with the discharge process. Although you may need a new discharge process, it is too early to implement something new and you certainly do not want to continue the process as it is currently.

One issue identified through your investigation is that surgeons have not been entering home wound care instructions, with the consequence that nurses are not triggered to educate the patient with anything specific on the discharge paperwork. The surgeons wonder if nurses can identify the wound care needs of each patient, place a nursing order for wound care, and then educate the patient on discharge.

4. As the CNL, you investigate whether this is an appropriate nursing task and within the nursing scope of practice by reviewing:
   A. The Joint Commission
   B. Centers for Medicare & Medicaid standards
   C. Your state's Nurse Practice Act
   D. Your hospital's policy and procedure manual

Answer C—Rationale: In order to determine what tasks a nurse can do in a certain state, the CNL must review that state's Nurse Practice Act. This is not found in any materials from the hospital, The Joint Commission, or the Centers for Medicare & Medicaid.

After this process, the discharge issues on your unit have improved.

5. As a trial CNL, whose buy-in will be the most important in fully implementing the CNL role in the hospital?
   A. The chief nursing officer (CNO)
   B. The unit manager

C. The members of the interdisciplinary team

D. The staff affected by your outcomes

Answer A—Rationale: The person who will have the most influence in your hospital on the implementation of the CNL role is the CNO. The unit manager, staff, and members of the interdisciplinary team are all important but will not have as much influence as the CNO.

Case Study 3

A 36-year-old Hispanic woman is pregnant with her third child. She has had one live birth and one stillbirth. She is 5′2″ tall and weighs 220 lb., and her BMI is 40.2. Her current blood pressure is 140/80 mmHg. Her past obstetrical history includes a cesarean section for a 9 lb. 5 oz. live female at 38 weeks gestation. She also had a vaginal stillborn birth at 36 weeks gestation weighing 7 lb. 2 oz. Both of these births were in Honduras. This patient presents to the clinic after recently arriving in the United States at 32 weeks gestation with complaints of headache, blurred vision, lethargy, and diaphoresis. The patient arrives with no record of her prenatal care. The following lab results are from today's visit: Urine dipstick 3+ glycosuria and no proteinuria, fasting blood sugar of 58 mg/dL, and a biophysical profile of 8/10. An oral glucose tolerance test (OGTT) was also done today with a result of 150 mg/dL.

1. Which of the following interventions is appropriate for the nurse to tell the CNL?

   A. The patient is experiencing hyperglycemia and should be given a protein snack.

   B. The patient is experiencing hyperglycemia and should be given insulin and 1 cup of milk.

   C. The patient is experiencing hypoglycemia and should be given insulin and 1 cup of orange juice.

   D. The patient is experiencing hypoglycemia and should be given 1 cup of skim milk.

Answer D—Rationale: The patient's fasting blood sugar is below 60 mm/dL and is symptomatic. She must be treated for hypoglycemia by drinking 1 cup of skim milk, or ½ cup of juice, or ½ cup of soft drink.

2. The patient's blood sugar should be repeated after the snack at what interval?

   A. 1 hour

   B. 15 minutes

C. 30 minutes

D. 2 hours

Answer B—Rationale: According to the American Diabetes Association, the blood sugar should be rechecked after 15 minutes of giving a snack.

3. What does the result of the 150 mg/dL from the OGTT signify?

   A. Based on a value greater than 140 mg/dL, the patient should have 3-hour 100-g OGTT within 1 week.

   B. The results are within normal limits and do not meet the threshold for the diagnosis of gestational diabetes.

   C. A fasting blood sugar should be checked as soon as possible.

   D. Based on this abnormal value, the 3-hour OGTT is not required.

Answer A—Rationale: If your blood glucose is higher than 140 mg/dL, the next step is the oral 3-hour glucose tolerance test. This test will determine if you have gestational diabetes.

4. What are the risk factors for this patient developing gestational diabetes?

   A. Obesity, advanced maternal age

   B. Previous infant with birth weight greater than 9 lb., stillbirth, hypertention, and proteinuria

   C. Obesity, advanced maternal age, Hispanic/Latina, previous infant with birth weight greater than 9 lb., and stillbirth

   D. Hispanic/Latina, stillbirth, and proteinuria

Answer C—Rationale: Risk factors for developing gestational diabetes include the following: Obesity, age greater than 25, nonwhite race, have had a stillbirth in previous pregnancy, and/or previous birth of larger for gestational age infant.

Case Study 4

You are informed by your nurse manager about a large clinical issue involving a patient that has occurred on another unit. In your role as the CNL, hospital leadership has asked for you to temporarily work on a new unit to investigate the issue and offer solutions to improve practice. The clinical incident involved a postoperative patient on patient-controlled analgesia (PCA) with a low-dose continuous infusion who became extremely oversedated during the night. When the nurse discovered the patient, he had a respiratory rate of 5, oxygen saturations in the 60s, and appeared grossly cyanotic.

1. How do you begin orienting to this new unit and the situation?
   A. Perform a 5P (persons, patients, professionals, processes, patterns) assessment of the unit
   B. Review hospital policy and procedures related to PCA use
   C. Perform a root cause analysis (RCA)
   D. Create an interdisciplinary team to address this issue

Answer A—Rationale: The first action of the CNL should be to assess and evaluate this microsystem.

2. As you begin to investigate the issue, what is one way you can present *a graphical* representation of the different factors that contributed to the issue?
   A. An RCA
   B. A fishbone diagram
   C. A concept map
   D. A clinical decision tree

Answer B—Rationale: A fishbone diagram is an appropriate way to diagram out the clinical issue and related causative factors.

3. What process do you use to fully investigate the clinical incident?
   A. Plan-Do-Study-Act (PDSA)
   B. 5P assessment
   C. An RCA
   D. Clinical decision tree

Answer C—Rationale: The RCA is the tool/process the CNL should use to identify the primary cause of the issue after it has occurred.

Through your analysis, you identify that this patient also had a diagnosis of obstructive sleep apnea (OSA). The patient was not placed on a continuous pulse oximeter. The nurse had last rounded on the patient approximately 1 hour prior to discovery.

4. You question the appropriateness of the PCA orders given the risks and patient's comorbidities. What information do you gather next?
   A. Discuss with the surgeons their rationale behind the order
   B. Review the current evidence on PCA use and oversedation
   C. Contact a peer in the sleep center to discuss risks and benefits of OSA and PCA use
   D. Examine the current hospital policy and procedure manual

Answer B—Rationale: Reviewing current evidence is the priority for the CNL to inform investigation of a clinical issue.

Your analysis indicates a need to change the hospital's current policy on PCA use, increase education on opioid use in conjunction with an OSA diagnosis, and improve the hospital policy regarding patient PCA monitoring.

5. What is one system the CNL can use to implement these changes?
   A. PDSA
   B. RCA
   C. Clinical decision tree
   D. Concept map

Answer A—Rationale: PDSA is a system to implement a QI project.

Case Study 5

Ms. Jones is a 35-year-old patient admitted to your microsystem. The patient has a history of obesity, hypertension, obstructive sleep apnea (OSA), type 2 diabetes, tracheostomy, and is on a ventilator at night. Ms. Jones is currently unemployed and waiting on her disability approval. The patient was living in an apartment with her 18-year-old daughter and three grandchildren. The 35-year-old mother was admitted into the hospital because of a power outage in her two-bedroom apartment.

1. As a CNL, what key stakeholders would you include to provide this patient with the best outcomes?
   A. Medical social worker, CCM, primary nurse, clinical nutritionist, CNL, respiratory therapist, and physician
   B. Physical therapist, occupational therapist, CNL, primary nurse, medical social worker, and laboratory technician
   C. Clinical care manager, primary nurse, medical social worker, and respiratory therapist
   D. Pharmacist, clinical care manager, medical social worker, occupational therapist, and physical therapist

Answer A—Rationale: Collaboration is an interdisciplinary process of problem solving that involves shared responsibility for decision making and execution of plan of care while working toward a common goal. Thus, the best team to collaborate would include the physician, primary care nurse, a clinical nutritionist for diabetes and obesity, a social worker to help with unemployment/disability approval, a respiratory therapist for ventilation associated with sleep apnea, a case manager for the complexity of the case, and the CNL as a facilitator and coordinator on this collaboration.

While reviewing your patient's chart, you notice that the patient has a 13.5 hemoglobin A1c. During rounds, you notice that the family brought the patient pasta with Alfredo sauce from home.

2. What would be the most appropriate next step as a CNL?
   A. Discuss the importance of following a diabetic diet with the patient and her family
   B. **Ask the physician to consult the diabetes educator and clinical nutritionist, and discuss the risk of diabetes with the patient and her family**
   C. Take the food out of the room and tell the patient that she needs to lose weight to be there for her grandchildren
   D. Ask the patient if she has been taking her insulin appropriately

Answer B—Rationale: As a CNL, you are responsible for clinical decision making on multiple perspectives including the client and/or family preferences. The CNL also understands the roles of the interdisciplinary team members. It is important to know how much knowledge the patient has and also work with them to come up with a meal plan they can actually follow.

While you are discussing discharge planning with Ms. Jones, you find out that she does not have the means to pay for the electrical work at her home. You ask Ms. Jones if she has any family to stay with her while she resolves the electrical issues and she says that there is no one available to help her.

3. What is the best statement from the CNL at this time?
   A. "Would you consider a short-term stay at a nursing facility until this problem is resolved?"
   B. "We cannot keep you in the hospital forever, Ms. Jones. It costs too much."
   C. "I will discuss this with the director for case management and see if she will pay for your electrical work."
   D. **"Let me refer you to the social worker and CCM."**

Answer D—Rationale: The social worker can help with financial planning/coverage options; the case manager can help with insurance/billing questions.

Ms. Jones has now been in the hospital for 2 months, and she develops shortness of breath and pain in her right leg. Your patient has developed a pulmonary embolus, which requires an admission to the intensive care unit.

4. As a CNL, what would be the most appropriate intervention after assuring quality care is provided for this patient?
   A. Form a multidisciplinary team to review the patient's plan of care and gather whether anything can be done to prevent this from occurring
   B. Perform a root cause analysis (RCA)
   C. Review this case with your nurse manager
   D. Review the chart to see if Ms. Jones was mobile during her hospital stay

Answer B—Rationale: RCA is performed to prevent future harm by eliminating the latent errors (hidden problems within the systems that contributed to adverse events).

Ms. Jones is better now and is ready for discharge. She will be going home on Lovenox injections twice a day and transitioning to Coumadin.

5. To ensure that Ms. Jones has the best possible outcomes, what key member of the team should the CNL consult with for follow-up?
   A. Home health nurse for lab draws, family, physician, diabetes telehealth, and medical social worker
   B. Nursing assistant, home health nurse, family, physician, physical therapist, and CNL
   C. Diabetes telehealth, CNL, medical social worker, and occupational therapist
   D. Home health nurse for lab draws, CNL, and family

Answer A—Rationale: A CNL understands the importance of collaborative and interdisciplinary communication as it relates to patient outcomes. The CNL must know the role of each team member as it relates to patient safety and patient outcomes.

Case Study 6

You are a CNL student contemplating a topic for your capstone project. You believe that patients transferred from the medical intensive care unit (MICU) to your medical unit are frequently transferred back to the intensive care unit (ICU) due to multiple rapid response team (RRT) calls.

1. You want to look further into whether this is truly a concern for your unit. What first step should you take as a CNL student?
   A. Assess the current rate of RRTs and transfers back; collect data to see how many patients are transfer-backs to the MICU
   B. Implement a process to reduce transfers back to the MICU

C. Perform a literature review on RRTs and transfers back

D. Design a study to decrease RRTs and transfers back to MICU

Answer A—Rationale: Prior to performing a literature review or implementing a process, the CNL should assess to identify the problem; therefore, assessing current numbers and collecting appropriate data are the first step.

After assessing your unit population, you find that the rate of RRTs and transfers back to the ICU is higher than the national mean.

2. What should be your next step?

A. Design a study and implement the best practice

B. Perform a literature review and create a team

C. Design a study and perform a literature review

D. Identify the problem and create a PICOT question

Answer D—Rationale: The first step to the EBP process is to identify a clinical problem. Creating a PICOT question will help the CNL in performing a literature review.

When performing a literature review, you stumble upon several articles from various websites. You are trying to determine the most reliable source to use for the literature review.

3. Which resource is the best choice for you to use to perform a literature review?

A. Google

B. Mayo Clinic

C. Cumulative Index Nursing and Allied Health (CINAHL)

D. Wikipedia

Answer C—Rationale: CINAHL is a resource the CNL can utilize to obtain the most updated articles. It is a research tool for nursing and allied health professionals with peer-reviewed articles.

You created a PICOT question: "Will the use of a CNL assessing potential patients to be transferred from the MICU to the medical unit prevent transfers-back and decrease RRTs within a 6-month period?" After performing a literature review, you found several results on your topic.

4. Which of the following demonstrates the strongest level of evidence?

A. A well-designed randomized control trial study about using an ICU rounding nurse to decrease RRT calls

B. An article discussing a quasi-experimental study that reduced the frequency of RRTs utilizing an educational intervention

C. **A meta-analysis of randomized control trial studies that demonstrated a significant improvement in reducing the number of bounce backs and RRTs to ICUs**

D. A descriptive study about the challenges of a medical unit using RRTs

Answer C—Rationale: According to the Melnyk and Fineout-Overholt recommendations of using a hierarchy, a systematic review or meta-analysis of RCTs and evidence-based clinical practice guidelines is level 1 of 6, making it the strongest level of literature review.

After synthesizing the data, you decide that the best practice is to perform an educational intervention for nurses about RRTs and transfers-back and assess patients prior to transferring them to a medical unit.

5. Prior to the implementation process, what is the best step for you to take next?

   A. Form a team of stakeholders

   B. Develop a comparison group

   C. Talk to the manager

   D. Start the implementation process

Answer A—Rationale: After performing the literature review and developing a PICOT question, you should create a team of stakeholders to ensure the intervention has the appropriate resources to make the study successful.

Glossary

Accountable care organizations: those organizations that, through the Affordable Care Act, will only be rewarded for improving quality and increasing cost savings. These are organizations in which physicians and hospitals work together to improve outcomes and share in cost savings.

Acuity: level of intensity of care required by patients.

Advocacy: the act of expressing or defending the rights or causes of another.

American Association of Colleges of Nursing (AACN): the national voice for baccalaureate and graduate nursing education. AACN's educational areas, research, federal advocacy, data collection, publications, and special programs work to establish quality standards for nursing education; assist deans and directors to implement those standards; influence the nursing profession to improve healthcare; and promote public support for professional nursing education, research, and practice.

Autonomy: the right of individuals to make their own decisions based on informed consent and the lack of coercion; personal freedom and self-determination.

Background statement: a brief scenario that provides the information necessary or useful in answering the question. This may be called the case event.

Benchmarking: in healthcare, it has been defined as the continual and collaborative discipline of measuring and comparing the results of key work processes with those of the best performers when evaluating organizational performance.

Beneficence: supporting actions that promote good.

Big data: refers to the volume, variety, and rapid accumulation of data, as well as to the analytics being used to evaluate that data for the discovery and communication of patterns within and between data. Also, an accumulation of data that is too large and complex for processing using traditional database management tools.

Case event: the heart of the multiple-choice question that provides the information that an individual needs to think about to answer the question. This may also be called the background statement.

Case mix: the mix (variety) of patients for whom care is delivered organized by specified characteristics (e.g., gender, diagnosis-related group [DRG], payer).

Chronic illness or disease: an illness or disease that has lasted 3 months or longer. They tend to become more common with age.

Client advocate: the CNL becomes competent at ensuring that clients, families, and communities are well informed and included in care planning. The CNL also serves as an informed leader for improving care and as an advocate for the profession and the interdisciplinary healthcare team.

Clinical decision support: a key functionality of health information technology encompassing a variety of tools including, but not limited to: computerized alerts and reminders for providers and patients; clinical guidelines; condition-specific order sets; focused patient data reports and summaries; documentation templates; diagnostic support; and contextually relevant reference information.

Clinical nurse leader (CNL): a role that evolved out of a partnership between nursing education and practice leaders to address the need for a nurse educated to address patient care needs in a complex, changing healthcare delivery environment.

Clinical Nurse Leader Association (CNLA): an association that provides a forum for CNLs to collaborate, network, share data, and promote the CNL role.

Clinician: the CNL is designer/coordinator/integrator/evaluator of care to individuals, families, groups, communities, and populations. He or she is able to understand the rationale for care and competently deliver this care to complex and diverse populations. The CNL provides care at the point of care with particular emphasis on health promotion and risk reduction services.

CMS: the Centers for Medicare & Medicaid Services. The Health and Human Services agency responsible for Medicare and parts of Medicaid. CMS is responsible for oversight of HIPAA administrative simplification transactions and code sets, health identifiers, and security standards. CMS also maintains the Healthcare Common Procedure Coding System (HCPCS) medical code set and the Medicare Remittance Advice Remark Codes administrative code set.

Coaching: an ongoing two-way process in which the CNL can share knowledge and experience to help other nurses achieve desired professional goals.

Codes of ethics: formal statements that serve to articulate the values and beliefs of a given discipline, serving as a standard for professional actions and reflecting the ethical principles shared by its members.

Collaboration: the process of working with a group of interdisciplinary providers in order to achieve a common goal.

Commission on Nurse Certification (CNC): an autonomous arm of AACN, governed by the CNC Board of Commissioners. CNC recognizes individuals who have demonstrated professional standards and knowledge through CNL certification. CNC promotes lifelong learning through CNL recertification.

Communication: the transmission of feelings, attitudes, and ideas between people through the exchange of verbal and written words as well as physical behaviors and tone of voice.

Complementary and alternative medicine (CAM): nonpharmacological medical treatments that are not part of mainstream medicine use (e.g., aromatherapy, art therapy, massage, and acupuncture).

Complexity theory: every complex system has a life of its own, and the theory considers the patterns of relationship in the system: how they are sustained, how they self-regulate and self-organize, and how outcomes emerge.

Computerized physician order entry (CPOE): a feature of the EHR that assures standardized, legible communication of the medical plan of care to other members of the healthcare team.

Coordination: the intentional organization of providers and the activities they provide through planned communication in order to yield the desired outcomes for the client.

Cost-benefit analysis: comparing the advantages of an intervention versus not using it.

Cost center: a microsystem responsible for providing services and monitoring the costs associated with such service provision.

Cost-consequence analysis: expense associated with illness beyond care.

Cost-effectiveness analysis: comparing two types of possible intervention.

Cost identification: summary of each expense.

Cost of illness: total expenses related to care.

Cost minimization: analysis of costs and possible reductions.

Critical listening: involves three major components: ethos, or speaker credibility; logos, or logical arguments; and pathos, or psychological appeal.

Cultural awareness: CNLs need to recognize their own individual values, beliefs, and prejudices. CNLs should reflect on their own cultural practices.

Cultural competence: conceptualized as the process in which CNLs continuously strive to achieve the skills, knowledge, and ability to work effectively within the cultural context of the patient.

Cultural interaction: CNLs will need to work with individuals from various cultural backgrounds to expand their understanding and become more at ease and self-assured.

Cultural knowledge: CNLs should stay unbiased and find information concerning other cultures to establish educational underpinnings.

Cultural sensitivity: CNLs will need to understand and accept the individual's values and beliefs. The CNL will need to show presence, support, empathy, flexibility, and tolerance.

Cultural skills: CNLs need to demonstrate the ability to communicate efficiently. Additionally, they should have the ability to identify, assess, and incorporate the values, beliefs, and cultural customs of the person under their care.

Cyber security: measures taken to protect a computer or computer system against unauthorized access or attack.

Dashboard: a graphic representation of essential information that highlights an organization's performance in a range of designated areas of quality.

Developmental tasks: a task that consistently occurs at a certain period in an individual's life.

Diagnosis-related group (DRG): group used by Medicare and other payers to determine reimbursement to organizations and providers.

Digital divide: the social, economic, and educational inequalities between those who have access to computers and online resources and those who do not.

Direct costs: costs that are directly related to the provision of a service; the cost can be specifically identified for an individual patient or activity.

Distractors: incorrect options listed as potential answers in the multiple-choice questions.

Educator: the CNL uses appropriate teaching principles and strategies as well as current information, materials, and technologies to teach clients, healthcare professionals, and communities.

Epidemiology: has been described as the sum of factors that influence the incidence and distribution of disease.

Ethics: involves the principles or assumptions underpinning the way individuals or groups should conduct themselves and is concerned with motives and attitudes, as well as the relationship of these attitudes to the individual.

Ethos: refers to the credibility of the speaker.

Evidence-based practice: is conducted when there are one or more best practices that can be applied to clinical practice. It is a broader concept than research or research utilization and includes using the best and current evidence, the patient's preferences, and the clinician's expertise or judgment.

Expenses: dollars owed as a result of both services delivered and organizational costs incurred in the delivery.

Failure mode effect and analysis (FMEA): a systematic method to proactively evaluate a process to identify how it may fail to assess the relative impact of possible failures.

First-party payers: individuals responsible for payment for services rendered.

Forming stage: the first stage of team formation in which team members share common goals that are understood, clearly articulated, and championed by team members. The team members are seeking a safe and trusting environment, where they can feel comfortable expressing their ideas and concerns.

Functional assessment tool: a tool utilized to assess an individual's ability to master activities of daily living.

Gap analysis: evaluates the strengths and weaknesses of a team in relation to the required outcomes. Analysis is performed of disciplines represented and skills possessed by members to support any additions or deletions needed for successful outcomes.

Gross domestic product: market value of all goods and services produced (created) within a country in a specific period.

Healthcare informatics: the collection, classification, storage, retrieval, and dissemination of recorded healthcare knowledge using computer technology.

Healthcare Information and Management Systems Society (HIMSS): a global nonprofit organization with a majority of its 44,000 individual members working in healthcare; it promotes the optimal use of information technology and management systems through its content expertise, professional development, research initiatives, and media vehicles.

Healthcare literacy: the capacity to obtain process and understand basic health information to make appropriate health decisions.

Health policy: generally denotes policy that impacts the health of the individual, families, or communities through production, provision, and financing of healthcare services.

Healthy People 2020: identifies nationwide health improvement priorities and sets directions for health policy. The Healthy People initiative provides science-based 10-year national objectives for improving the health of all Americans. See www.healthypeople.gov.

HIEs: organizational or geographical entities that manage health information electronically across organizations or regions.

Holistic health: the integration of the physiological, psychological, and spiritual aspects of an individual's health.

Horizontal leadership: situation in which there may be multiple individuals who assume leadership of a team or teams in order to achieve a common goal.

Horizontal organization: an organization with decentralization of power and/or control, at least within specific departments. The emphasis is placed on horizontal collaboration.

Hospice/end-of-life care: provides quality care to people in the last months of their life who have decided to stop curative treatments.

Hospital-acquired condition (HAC): reasonably preventable conditions that develop during the hospital stay that were not present on admission.

Hospital Consumer Assessment of Healthcare Providers and Systems (HCAHPS): a standardized tool being utilized that measures patient perception of the quality of care received. This measure of quality is part of the value-based purchasing initiative by CMS and had a great impact on hospital processes.

Human–computer interface: includes both the study of how humans interact with computers, and the extent to which technology systems are developed for successful interaction with humans.

ICD-9-CM: *International Classification of Diseases, Ninth Revision, Clinical Manifestations;* used for documentation of diagnoses and procedures; in turn, used to assign a DRG and create patient charges.

Indirect costs: those costs of doing business that are not directly related to a specific individual, such as heat, electricity, overhead, water, and some administrative personnel.

Individual level of prevention: the level which includes healthcare interventions like counseling on healthy lifestyles, such as dietary counseling for people at risk of colorectal cancer.

Informatics nurse specialist (INS): individual who must be able to understand and use the integrated knowledge of many elements including nursing science, information science, computer science, cognitive science, and others appropriate to specific issues.

Information manager: the CNL is proficient in using information systems and technology to improve healthcare outcomes.

Institute of Medicine (IOM): organization whose purpose is to provide national advice on issues relating to biomedical science, medicine, and health; its mission is to serve as advisor to the nation to improve health. It works outside the framework of the U.S. federal government to provide independent guidance and analysis and relies on a volunteer workforce of scientists and other experts, operating under a formal peer-review system. The institute aims to provide unbiased, evidence-based, and authoritative information and advice concerning health and science policy to policy makers, professionals, leaders in every sector of society, and the public at large.

Institutional review board: a committee that has been formally designated to approve, monitor, and review biomedical and behavioral research involving humans at healthcare institutions.

Interdependence: the interaction of staff that is characterized by trust, collaboration, willingness to help each other, appreciation of complementary roles, respect, and recognition that all contribute individually to a shared purpose.

Interdisciplinary: refers to nurses, physicians, mid-level providers, and all others associated with the medical care of a patient.

Interdisciplinary collaboration: healthcare providers of different disciplines collaborating as colleagues to provide team-focused patient care.

Interdisciplinary communication: communication, in the sense of cross-fertilization of ideas, involving two or more healthcare disciplines caring for patients.

Interoperability: the ability of computer software, or a computer system, to work with another system.

The Joint Commission: an accreditation group that develops and upholds patient safety and care standards for hospitals and other healthcare organizations. It accredits more than 20,000 healthcare organizations and programs in the United States. A majority of state governments recognize Joint Commission accreditation as a condition of licensure and the receipt of Medicaid reimbursement.

Justice: the concept that all people should be treated fairly.

Keyed response: the correct answer among the options or potential answers in a multiple-choice question.

Lateral integration: the combination of knowledge, skills, and services provided by interdependent and independent disciplines to unified care across multiple transitions and environments. Lateral integration is also when care is provided that integrates multiple disciplines across the continuum of care.

Leading health indicators: a small set of Healthy People 2020 objectives which have been selected to communicate high-priority health issues and actions that can be taken to address them.

Lean: a systematic method for the elimination of waste within a process.

Length of stay: time spent (number of days) in an organization receiving healthcare services.

Lifelong learner: recognizes the need for and actively pursues new knowledge and skills as one's role and needs of the healthcare system evolves.

Logos: logical arguments or inquiring whether a speaker makes errors in logic.

Macrosystems: bigger systems made of smaller systems (microsystems).

Medicaid: a program sponsored by states and the federal government for low income and/or disabled individuals; services and payment are provided.

Medical home: a concept initially designed in 1969 and now used to coordinate medical care among multiple providers.

Medicare: a government program related to Social Security for the elderly.

Member of a profession: the CNL remains accountable for the ongoing acquisition of knowledge and skills related to his or her profession and to effect change in healthcare practice and outcomes and in the profession.

Mentoring: mentoring involves a long-term relationship oriented toward nurses who are focused on advancing clinically.

Microsystem: smaller systems that are functional, frontline units that provide the most healthcare to the most people; it is the place where patients, families, and healthcare teams meet. These smaller systems produce quality, safety, and cost outcomes at the frontline of care.

Modifiable risk factors: factors that could be changed if the individual is willing to change through lifestyle, habits, and diet.

Moral stress: most often occurs when faced with the situations in which two ethical principles compete.

Mourning: stage in a process in which team members have achieved the group's mission or goals that were set forth. This stage involves termination of the group.

National Database for Nursing Quality Indicators® (NDNQI): the only national nursing database that provides quarterly and annual reporting of structure, process, and outcome indicators to evaluate nursing care at the unit level.

National Healthcare Safety Network® (NHSN): an Internet-based surveillance system that integrates and expands a facility's own surveillance program of diseases/infections to a national level.

National Quality Foundation (NQF): provides national leadership to establish national priorities and goals ensuring that healthcare delivery is safe, effective, patient centered, timely, efficient, and equitable.

Nonmaleficence: the concept that one should not do harm.

Nonmodifiable risk factors: any risk factor, like heredity, for a particular condition, such as breast cancer, which cannot be modified.

Norming: the third stage of team formation in which team members feel they are working in a safe environment, where everyone's opinions and ideas are shared openly and valued.

Ongoing evaluation: the assessment of current processes, systems, and outcomes compared against identified metrics in order to meet changing needs and optimize efficiency, efficacy, safety, and quality of care.

Options: all the potential answers presented with the question.

Outcome: the end product of an action.

Outcomes manager: the CNL who regularly synthesizes data, information, and knowledge to evaluate and achieve optimal client outcomes.

Palliative care: focuses on improving the symptoms, dignity, and quality of life for individuals who are suffering with a serious illness or disease.

Pathos: the psychological or emotional element of communication that is often overlooked or misunderstood.

Patient-focused interventions: those interventions that recognize the role of patients as active participants in the process of obtaining appropriate, effective, safe, and responsive healthcare.

Patient Protection and Affordable Care Act (PPACA or ACA): legislation with the intent to improve access, decrease waste and costs, and support quality through process changes and improved outcomes.

Patient safety: the prevention of harm to patients. Emphasis is placed on the system of care delivery that (a) prevents errors; (b) learns from the errors that do occur; and (c) is built on a culture of safety that involves healthcare professionals, organizations, and patients.

Patient Safety and Quality Improvement Act: law enacted in 2005 to increase protection for those who report errors. The intention of this act is to encourage reporting of medical errors to enable healthcare professionals to become more aware of problems, trend issues, and work to make system and process changes quickly to avoid error recurrence.

Performance improvement: an atmosphere for learning and redesign that is supported by the continuous monitoring of care, use of benchmarking, frequent tests of change, and a staff that has been empowered to innovate.

Performance results: focuses on improving patient outcomes, reducing avoidable costs, streamlining delivery, using data feedback, promoting positive competition, and engaging in frank discussions about performance.

Performing: the fourth stage of formation in which tasks are being completed. Team members are working together or independently in their assigned roles collaboratively. Team members are focused on problem solving, seeking solutions, and long-term outcomes.

PICOT: a method for developing a clinical question for EBP or research. It uses the letters for the following: (a) **p**atient population/disease, (b) **i**ntervention or issue of interest, (c) **c**omparison intervention, (d) **o**utcome, and (e) **t**ime.

Plan-Do-Study-Act (PDSA): the change process that includes implementing and testing the change; created by Deming and Shewhart.

Politics: the process of influencing the allocation of scarce resources.

Population level of prevention: includes policies and environments that promote health. Examples are: publicity campaigns alerting the public to the benefits of lifestyle changes in preventing colorectal cancers; promotion of high-fiber diets; subsidies to help people access exercise programs; and anti-smoking campaigns.

Predictive modeling: a process used to create a statistical model of future behavior. It allows the forecasting of probabilities and trends.

Primary prevention: involves measures to prevent illness or disease from occurring.

Private insurance: third-party payers in the private marketplace that are not funded by government sources.

Protected health information (PHI): information that resides in one central location, making it available to all providers of care requesting that information at any point in time.

Qualitative studies: involve the collection of data in nonnumeric form (e.g., using words in forms such as person interviews, observations). These are different than quantitative studies.

Quality of care: the extent to which healthcare services for individuals and the population increase the likelihood of preferred outcomes that are consistent with current knowledge.

Quality improvement: ensures that an organization, product, or service is consistent. It is focused not only on product and service quality, but also on the means to achieve it.

Quantitative studies: investigate clinical questions that involve the collection of data in numeric form. These are different than qualitative studies.

Question query: follows the case event; it asks something specific about the case event. It may be called the stem.

Reimbursement: dollars received by an organization or provider for services rendered.

Research: data collection conducted when there is a gap in knowledge.

Research utilization: refers to the review and critique of scientific research and then the application of the findings to clinical practice.

Respect for others: acknowledgment of the rights of individuals to make decisions and live or die on the basis of those decisions.

Retrospective/prospective payment: prior to 1994, retrospective payment was a system used to reimburse hospitals for services delivered on the basis of cost without any foreknowledge; since 1994, prospective payment is a system wherein reimbursement to hospitals or other organizational entities is based on a DRG or ambulatory patient classification (APC).

Revenue: money received through the delivery of services.

Risk anticipation: the ability to critically evaluate and anticipate risks to client safety.

Risk reduction: a decrease in the probability of an adverse outcome. Also any lowering of factors considered hazards for a specified disease.

Role conflict: when the role is different from what the new CNL has expected.

Root cause analysis (RCA): a structured method used to analyze the occurrence of serious adverse events. It involves the investigation of the systems and factors that converged to cause the event. Initially developed to analyze industrial accidents, RCA is now widely deployed as an error analysis tool in healthcare. A central tenet of RCA is to identify underlying problems that increase the likelihood of errors while avoiding the trap of focusing on mistakes by individuals. RCA thus uses the systems approach to identify both active errors and latent errors.

SBAR: communication format used in healthcare that is clear, concise, and effective. SBAR refers to the situation, background, assessment, and recommendation. Using SBAR is a prime example of bridging the way medical professionals communicate with each other. When there is a patient concern, communication that is clear, concise, and to the point when making a recommendation for action is valued and respected.

Second-party payers: reimbursement method in which the agency providing the services also pays for the service.

Secondary prevention: refers to methods and procedures used to detect the presence of disease in the early stages so the effective treatment can be initiated and complications decreased.

Self-determination: the ability to make one's own choices without interference from others.

Six Sigma: a disciplined, data-driven approach and methodology for eliminating defects (driving toward six standard deviations between the mean and the nearest specification limit) in any process.

Social justice: the idea that individuals or groups should have equal access to economic, social, and political opportunities.

Stem: follows the background statement or case event. This element contains the specific problem or intent, and may also be called the question query.

Storming: second stage of team formation; a potentially tumultuous stage in which conflict may occur. There may be a lack of unity, as well as struggles over leadership and power, in the group.

SWOT analysis: evaluation in which the intent is to determine the readiness of implementing a teamwork initiative within your facility.

Systems analyst/risk anticipator: the CNL participates in systems review to improve the quality of nursing care delivered and, at the individual level, to critically evaluate and anticipate risks to client safety with the aim of preventing medical error.

Team manager: the CNL properly delegates and manages the nursing team resources and serves as a leader in the interdisciplinary healthcare team.

Technology Informatics Guiding Education Reform (TIGER): collective formed by a group of nurses who believe in the importance of nursing's role in the implementation of information technology.

Telehealth: the practice of healthcare when the healthcare provider and patient are widely separated, using two-way voice and visual communication (e.g., satellite or computer).

Tertiary prevention: refers to prevention strategies needed after a disease or condition had been diagnosed in an attempt to return the client to an optimum state of health.

Test anxiety: a type of performance anxiety that can cause stress when one is preparing for an exam.

Therapeutic relationship: a helping relationship between nurse and patient that is based on mutual trust and respect, the nurturing of faith and hope, being sensitive to self and others, and assisting with the gratification of a patient's physical, emotional, and spiritual needs through the nurse's knowledge and skill.

Third-party payers: governmental or private insurance entities who pay for all or some of the services provided.

Traditional systems thinking: the theory that leaders can control the evolution of complex systems by intentions and clear thinking; this thinking leads to a perpetual cycle in which a system eventually does not act as predicted, and a need is formed for a new system.

Transactional leadership: promotes a task-oriented environment based on individuals working at an agreed level of performance in return for a reward.

Transformational leadership: allows charismatic leaders to inspire and broaden their followers' interests as well as generate a sense of awareness and acceptance into the mission, vision, and goals of the organization.

Transtheoretical model of change: classic modes of how people intentionally change behaviors, which include the stages of change (precontemplation, contemplation, preparation, action, and maintenance).

Value-based purchasing: the method of payment by CMS for in-hospital stays, which began in 2012; it pays on the basis of hospital scores in patient experience or the HCAHPS, the processes of care (clinical guidelines, order sets, etc.), and outcomes, such as core measures, as well as morbidity and mortality rates.

Values: personal beliefs about the truths and worth of thoughts, objects, or behaviors.

Values clarification: a process used to promote clarity regarding personal and professional values that will intersect thoughts and actions in relation to policy and politics.

Volume: the number of beds occupied, procedures done, cases received, visits made, or other description of amount of services provided.

Appendix A

Clinical Nurse Leader (CNL®) Certification Exam Blueprint as of Spring 2017

(For CNL Exams administered beginning April 2017)

Domains and Subdomains	Weight (%)
I. Nursing Leadership	32%
A. Horizontal Leadership	
B. Healthcare Advocacy	
C. Implementation of the CNL Role	
D. Lateral Integration of Care Services	
E. Patient Assessment	
F. Ethics	
II. Clinical Outcomes Management	23%
A. Illness/Disease Management	
B. Health Promotion and Disease Prevention & Injury Reduction/Prevention Management	
C. Healthcare Policy	
III. Care Environment Management	45%
A. Knowledge Management	
B. Healthcare Systems/Organizations	
C. Interprofessional Communication and Collaboration Skills	
D. Team Coordination	
E. Quality Improvement and Safety	
F. Evidence-Based Practice	
G. Healthcare Finance and Economics	
H. Healthcare Informatics	

TABLE A.1 Clinical Nurse Leader® Certification Exam—Detailed Blueprint

I. Nursing Leadership	**32% of exam**
A. Horizontal Leadership	
1. Apply leadership change and complexity theories	
2. Apply Strategies to guide the collaborative team to use clinical judgement to make safe patient care decisions	
3. Facilitate delegation of patient care coordination activities	
4. Appraise and evaluate coordinated care activities	
5. Demonstrate accountability for microsystems healthcare outcomes	
6. Practice as a role model for other healthcare providers, including coaching and mentoring the healthcare team	
7. Coordinate evaluation and update plans of care at an advanced level collaboratively with the interprofessional team and the patient	
8. Organize a framework for systematic collaborative team practices to address the complexity of patient care issues	
9. Serve as a partner and leader in the interprofessional health team	
10. Manage and lead group processes to meet care objectives and complete healthcare team responsibilities	
11. Develop effective working relationships within an interprofessional team to influence microsystem outcomes	
12. Demonstrate higher order critical thinking and problem solving skills	
B. Healthcare Advocacy	
1. Initiate partnerships to identify health disparities, establish health promotion goals, and implement strategies to address those concerns	
2. Interface between the patient and the healthcare delivery system to protect the rights of patients and to effect quality outcomes; knowledge of patient rights and responsibilities	
3. Ensure that patients, families, and communities are well informed in creating a patient-centered plan of care	
4. Negotiate and advocate for the nursing profession, the CNL role, and the interprofessional team to healthcare providers, policy makers, and consumers	
5. Identify and propose microsystem resources to meet the needs of target populations	
6. Explain healthcare issues and concerns to key stakeholders including elected and appointed officials, policy organizations, and to healthcare consumers	
7. Translate appropriate healthcare information to advocate for informed healthcare decision making	
8. Recommend improvements in the institution or healthcare system and the nursing profession	
9. Advocate for patients, particularly the most vulnerable	

(*continued*)

TABLE A.1 Clinical Nurse Leader Certification Exam—Detailed Blueprint (*continued*)

C. Implementation of the CNL Role
1. Demonstrate professional identity and practice in developing the CNL role
2. Explain the capacity of CNL practice to improve healthcare processes and outcomes
3. Exhibit qualities of a microsystem leader within and across interprofessional teams
4. Appraise and apply current and new CNL evidence, competence, and practice
5. Synthesize CNL practice outcomes for dissemination at system, regional, national, or international level
6. Collaborate with a network of CNL professionals at the system, regional, national, or international level
D. Lateral Integration of Care Services
1. Coordinate the healthcare of patients across the care continuum
2. Integrate an interprofessional approach to discuss strategies to identify and acquire resources for patient populations
3. Coordinate and perform risk analysis using appropriate evidence-based tools to predict patient risk and safety issues within and across microsystems
4. Apply care management skills and principles to provide and coordinate patient care within and across specific episodes of illness and throughout the care continuum
5. Manage, monitor, and influence the microsystem environment to foster health and quality of care across the care continuum
6. Apply systems and organization theory in the design, delivery, and evaluation of healthcare delivery across the care continuum
E. Patient Assessment
1. Perform an advanced comprehensive assessment of the patient across the lifespan (e.g., health history, culture, socioeconomic status, spirituality, health literacy)
2. Perform an advanced assessment of microsystems across the care continuum to determine patient population care needs
F. Ethics
1. Apply patient-centered ethical decision-making framework to clinical situations that incorporates moral concepts, professional ethics, and law
2. Apply legal and ethical guidelines to advocate for patient well-being and preferences
3. Identify and analyze common ethical dilemmas including the impact on patient care and outcomes
4. Evaluate ethical decision making from both a personal and organizational perspective and analyze how these two perspectives may create conflicts of interest
5. Collaborate with the ethics committee and recognize their role in healthcare delivery

(*continued*)

TABLE A.1 Clinical Nurse Leader Certification Exam—Detailed Blueprint (*continued*)

II. Clinical Outcomes Management	**23% of exam**
A. Illness/Disease Management	
1. Coordinate the provision and management of care at the microsystem level and across the care continuum	
2. Evaluate care for patients across the lifespan with particular emphasis on health promotion and risk reduction services	
3. Identify patient problems that require intervention, with special focus on those problems amenable to nursing intervention	
4. Evaluate and determine readiness, needs, and interventions for safe transition of care	
5. Design and modify patient care based on analysis of outcomes, evidence-based knowledge, and patient's goals of care	
6. Analyze microsystems of care and outcome datasets to anticipate patient risk and improve quality of care delivery	
7. Apply theories of chronic illness care and population health management to patient and families	
8. Integrate community resources, social networks, and decision support mechanisms into care management	
9. Recognize differences in responses to illness and therapies based on patient's cultural, ethnic, socioeconomic, linguistic, religious, and lifestyle preferences	
10. Identify disease patterns and their implications on patient's activation for self-care and on-going care	
11. Use advanced knowledge of pathophysiology, assessment, and pharmacology to anticipate illness progression, response to therapy and to guide, teach, and engage patients and families regarding care	
12. Use knowledge of cost and affordability issues in managing patient illness/disease across the care continuum	
13. Synthesize literature and research findings as the foundation for the design of interventions for illness and disease management	
14. Coordinate and implement education programs for patients and health professionals	
15. Identify and interpret epidemiological patterns in order to manage illness and disease	

(*continued*)

TABLE A.1 Clinical Nurse Leader Certification Exam—Detailed Blueprint (*continued*)

B. Health Promotion and Disease Prevention & Injury Reduction/Prevention Management
1. Collaborate with interprofessional team members to promote health and/or prevent disease
2. Employ strategies to engage patients in therapeutic partnerships with interprofessional team members for disease management and self-care activation
3. Identify and/or modify interventions based on evidence to meet specific patient needs for health promotion and disease prevention
4. Design and implement interventions to modify risk factors and promote engagement in healthy lifestyles for diverse populations
5. Assess protective, predictive, and genetic factors that influence the health of patients
6. Develop clinical and health promotion programs for patient populations to reduce risk, prevent disease, and prevent disease sequelae, particularly related to chronic illness
7. Recognize the need for and develop community partnerships to establish risk reduction strategies to address social and public health issues
8. Incorporate cultural definitions of health into health promotion and disease prevention strategies
9. Incorporate theories and research in creating patient engagement strategies to promote and preserve health and healthy lifestyles
C. Healthcare Policy
1. Recognize the effect of healthcare policy on health promotion, risk reduction, and disease and injury prevention with emphasis on vulnerable populations
2. Recognize the interactive effect of economics on national/global health policy related to health outcomes
3. Analyze the effect of local, state, and/or national healthcare policy as they apply to the standards of care and scope of practice in the microsystem
4. Identify the influence of regulatory guidelines and quality controls within the healthcare delivery system

(*continued*)

TABLE A.1 Clinical Nurse Leader Certification Exam—Detailed Blueprint (*continued*)

III. Care Environment Management	**45% of exam**
A. Knowledge Management	
1. Collect data that documents the characteristics, conditions, and outcomes for various patient groups	
2. Apply knowledge of technology, equipment, treatment regimens, or medication therapies to anticipate risk	
3. Compare and evaluate trends of institutional and unit data to national benchmarks	
4. Identify variations in clinical outcomes among various groups to determine where nurses have the greatest impact at the microsystem level	
5. Synthesize data, information, and knowledge to evaluate and achieve optimal patient outcomes	
6. Integrate assessment data into information management systems for decision support	
7. Analyze and disseminate microsystem data that impacts health outcomes	
8. Employ strategies to engage the interprofessional team to impact healthcare outcomes	
9. Distinguish the impact of health literacy of patient engagement and activation for self-care	
B. Healthcare Systems/Organizations	
1. Apply knowledge of teamwork to manage change and disseminate information at the systems level	
2. Critique and/or modify existing policies and procedures based on current evidence	
3. Implement system-based strategies that decrease healthcare disparities	
4. Apply theories of systems thinking to address problems and develop solutions	
5. Distinguish how healthcare delivery systems are organized and their effect on patient care	
6. Identify the economic, legal, and political factors that influence healthcare delivery	
C. Interprofessional Communication and Collaboration Skills	
1. Analyze patterns of communication and chain of command that impact care within the interprofessional team and across settings	
2. Apply concepts of communication skills including critical listening during assessment, intervention, evaluation, and education of patients, families, and the healthcare team	
3. Employ effective negotiation skills	
4. Employ appropriate communication techniques and strategies that address social, political, economic, environmental, technological, and historical issues	

(*continued*)

TABLE A.1 Clinical Nurse Leader Certification Exam—Detailed Blueprint (*continued*)

5. Utilize interprofessional communication, collaboration, and group process concepts to meet care objectives and complete healthcare responsibilities
6. Translate and interpret data for the patients, families, and the healthcare team
7. Communicate effectively in a variety of written and spoken formats
8. Construct relationships with interprofessional team including management and administration
9. Incorporate knowledge of cultural differences to bridge cultural and linguistic barriers
10. Integrate emotional intelligence in communication and collaboration with patients, families, and the healthcare team
11. Recognize and utilize the roles and responsibilities of the interprofessional team

D. Team Coordination

1. Perform, teach, delegate, and manage skilled nursing procedures in the context of safety
2. Demonstrate effectiveness in group interactions, particularly in skills necessary to interact and collaborate with other members of the interprofessional team
3. Evaluate underlying assumptions and relevant evidence that influence patient and interprofessional team behavior
4. Establish and maintain effective working relationships within an interprofessional, multicultural team to make ethical decisions
5. Facilitate group processes to meet care objectives to ensure completion of interprofessional team responsibilities
6. Identify areas in which a conflict of interest may arise and propose resolutions or actions to resolve/prevent the conflict
7. Promote a positive and healthy work environment and a culture of retention
8. Incorporate patient/family/interprofessional team input to design, coordinate, and evaluate plans of care

E. Quality Improvement and Safety

1. Employ quality improvement methods in evaluating individual and aggregate patient care
2. Evaluate healthcare outcomes through the acquisition of data and the questioning of inconsistencies
3. Develop and implement the redesign of patient care utilizing assessment methodologies including but not limited to: gap analysis, Failure Modes Effect Analysis (FMEA), Root Cause Analysis (RCA), Plan-Do-Study-Act (PDSA) Cycles, and microsystem assessment
4. Gather, analyze and synthesize data related to risk anticipation to reduce risk and maintain patient safety
5. Employ strategies to guide the interprofessional team in quality improvement activities within the microsystem to impact the meso- and macrosystems

(*continued*)

TABLE A.1 Clinical Nurse Leader Certification Exam—Detailed Blueprint (*continued*)

F. Evidence-Based Practice
1. Create framework within the microsystem to integrate patient and family preferences, interprofessional clinical expertise, and best evidence into clinical decisions
2. Develop foundations for assessment and clinical decisions by applying evidence-based practice
3. Synthesize quantitative or qualitative evidence for critical thinking and decision making to achieve optimal patient outcomes
4. Select relevant sources of evidence to meet specific needs of patients, microsystems, or communities when planning care
5. Use current evidence to improve patient care
6. Identify relevant outcomes and measurement strategies that will improve patient outcomes and promote cost effective care
G. Healthcare Finance and Economics
1. Propose cost effective strategies and/or interventions to the interprofessional team that improve efficiency and patient care outcomes
2. Serve as a steward for the environmental, human, and material resources while coordinating patient care
3. Evaluate the fiscal context in which practice occurs
4. Identify high cost /high volume activities, to benchmark costs nationally and across care settings
5. Apply ethical principles in regard to healthcare delivery relating to healthcare financing and economics
6. Identify the impact of financial policies on healthcare delivery and patient outcomes
7. Interpret the impact of both public and private reimbursement policies that may affect patient care decisions
8. Evaluate the effect of healthcare financing on access to care and patient outcomes
9. Examine current healthcare economic concepts including but not limited to: Return on Investment (ROI), Value-Based Purchasing (VBP), bundled payments, and basic marketing strategies

(*continued*)

TABLE A.1 Clinical Nurse Leader Certification Exam—Detailed Blueprint (*continued*)

H. Healthcare Informatics
1. Assess, critique, and analyze information sources
2. Design care utilizing informatics and patient care technology
3. Apply multiple sources of systems data in designing processes for care delivery
4. Evaluate clinical information systems in order to provide feedback related to efficient and accurate documentation
5. Apply ethical principles in the use of information systems
6. Evaluate the impact of new technologies on patients, families and healthcare delivery
7. Identify and assess the relationships between information systems, accurate communication, error reduction, and healthcare system operation
8. Analyze and disseminate healthcare information among the interprofessional team and across the care continuum
9. Validate accuracy of consumer-provided information regarding culturally relevant health issues from multiple sources
10. Utilize technology for health promotion and disease prevention
11. Collaborate with quality improvement and information technology teams to design and implement processes for improving patient outcomes
12. Utilize current technology to anticipate patient risk
13. Demonstrate to other healthcare providers the efficient and appropriate use of healthcare technologies to maximize healthcare outcomes
14. Access, critique, and analyze information from multiple sources

Resource

Commission on Nurse Certification (2016). *Clinical Nurse Leader* (CNL®). Job analysis summary & certification examination blueprint. Retrieved from http://www.aacn.nche.edu/cnc/job-analysis-study. Used by the Permission of American Association of Colleges of Nursing.

Appendix B

Reflection Questions for the Chapters

Chapter 5

1. How would you describe horizontal leadership?
2. How does horizontal leadership differ from other types of leadership?
3. Which of the change theories do you expect to use in your practice as a CNL?
4. What is the difference between coaching and mentoring, and how would you use them once you are a CNL?

Chapter 6

1. As a CNL, what is your responsibility to your microsystem when change in practice becomes necessary to provide better patient care?
2. How do you see the role of CNL in your microsystem as it relates to interdisciplinary communication and patient outcomes?
3. How do you see the role of CNL in relation to bedside nursing and the therapeutic relationship with the client as an advanced generalist?
4. How will you use conflict resolution in your microsystem to facilitate effective communication between disciplines?

Chapter 7

While reflecting on a situation where you, as a CNL, had to act as the patient/family advocate:

1. What are two ways CNLs incorporate social justice into practice?
2. Describe two ways that CNLs can advocate for nursing in general and, more specifically, two ways to advocate for CNLs.

3. What are other disciplines that CNLs can seek as resources for advocacy issues?
4. Why should patients be allowed to change or end healthcare treatments?

Chapter 8

1. Describe the eight aspects of the CNL role that a new CNL must integrate into practice.
2. Reflect on and describe a situation where a CNL is able to enhance both high-quality, cost-effective healthcare, as well as the advancement of the profession.
3. Identify two ways a CNL can help to integrate his or her role into the practice setting.
4. What resources might a CNL choose to help with the integration of his or her role into practice?

Chapter 9

1. Describe the role of the CNL called lateral integration.
2. What are the four components of lateral integration?
3. How can a CNL promote communication?
4. Identify potential stakeholders who may be involved with the CNL in lateral integration, and note how they might help patient outcomes.

Chapter 10

1. What are some of the prevalent illnesses and diseases in your specialty area? Are these diseases preventable? Are the illnesses and diseases amenable to nursing interventions?
2. What factors should be taken into account when assessing readiness for discharge to the next level of care?
3. What are some key aspects to consider when assessing an individual's level of pain?
4. What are some of the differences in individuals' responses to illness, considering their cultural, ethnic, socioeconomic, religious, and lifestyle preferences?

Chapter 11

1. Describe how a CNL might incorporate summaries of outcomes data to direct caregivers into the routine operations of a microsystem.

2. The amount of knowledge required by all members of the healthcare team in today's work environment is overwhelming to many. Describe organizational resources a CNL might utilize to best plan a strategy for improving knowledge management in a microsystem.
3. Compare and contrast the role of a root cause analysis (RCA) and a failure mode effect analysis (FMEA), and how a CNL can maximize the use of these strategies.
4. Consider how the role of the CNL is key to prioritizing the communication of new knowledge to direct caregivers.

Chapter 12

1. How could a CNL working on Mrs. Louis's unit initiate a change project related to her experience and the coordination of patient care?
2. What type of team would a CNL organize to make improvements?
3. What type of data and outcomes could be measured in the team's project?
4. How would the challenges of health promotion impact the work of the team, for example, healthcare literacy?

Chapter 13

1. What are key aspects of the definition of evidence-based practice (EBP) that the CNL can use to teach other professional nurses about this important topic?
2. Explain two ways that a CNL can implement EBP into the practice setting.
3. How does a CNL know what is the current best practice related to a clinical topic?
4. What are two key databases or websites that a CNL might use to search for evidence to support practice?

Chapter 14

1. What are the important data that should be collected in an initial clinical assessment?
2. How can the CNL use the Healthy People 2020 leading health indicators to coordinate client care?
3. Explain why a therapeutic relationship is important for the CNL in the clinical assessment process.

4. Why is a functional assessment a valuable tool for the CNL to use during a patient assessment?

Chapter 15

1. At what stage of Tuckman and Jensen's group process may team members experience conflict and struggle over power in the group? How can a CNL support this phase of group development?
2. As a CNL, you have identified an issue with near misses in patient home medication dosing and in hospital medication dosing. How would you go about building an effective team to address this issue? What interprofessional team members would you include when coordinating care?
3. Identify any reason a collaborative interprofessional team may be formed in your unique healthcare setting.
4. What resources can a CNL seek out to deal with conflict among teams? How can friction among a group impact the outcomes of the group in a negative and positive way?

Chapter 16

1. Describe the concept of patient volume and the related impact of this key variable on the financial structure of the microsystem.
2. Utilization of services and supplies has a great impact on the microsystem and also the mesosystem/organization as a whole. Consider multiple ways that the CNL can be a driving force in the most efficient utilization of services and supplies.
3. Discuss how issues of staffing mix, productivity, and design of the staffing matrix affect the work of the CNL within the microsystem.
4. Why is it relevant for the CNL to understand factors related to staffing, budgets, and skill mix?

Chapter 17

1. The role of CNL was created to directly impact patient safety at the point of care. Describe how the CNL's knowledge of the healthcare system is integral to the success of CNL outcomes.
2. Apply elements of complexity theory to a current healthcare initiative that involves CNLs and interprofessional teams. Relate how the concepts of open-ended, adaptable systems play a role in the work of improvement teams.

3. Discuss the benefits of a thorough microsystem's assessment in relation to implementing care in a complex healthcare system.
4. Consider competencies of the CNL role that support the translation of emerging nursing science into the microsystem and throughout the complex healthcare system.

Chapter 18

1. What are the three things that would help CNLs increase their influence in organizations, communities, and in national and international healthcare?
2. How is a political analysis similar to a clinical assessment?
3. What skill sets do clinical nurses have that enable them to work at the unit level to sort out the actions that are needed to comply with HCAHPS, core measures, and other scoring procedures?
4. How do clinical nurse leaders use evidence-based research to inform their practice? What are some of the ways in which this same approach would apply in public health policy and health services research?

Chapter 19

1. Discuss the current and future role of frontline nurses in the rapidly advancing field of quality improvement. Consider the role of the CNL in supporting this engagement of nursing critical voice.
2. Develop a systematic process to organize the vast resources available on healthcare improvement topics.
3. How would you critically review publications, best practice guidelines, and related information on the topic and share it with the improvement team?
4. How does the CNL function as an integrator of lateral care in quality improvement and patient safety initiatives within a healthcare system?

Chapter 20

1. Consider those human factors that might impede the development of health information technologies in the workplace and address how you would manage those factors.
2. There are concerns about privacy and confidentiality in the use of health information exchanges. Knowing the definitions of privacy and

confidentiality and anticipating resistance by both staff and patients on the basis of their concerns, make a case about why organizations and patients should embrace the use of HIEs—what is in it for them?

3. How might you encourage clinicians to become engaged in the development and implementation of clinical decision support systems, both passive and active, on the basis of current evidence and experiential knowledge?
4. Identify questions/problems related to health information technology that should be a priority for those developing information technology.

Chapter 21

1. How can the CNLs best equip themselves with the skills and knowledge needed to address ethical concerns in healthcare? Discuss general and specific strategies.
2. How can the CNL best support direct care nurses as they are confronted with moral stress?
3. What areas of healthcare have classically been associated with ethical challenges in patient care and what emerging issues are presenting ethical concerns?
4. Consider the varied work environments across the healthcare systems. Discuss ways that CNLs can help direct caregivers to seek out support for appropriate resources when they feel a patient/family is being unjustly treated.

Index